In Clinical Practice

Taking a practical approach to clinical medicine, this series of smaller reference books is designed for the trainee physician, primary care physician, nurse practitioner and other general medical professionals to understand each topic covered. The coverage is comprehensive but concise and is designed to act as a primary reference tool for subjects across the field of medicine.

More information about this series at
http://www.springer.com/series/13483

Sam D. Hutchings

Editor

Trauma and Combat Critical Care in Clinical Practice

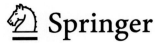 Springer

Editor
Sam D. Hutchings
Royal Navy and King's College Hospital
London
UK

ISSN 2199-6652   ISSN 2199-6660   (electronic)
In Clinical Practice
ISBN 978-3-319-28756-0   ISBN 978-3-319-28758-4   (eBook)
DOI 10.1007/978-3-319-28758-4

Library of Congress Control Number: 2016948863

Printed on acid-free paper

This Springer imprint is published by Springer Nature
The registered company is Springer International Publishing AG Switzerland

To the men and women of the military medical services involved in the Iraq and Afghanistan conflicts. You made the unsurvivable survivable.

Foreword

Trauma and combat medicine exemplifies perfectly the juxtaposition of the destructive and creative capacities of human beings. As it seems unlikely that the former element will be tamed, creativity and commitment in trauma research and clinical practice will be needed for the foreseeable future. *Trauma and Combat Critical Care in Clinical Practice* demonstrates effectively how civilian and military trauma research cross-fertilise each other to provide evidence-based practical guidance to maximise recovery from life-threatening injury. This book distils research evidence and wisdom acquired the hard way – from caring for victims of trauma often in the most difficult circumstances, as captured by the clinical vignette in the opening chapter.

The recent military experience in Afghanistan in particular has brought unique expertise in immediate resuscitation, stabilisation and surgery of soldiers suffering profoundly destructive injuries. Once stabilised, the critical care odyssey of evacuation by air – a feat of endurance by the attending clinical staff of up to 36 h – has made it possible for these patients to receive continuing multidisciplinary care in a major trauma centre and to be reunited with their families. Improvements in survival achieved by advances in the early stages of trauma care must now be accompanied by a better understanding of the immuno-inflammatory and endocrine responses to tissue injury and a focus on improving long-term outcomes.

Intensive care medicine has an increasingly important role in this complex recovery pathway though minimisation of secondary complications such as remote organ injury, infection and sepsis, muscle loss, scarring and ectopic calcification; and enhanced regeneration of tissue, restoration of function and psychological support. The bimodal distribution of trauma – the young and the old – provides an opportunity to study how the youthful capacity for regeneration and resilience may be promoted in the elderly, with the opportunity for translation into non-trauma critical illness. Many recent advances in the care of acutely and critically ill patients have come through better organisation and implementation of existing knowledge, and here again the trauma experience is invaluable in informing all aspects of acute care practice. This book provides valuable guidance not just for trauma care but for critical care management in general.

Brigadier Professor Tim Hodgetts CBE PhD
FRCP FRCSEd FRCEM
Medical Director, Defence Medical Services
Professor Julian Bion FRCP FRCA FFICM MD
Professor of Intensive Care Medicine
University of Birmingham

About the Editor

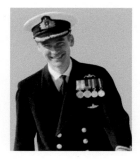

Surgeon Commander Sam D. Hutchings is the Royal Navy's head of specialty for Intensive Care Medicine and undertakes his clinical practice at King's College Hospital, London. He is also a clinical academic with areas of research interest covering resuscitation endpoints in traumatic haemorrhage and the use of novel point of care perfusion assessment tools. He has deployed operationally to Iraq, Afghanistan and Sierra Leone.

Preface

In the early 1980s, Trunkey[1] described a pattern of trauma mortality that is still widely referred to today. His tri-modal distribution model considered that death could occur in one of three peaks. The early peak (death within minutes) is caused by catastrophic injuries with severe anatomical disruption. These injuries were, and still are, difficult or impossible to treat, although preventative measures such as car seat belts and military combat body armour have reduced the frequency. The middle peak consists of deaths occurring within the first hours following injury and mainly results from profound disruption of homeostasis and physiology. Examples include uncontrolled blood loss leading to traumatic haemorrhagic shock or failure of respiration secondary to an obstructed airway or intrinsic lung damage. A vast amount of clinical academic endeavour has been spent on reducing this second peak. Some of the multitude of examples include the adoption of standardised ATLS teaching highlighting the importance of the "Golden Hour", the development of dedicated major trauma networks, physician-delivered pre-hospital care, and changes to resuscitation paradigms that emphasise the importance of physiological damage control rather than anatomical restoration and the adoption of point of care devices to prevent catastrophic haemorrhage. Many of these advances have been driven forward at pace by the Defence Medical Services of nations involved in combat operations during the first two decades of the twenty-first century, and there is no doubt that many military casualties

---

[1] Trunkey DD. Trauma. Sci Am. 1983;249(2):28–35.

have recovered from injuries that would have been deemed un-survivable just a few years earlier.

But what of the third peak? Trunkey attributed these late deaths to multiple organ failure occurring days or often weeks after the initial injury. However, an examination of the demographics of trauma deaths today shows that this third peak has been substantially reduced. Of the 518 British military casualties of the war in Afghanistan who received a massive transfusion at the Role 3 hospital in Camp Bastion, over 91 % survived.[2] This occurred despite an average injury severity score of over 30. Much of this success was due to a reduction in the second (early) mortality peak but not all. Of the 441 British military personnel who died from combat related injuries in the Iraq and Afghanistan conflicts, 83 % died prior to hospital admission, reflecting the persistence of Trunkey's first peak. Of the 17 % who died after reaching hospital, 53 % died in the first 24 h, meaning that those that survived beyond 24 h had a 93 % chance of long-term survival.[3] Those 7 % who suffered late deaths can be compared with around 20 % of deaths occurring during the late peak of the original Trunkey study, many of whom were also much less severely injured.

This trend of falling late mortality is also found when examining modern civilian trauma systems. A recent randomised study[4] examining the optimal ratio of packed cells to plasma in American trauma patients who received a massive transfusion showed a lower mortality than predicted pre-study (24 % vs. 35 %) but also a low incidence of death from multiple organ failure (12.8 % of those who died and 3 % of those who were enrolled).

Certainly more effective early resuscitation strategies play a key role in reducing late deaths However, the often unrecognised success story in these improvements in trauma

[2] Data from Defence Statistics (Health): Recovery rates for UK Service Personal admitted to Camp Bastion Field Hospital. 25 September 2013.
[3] Keene DD, Penn-Barwell JG, Wood PR, et al. Died of wounds: a mortality review. J R Army Med Corps. October 2015:jramc–2015–000490.
[4] Holcomb JB, Tilley BC, Baraniuk S, et al. Transfusion of Plasma, Platelets, and Red Blood Cells in a 1:1:1 vs a 1:1:2 Ratio and Mortality in Patients With Severe Trauma. JAMA. 2015;313(5):471–12.

mortality over the past three decades is the role of intensive care medicine.

Effective intensive (or critical) care underpins initial trauma resuscitation with intensivists often adopting key roles in the pre-hospital and emergency department environment. However, it is the dramatic changes that have occurred within intensive care units that have arguably had the most impact in reducing late mortality following traumatic injury. Examples are too numerous to detail in full, but the adoption of lung protective ventilation, advanced haemodynamic monitoring, targeted fluid management and protocol based sedation are but four examples where practice is radically different to that seen in the 1980s.

Perhaps more important than individual changes in treatment is the development of systems and guidelines based on robust evidence. This approach to management has been widely embraced by the new specialty of intensive care medicine. This book has its origins in one such set of guidelines, developed by the United Kingdom Defence Medical Services to support the delivery of critical care during the 2001–2014 Afghanistan conflict and subsequently adapted to other deployed environments. Many of the authors involved in that work have contributed to this book.

Finally, but crucially, is the role of the intensive care specialist themselves. This relative new comer to the hospital scene is a key facilitator in the management of critically injured patients. Intensivists not only provide organ system support to their patients but crucially act as links between the multitude of other specialties involved in the management of severely injured patients, constantly ensuring joined up management across the multi-specialty and multi-disciplinary team.

As alluded to earlier many recent advances in trauma critical care have been driven by recent military conflict. This book aims to provide an overview of trauma critical care, but it has a distinct military feel and focus. Almost all the chapter authors are military clinicians, from Britain and Australia, who have served in the recent Iraq and Afghanistan conflicts. Despite this, all of the chapters have relevance to the practice of trauma critical care in any environment. The first chapter of this book describes a patient journey, for a British military casualty of a hypothetical future conflict, from injury to tertiary care. Many of the early themes from this chapter are subsequently developed later in this book. Although the early chapters set the scene by describing the initial stages of the trauma patient pathway, the bulk of this book focuses on decisions faced by the intensivist once the patient has arrived within the intensive care unit. The whole book is laid out in a question-and-answer format and aims to provide useful guidance to some of the common questions that intensivists caring for trauma patients are faced with every day. Wherever possible, the evidence base behind the suggested answers is discussed, and where uncertainty exists over best practice, this is acknowledged and discussed.

It is my hope that the experience gained in recent conflicts, and reflected in this book, can continue to provide benefit for both civilian and military trauma patients in the years and decades ahead and that they may go some way to further flattening Trunkey's third peak.

Finally the views and opinions expressed in this book represent the personal experience of the authors and editor and should not be taken to represent the official view of the UK Ministry of Defence.

London 2016   Sam D. Hutchings

Acknowledgements

The production of this book has taken longer than expected, principally as the West African Ebola crisis of 2014/15 led to the unexpected and rapid deployment of myself and several of the key chapter authors, I would like to thank Julia Megginson and Melissa Morton at Springer for their exceptional patience during this time. Dr. Amarjit Samra, Director of Research at the Royal Centre for Defence Medicine, and Colonel Tom Woolley, Defence Professor of Anaesthesia & Critical Care, approved the manuscript for publication, and I am grateful for their efforts. I am indebted to Colonel Peter Mahoney, Emeritus Defence Professor, who persuaded me to take on this project and provided an introduction to the publisher. Surgeon Captain Jason Smith, Clinical Director of the PCRF, reviewed and improved the content of the first chapter. My father, David Hutchings, freely gave of his time to proof read the manuscript, correcting many errors I had overlooked and often adding a vital lay perspective. Finally, my heartfelt thanks to my wife Philippa and two sons Henry and Tom; time spent on this project has meant less time spent with them. For that my apologies and gratitude.

Contents

Contributors

Editor

Surgeon Commander Sam D. Hutchings, MRCS, FRCA, FFICM, DICM, DipIMC, Royal Navy Department of Military Anaesthesia and Critical Care, Royal Centre for Defence Medicine, Kings College Hospital, London, UK

Contributors

Jonathan Crighton, MBBS, FRCR Derriford Hospital, Plymouth, Devon, UK

Major William R.O. Davies, MBChB, MRCP, FRCA, FFICM Intensive Care, Royal Sussex County Hospital, Brighton, UK

Surgeon Commander Catherine M. Doran, BA, MB BCh, BAO, MD, FRCS, Royal Navy General Surgery, Royal Centre for Defence Medicine, Queen Elizabeth Hospital, Birmingham, UK

Squadron Leader George Evetts, MBBS, BSc, MRCP, FRCA, RAF Imperial School of Anaesthesia, London, UK

Wing Commander Ian Ewington, MBChB, MML, MRCP, FRCA, FFICM, RAF Royal Centre for Defence Medicine, Queen Elizabeth Hospital Birmingham, Birmingham, UK

C. Andrew Eynon, MBBS, MD, FRCP, FRCEM, FFICM Wessex Neurological Centre, University Hospital Southampton NHS Foundation Trust, Southampton, UK

Karen Friend, BSc, PgDip Department of Critical Care, King's College Hospital NHS Trust, London, UK

Surgeon Commander David A.T. Gay, MBBS, FRCR, PGCE, Royal Navy Derriford Hospital, Plymouth, Devon, UK

Commander Anthony D. Holley, MBBCh, DipDHM, FACEM, FCICM Department of Intensive Care Medicine, Royal Brisbane and Women's Hospital, Brisbane, Australia

Emrys Kirkman, OBE, PhD Defence Science and Technology Laboratory, Porton Down, Salisbury, UK

Lieutenant Colonel Stephen Lewis, Royal Army Medical Corps Department of Critical Care, King's College Hospital, London, UK

Surgeon Commander Simon J. Mercer, FRCA, Royal Navy Department of Anaesthesia, Aintree University Hospital, Liverpool, UK

Mark Midwinter, CBE BMedSci, MB BS, Dip App Stats, MD, FRCS Wide Bay Hospital and Health Services, Queensland Health, Brisbane, Australia

Major David N. Naumann, MA, MB, BChir, DMCC, MRCS, Royal Army Medical Corps NIHR Surgical Reconstruction and Microbiology Research Centre, Queen Elizabeth Hospital, Birmingham, UK

Academic Department of Military Surgery and Trauma, Royal Centre for Defence Medicine, Queen Elizabeth Hospital, Birmingham, UK

Surgeon Commander Kate Prior, FRCA, Royal Navy Department of Anaesthesia, King's College Hospital, London, UK

Colonel Michael C. Reade, MBBS, MPH, DPhil, FANZCA, FCICM Joint Health Command, Australian Defence Force, Canberra, ACT, Australia

The Burns, Trauma and Critical Care Research Centre, University of Queensland and Royal Brisbane and Women's Hospital, Brisbane, QLD, Australia

Surgeon Commander Paul S.C. Rees, MD, FRCP, DipIMC, Royal Navy School of Medicine, University of Saint Andrews and Ninewells Hospital Dundee, Dundee, UK

Squadron Leader Edward Spurrier, BM MD (Res) MRCS FRCS (Tr&Orth) Defence Medical Services, Birmingham, UK

Surgeon Captain Sarah A. Stapley, MB ChB FRCS FRCS (Tr&Orth) DM Trauma and Orthopaedics, Portsmouth NHS Trust, Royal Centre for Defence Medicine (Research and Academia), Birmingham, UK

Stephanie R. Strachan, MBBS, MMedEd, MRCP, FRCA, DICM Department of Critical Care, King's College Hospital NHS Trust, London, UK

Chapter 1
Treating the Critically Injured Military Patient

Sam D. Hutchings

Abstract Injuries sustained during armed conflict are often
of a magnitude not seen in civilian practice, frequently occurring as a result of high velocity projectiles and explosives. The
environment in which military healthcare providers operate
is often remote and austere and treatments must be adapted
accordingly. This chapter describes, using a fictional account
of one possible future scenario, the pathway from wounding to strategic evacuation for an injured UK serviceman. It
also outlines the critical care facilities provided by the UK
Defence Medical Services on deployed operations.

Keywords Armed conflict • Major trauma • Military
healthcare • Pre-hospital care • Critical care

S.D. Hutchings, MRCS, FRCA, FFICM, DICM, DipIMC
Department of Critical Care, Kings College Hospital,
Denmark Hill, London SE5 9RS, UK
e-mail: sam.hutchings@kcl.ac.uk

S.D. Hutchings (ed.), *Trauma and Combat Critical Care*
in Clinical Practice, In Clinical Practice,
DOI 10.1007/978-3-319-28758-4_1,
© Crown Copyright 2016

1

The following is a work of fiction based on one hypothetical future combat medical scenario. The medical capabilities described are either in current use, or proposed for use by the UK Defence Medical Services. Some of the treatments described are currently undergoing evaluation, and are not yet supported by robust evidence. They may, or may not, prove to be of use in severely injured patients in the future.

160400Z JUN 20[1]: Somewhere on a Distant Ocean

From the bridge of HMS *Queen Elizabeth* the officer of the watch could see the shapes of the other ships in the joint allied taskforce illuminated by the first rays of the sun as it inched over the horizon. Centred on the new British aircraft carrier the task force consisted of the French amphibious assault ship *Mistral* and her Royal Navy equivalent HMS *Albion*; these two vessels were currently close in to the coast, in preparation for the amphibious assault, planned to coincide with the first light of day. The remainder of the central core of the task force comprised two large replenishment ships and the Primary Casualty Receiving Ship, RFA *Argus*, herself a veteran of three previous conflicts and now in her 35th year of service. Further out, two Royal Navy Type 45 destroyers, along with a US Navy *Aegis* equipped cruiser provided air cover for the group. The young lieutenant looked at his watch; as the hand passed 0400, a flight of F35 fighters swept overhead. Over the distant horizon the first wave of landing craft were approaching the hostile enemy coast.

---

[1] This nomenclature is termed a date time group and is used by NATO and other military organisations. The time here is 0400 on 16 June 2020 and is given as Zulu (Z) time, which is GMT.

160500Z JUN 20: *Sabre* Beach

The young Royal Marine commando didn't even see the flash of the rocket propelled grenade as it launched from a concealed firing position in the treeline that fringed the beach. The warhead exploded less than half a metre away, kicking up a cloud of shrapnel that peppered the marine. The blast wind physically picked him up and threw him several feet in the air. Although the damage from most of the RPG fragments were absorbed by his Osprey body armour, one penetrated his upper thigh lacerating the femoral vein and puncturing the femoral artery. In addition, the physical force of the explosion and the impact of his landing fractured his left humerus, now bent at an unnatural angle. Still under hostile fire from the tree line his colleagues were prevented from reaching him to provide immediate assistance. However, his section commander was able to report the incident and a 'nine liner' casualty report[2] was sent to the task force.

160505Z JUN 20: 820 Naval Air Squadron Merlin, *Piranha 1*

The Maritime in Transit Care (MiTC) team, strapped into their seats in the back of the aircraft, consisted of a Royal Navy consultant in pre-hospital medicine, an emergency nurse and a medical assistant. They were equipped with a range of resuscitation equipment and monitoring devices, enough blood products to facilitate the first phase of resuscitation and a novel device for stopping blood loss from the lower body that was about to be tested for the first time on the battlefield. Within minutes of receiving the 9 liner they lifted from the flight deck of RFA *Argus* and sped towards the distant shoreline.

---

[2] A '9 liner' report includes information such as location, number of casualties, and their priority for evacuation.

160510Z JUN 20: *Sabre* Beach

A series of section attacks had driven back the enemy, who had been pouring suppressing fire onto the beachhead. With the area secured a commando trained Royal Naval Medical Assistant raced forward towards the injured marine. Performing an abbreviated primary survey, he focused his initial actions on controlling the potentially catastrophic haemorrhage flowing from the wound in the Marine's groin. The injury was too proximal for the application of a tourniquet so he quickly packed the wound with a haemostatic dressing. After ensuring that the casualty's airway was patent and his respiratory rate acceptable, he moved on to assess his circulation. A significant amount of blood had already been lost and the casualty's pulse was weak and rapid, his extremities cool. In the distance the sound of the Merlin's rotors could be heard over the crash of the waves.

160520Z JUN 20: *Sabre* Beach

With the Merlin still "burning and turning"[3] the pre-hospital team ran down the stern ramp. The team had many years of experience in the pre hospital arena, some of it gained during previous conflicts and kept up to date working within civilian pre hospital care systems. They quickly ascertained that the young marine had lost a significant proportion of his circulating blood volume. Wasting no time, they moved him to the back of the aircraft, which then lifted and turned back over the ocean.

---

[3] A phrase indicating that the aircraft had landed but not shut down it's rotors or engines in anticipation of the requirement for a quick departure.

160525Z JUN 20: 820 Naval Air Squadron Merlin, *Piranha 1*

In the back of the aircraft the team worked on the casualty. After securing intraosseus access into the undamaged contralateral humerus, the team rapidly infused two units of blood and two units of plasma. However, the ongoing blood loss had caused his brain perfusion pressure to fall and he was becoming increasingly agitated. The team moved on to induce anaesthesia using the intraosseous route for drug delivery, before undertaking endotracheal intubation and ventilation. The critical decision now was whether there was enough time to get the casualty to the nearest medical treatment facility on RFA *Argus* before the blood loss led to hypovolaemic cardiac arrest.

With the casualty's blood pressure now barely recordable the team made the decision to institute Resuscitative Endovascular Balloon Occlusion of the Aorta (REBOA) treatment.

After accessing the casualty's femoral artery on the contralateral side to the injury, the pre hospital consultant inserted the balloon occlusion catheter over a wire. An ultrasound transducer on the tip of the catheter attached to a small portable monitor allowed the catheter to be precisely placed in the distal aorta, avoiding occlusion of the renal arteries. The balloon was then inflated under ultrasound guidance until flow was just occluded. With blood loss controlled, the team continued aggressive volume resuscitation using the remaining blood products in their shock pack[4] as the aircraft touched down on *Argus's* flight deck.

---

[4] A pack of blood products, usually containing four units of O negative packed red cells and 4 units of plasma.

160600Z JUN 20: Emergency Department, Primary Casualty Receiving Facility, RFA *Argus*

The casualty was transferred into the Emergency Department (ED) after rapidly travelling down four decks in a huge purpose built lift that penetrated the cavernous hull of the ship. The purpose built facility was full of medical staff but the atmosphere remained calm and quiet. The pre-hospital consultant delivered a brief AT – MIST handover[5] to the trauma team. At the head end of the patient one anaesthetic specialist connected the patient to a ventilator whilst another inserted a large sheath into the subclavian vein. This 'trauma line' was connected to a rapid infusion device through which further boluses of blood and plasma were delivered, at a rate of up to 1000 ml/min. Concurrently a radiology consultant performed a rapid focussed ultrasound scan to exclude intra-abdominal haemorrhage and a digital chest X Ray was obtained at the outset of the primary survey. As the primary survey progressed the trauma team leader, a consultant in Emergency Medicine, had a critical decision to make; should the casualty go straight to the operating theatre or would advanced imaging enable further definition of the injuries sustained? In conjunction with the surgical specialists he decided that, although blood loss was currently controlled, the casualty required immediate surgery in order to obtain proximal vascular control, release the REBOA balloon and restore distal perfusion as soon as possible. Further imaging would be performed at the conclusion of this damage control surgery.

---

[5] A didactic handover format comprising information on patient **A**ge, **T**ime and **M**echanism of injury, **I**njuries, vital **S**igns and **T**reatments administered.

160615Z JUN 20: Operating Theatre, PCRF

The operating theatre in the PCRF is directly adjacent to the ED and the casualty was swiftly transferred onto the operating table. Three surgical teams were prepared to receive the patient, including specialists in general, orthopaedic and plastic surgery. A team of specialist theatre nurses prepared the patient and exposed the operative field. When the team was ready and a brief summary of priorities given by the lead surgeon and lead anaesthetist, the surgery commenced with the general surgeon obtaining proximal vascular control, after which the aortic balloon was deflated. The surgeons commenced the repair of the lacerated femoral vessels, inserting a jump graft to bypass the areas of injury and restore perfusion. Whilst this was underway the anaesthetic team undertook further volume resuscitation. Blood products including packed red blood cells, plasma, platelets and cryoprecipitate were provided from the on-board blood bank, and were tailored to meet the individual requirements of the patient's coagulopathy, guided by near patient thromboelastometry. The main objective of surgery was to obtain surgical haemorrhage control, and to restore perfusion to the lower extremities as quickly as possible, in order to minimise the subsequent ischaemia re-perfusion injury. Definitive surgical repair would be performed at a later time. The complex fracture of the humerus was expeditiously treated by the orthopaedic surgeon by the application of an external fixator.

160730Z JUN 20: CT Scanner, PCRF

After the operation concluded, the patient was moved to the CT scanner, located on the other side of the ED. His whole body was imaged to exclude other injuries, such as occult spinal fracture, and to confirm the integrity of the surgical repair. The radiology consultant reported the images in real time alongside the other members of the multi-specialty trauma team. The scan showed that flow through the arterial jump graft was adequately perfusing the lower limb and that in addition to the already noted injuries the casualty had sustained some rib fractures and associated areas of lung contusion. However, brain imaging and spinal reconstructions were reassuringly normal and there were no significant pelvic or abdominal visceral injuries.

160745Z JUN 20: Intensive Care Unit, PCRF

Less than 3 hours after he was first injured, the casualty arrived in the PCRF intensive care unit. The anaesthetist handed over to the intensive care consultant who continued the resuscitation, using focused transthoracic echocardiography to optimise the patient's volume status and thromboelastography to target on-going haemostatic resuscitation. The goal now was to ensure that tissue perfusion was normalised as quickly as possible and to aid in this a point of care videomicroscope was employed to assess flow through the sublingual microcirculation.

181500Z JUN 20: Royal Air Force C17 Transport Aircraft

The patient went on to develop a marked systemic inflammatory response and vasoplegia following reperfusion, and this necessitated ongoing organ support on the ICU. Given the operational situation, there was a delay of several days until the patient could be evacuated to a land based airhead and repatriated to the UK. He was transferred from *Argus* and met at the airhead by a dedicated Royal Air Force Critical Care Air Support Team (CCAST). This specialist team of intensivists and critical care nurses were able to provide ongoing organ support during the transfer within a C17 aircraft. Four days after injury the patient arrived at a large tertiary hospital within the United Kingdom. After further definitive surgery he was weaned from ventilatory and cardiovascular support and made a full recovery from his injuries.

The Challenges of Treating Critically Injured Patients During Military Operations and the Contribution of Critical Care Services

Patients like the Royal Marine in our fictional example who sustain injuries during conflict present with a constellation of injury patterns unlike anything commonly encountered in civilian medical practice. The use of explosives and high velocity ballistic rounds often produce catastrophic injury patterns that can be rapidly fatal without appropriate management. Furthermore patients often sustain these injuries in parts of world without any modern medical, let alone specialist critical care, facilities. The point of injury may be exposed to hostile enemy fire and be many miles away from the nearest allied medical treatment facility. Although the initial treatment for these patients will usually be provided by specialists in Emergency Medicine, Surgery and Anaesthesia, without the intensive monitoring and on going resuscitation provided by a deployed critical care unit, these patients are at risk of early mortality and significant morbidity. Critical care specialists and services will play an increasingly vital role as patients move onwards following initial resuscitation and surgery.

Figure 1.1 shows the "Pathway to Recovery" for a serviceman or woman injured during military operations. As outlined in the fictional account above, each step is a vital link in the pathway from injury to eventual recovery and the absence of any of these components may lead to increased mortality or morbidity. Critical care support comes relatively late in the pathway but is often necessary for a far longer period than the other components. There are a variety of environments where deployed critical care services can be delivered.

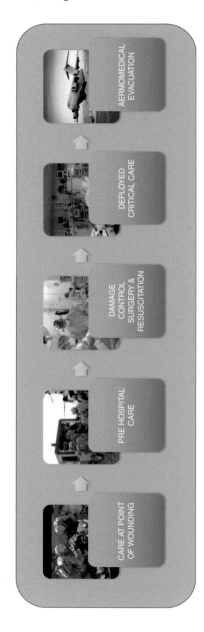

FIGURE 1.1 Pathway to recovery for critically injured UK service personnel. Each link in the chain performs a vital function but patients will often spend the majority of their time prior to strategic evacuation within deployed critical care facilities

What Types of Critical Care Services Are Provided Within Deployed Medical Treatment Facilities?

There are a variety of medical treatment facilities that can be deployed to support military operations. Those that have provision to support critically ill patients are detailed here. As discussed in the Preface, this book has a particular UK focus, but similar structures are systems are used by other NATO and allied nations.

Forward Medical Treatment Facility (Ashore or Afloat)

Smaller facilities will often be used to support more mobile operations or where there is a very long chain of evacuation back to a larger facility. They can be land based, often deliverable entirely from the air at short notice, or maritime. In the latter case a small critical care facility can be placed on a variety of existing warships or auxiliary vessels. These facilities have the capacity to hold ventilated patients for a limited time (usually up to 48 hours) prior to evacuation to a higher scale deployed medical treatment facility or the home base. However, they lack many of the services available at larger facilities. In addition to lack of imaging (which may include mobile x-ray and ultrasound rather than CT), and reduced pathology services (limited blood tests and transfusion services without platelets or cryoprecipitate), the equipment is often more basic. In the lighter scale facilities, the intensive care ventilator is no more than a simple transport ventilator. The intensive care beds are light-weight frames with issues for pressure area care. Monitoring is, however, similar, and the majority of drugs required for critical care are available, albeit in smaller quantities. An example of the critical care area within such a facility is shown in Fig. 1.2.

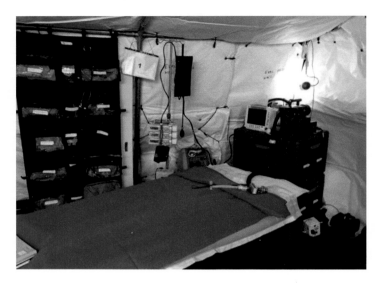

Figure 1.2 The critical care area within the Commando Forward Surgical Group (CFSG) forward medical treatment facility. Designed to support the UK Royal Marines close to the forward edge of the battle space it is staffed by surgeons, anaesthetists and intensive care nurse specialists (Photograph courtesy of Surgeon Commander Barrie Decker Royal Navy)

Vanguard Field Hospital

Newly deployed land based field hospitals will usually be designed to stay in one location, further removed from the area of battle. They will typically utilise tented accommodation and the physical infrastructure may be relatively austere. There will be less physical space than in a mature hard standing facility and this may impact on some of the interventions that can be delivered. The working environment may be harsher and supply of essentials such as lighting, temperature control and medical gases will be harder to guarantee. The impact of the environment can be more pronounced and this may produce effects on staff and service delivery. Despite this the range of clinical and support services available are not dissimilar to those in a more mature deployed treatment

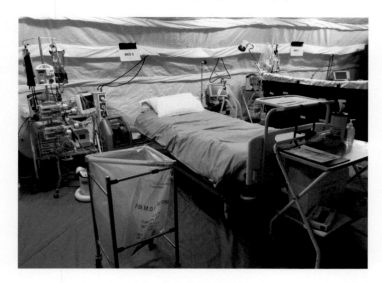

FIGURE 1.3 A bed space within the intensive care unit of a land based field hospital, taken during an exercise (Photograph courtesy of Lieutenant Colonel Stephen Lewis RAMC)

facility. There will be a laboratory service capable of supplying blood products and supporting a massive transfusion protocol. Near patient testing in the form of ROTEM and iStat will also be available. CT scanning facilities will be available in more established facilities but not necessarily during the initial, insertion phase. An example of the critical care area in such a facility is shown in Fig. 1.3

The Mature Deployed Medical Treatment Facility

This type of unit would be very familiar to a civilian intensivist. It is usually contained within a hard standing facility and is well lit and temperature controlled. Bed spaces are large and equipped with modern electronic beds. There are usually adequate supplies of high pressure oxygen, although this will be delivered by cylinders rather than pipelines from a remote source. Electricity generation is reliable and capable of delivering an uninterrupted supply under most circumstances. There are dedicated areas for administration and staff downtime. Resupply is not normally a problem with an air bridge delivering timely resupply of consumables and equipment. Strategic aeromedical evacuation is usually conducted from a co-located airhead, reducing the requirement for a secondary transfer. Examples of this type of facility, operated by the UK DMS, include the latter build critical care areas within the Role 3 Hospital at the Contingency Operating Base, Basra, Iraq (maximum 4 beds) and the Role 3 Hospital at Camp Bastion, Afghanistan (maximum 16 beds). Figure 1.4 shows an example of such a facility.

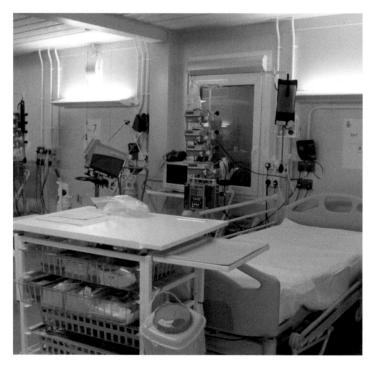

FIGURE 1.4 A bed space within the intensive care unit at the Role 3 Hospital, Camp Bastion, Afghanistan

Primary Casualty Receiving Facility (PCRF)

The PCRF is housed within RFA Argus, shown in Fig. 1.5.

Within this ship is a modular hospital, which contains a ten bed critical care facility, shown in Fig. 1.6. The critical care facility is one part of a complex that includes a four resuscitation bay emergency department, a CT scanner and a two table operating theatre as well as dedicated support from laboratory services.

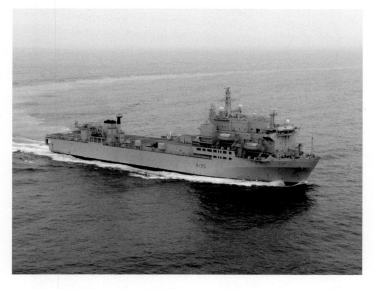

FIGURE 1.5 RFA Argus, a 28,000 tonne multi role vessel of the Royal Fleet Auxiliary. Her primary role is to deploy and operate the Primary Casualty Receiving Facility. She is a veteran of the Falklands Conflict (as the MV Contender Bezant), the Gulf conflicts of 1991 and 2003 and most recently the operation to provide assistance to Sierra Leone during the 2014/15 Ebola crisis

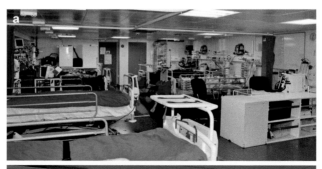

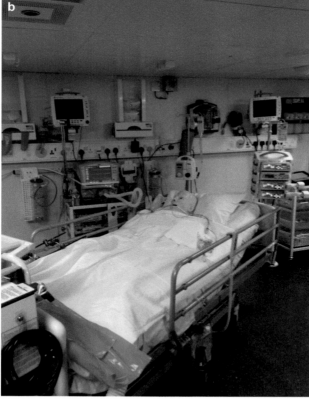

FIGURE 1.6 One half of the PCRF intensive care unit, showing half of the ten bed spaces. A bed space with a simulated patient from a recent exercise is also shown

Critical Care Air Support Teams (CCAST)

Evacuation of critically ill patients to home base facilities is undertaken by specialist teams of clinicians and nurses from the Royal Air Forces Critical Care Air Support Teams. These teams are consultant lead and can continue virtually all critical care interventions throughout the transfer period, thus providing a critical care air bridge between deployed and home nation facilities. Teams are on standby 24 hours a day and the mean time from hospital admission to patient evacuation during recent operations in Afghanistan was less than 18 hours. A fuller account of the CCAST service is provided in Chap. 19.

Chapter 2
Evolution and Organisation of Trauma Services

C. Andrew Eynon

Abstract Traumatic injury is a significant worldwide public health problem. It is a major cause of death across the ages, with many survivors having life-long disabilities. The social and economic costs resulting from trauma amount to 1–2 % of gross national product. Over the last 40 years considerable progress has been made in the management of major trauma. Better education and training combined with alterations in the systems of trauma care have resulted in considerable improvements in hospital mortality rates. Many of the developments in civilian trauma care have originated from changes initiated during military conflicts. Recognition of trauma as a disease has also focused attention and resources on prevention of injury and recovery from illness, and the assessment of the trauma system as a whole.

C.A. Eynon, MBBS, MD, FRCP, FRCEM, FFICM
Wessex Neurological Centre, University Hospital
Southampton NHS Foundation Trust, Tremona Road,
Southampton SO16 6YD, UK
e-mail: andy.eynon@uhs.nhs.uk

S.D. Hutchings (ed.), *Trauma and Combat Critical Care
in Clinical Practice*, In Clinical Practice,
DOI 10.1007/978-3-319-28758-4_2,

Keywords   Regional trauma networks • Major trauma centre • Trauma unit • Injury demographics • Quality improvement • Trauma outcomes

What Are the Demographics of Traumatic Injury and How Are These Evolving?

Injuries are the cause of nearly six million deaths or 10 % of all worldwide deaths each year [1]. The causes of trauma death by mechanism of injury are shown in Fig. 2.1.

The WHO divides injuries into either intentional or unintentional. Intentional injuries include those that are self-inflicted or those resulting from interpersonal violence or warfare. Unintentional injuries include those sustained though road-traffic collisions, poisoning, falls, fires or drowning. In 2004, deaths from road traffic accidents and falls were the 9th and 20th commonest causes of death, accounting for 1.3 million and 700,000 deaths respectively [2]. About half of trauma deaths are in people of working age, between 15 and

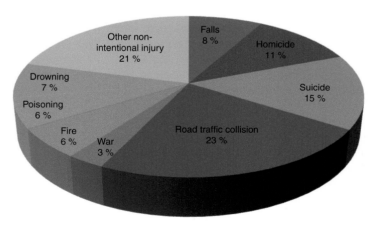

FIGURE 2.1 Causes of injury deaths worldwide (Adapted from World Health Organization. Injuries and violence: the facts. Geneva: WHO; 2010)

45 years, and it is the leading cause of death in this age group [1]. Injury affects more males than females; over two thirds of injuries occur in males and death from trauma is twice as common in males as it is in females [1]. Although the elderly are less likely to be injured, morbidity and mortality are higher for comparable severities of injury and trauma remains one of the commonest causes of death in those over 60 years of age [3]. The incidence of major trauma in the elderly is increasing. Approximately 30 % of people aged over 65 years fall each year, increasing to 40 % for those over 75 years [4, 5]. In Victoria State, Australia, in 2010–2011, a third of adult major trauma patients were aged 65 years and over compared to 24 % in 2005–2006, with the most rapid increase in incidence occurring in patients aged 85 years and over [6]. In the USA, the mortality rate for drivers 85 years and over is nine times that for drivers 25–69 years [7]. Older drivers are the most rapidly growing section of the driving population in the USA.

The majority of all injury deaths occur either at the scene or before hospitalisation. In high income countries there are up to nine pre-hospital deaths for each hospital death [8]. This figure is likely to be even higher in low or middle income countries. The trauma epidemic is only increasing. Globally, road traffic fatalities are predicted to increase to 2.6 million by 2030 with an increasing divide between developed countries, where road traffic deaths are falling, and the developing nations, where increasing vehicle numbers are expected to result in a 92 % rise in road traffic deaths in China and 147 % in India [9].

An estimated 16 % of all disabilities worldwide are the result of injuries [1, 2]. Each year, around 50 million people suffer moderate or severe disability as a result of trauma. The World Health Organisation (WHO) estimates the number of years lost through premature deaths and the years an individual lives with disability. These are combined to give the number of disability adjusted life years (DALYs); estimated to be around 180 million [2]. This loss of working lives, either through death or disability in people of working age, presents an enormous socioeconomic burden. Road traffic accidents are estimated to cost $518 billion globally per year [1]. This equates to 1 % of gross national product in low-income countries, 1.5 % in middle-income countries and 2 % in high-income countries [2, 10].

Trauma care has developed enormously over the last 40 years, initially with the designation of major trauma centres in the USA in the 1970s. More recently there has been a shift towards the development of major trauma systems that encompass the entire patient journey from injury to rehabilitation and also including preventive measures. Performance measures have also started to shift from those solely concerned with hospital care to measures that assess the whole of the patient's journey.

What Factors Have Lead to Changes in the Provision of Trauma Critical Care Over the Past 40 Years?

In 1966, the National Academy of Sciences in the United States published 'Accidental death and disability: the neglected disease of modern society' [11]. This highlighted the differences in the quality of care provided to civilian victims of trauma in the USA compared to military personnel in Vietnam. Over subsequent years, regionalised trauma systems were developed incorporating pre-hospital care, communications and networks of hospitals. In 1976, the American College of Surgeons Committee on Trauma published criteria to categorize hospitals according to the resources available to treat trauma patients [12]. Health Authorities in many states used these to designate hospitals into one of four levels for trauma care depending on their capabilities. Regional trauma systems and centres were also designed to improve the preparedness for major incidents. Implementation has not been universal 'because of questions of need, efficacy, cost and possibly political intervention' [13]. In the USA the focus has appeared to be primarily on the trauma centre with a lesser emphasis on the trauma system as a whole.

In Australia a systems approach to trauma care was first proposed in New South Wales in 1988. Since that date, similar systems have been developed across the country [14]. In 2011, all of Australia's 26 designated trauma centres and 4 established state-based trauma registries joined in partnership to develop an Australian Trauma Quality Improvement Program (AusTQIP) underpinned by the Australian Trauma Registry (ATR) [15]. The annual cost for traumatic injury related health care in Australia exceeds $3.4 billion, over 7 % of total health costs, and it is likely these costs are underestimated. The annual cost of traumatic injury to the Australian economy has been estimated to be $18 billion [15]. For the more than 1200 people who suffer traumatic brain or spinal cord injuries in Australia every year, the overall cost (including health care, equipment and life-time care) exceeds $3 billion per year. The disproportionate impact on younger people means that traumatic injury is also the leading cause of loss of economically productive years of life.

In the UK, there have been a series of publications over the last 30 years, highlighting the deficiencies in trauma care. The first of these, in 1988, studied 1000 injury-related deaths and found that of 514 patients admitted to hospital alive, 170 deaths were considered preventable by three or more assessors [16]. In 2007, the NCEPOD report *'Trauma, who cares?'* highlighted deficiencies in both organisational and clinical aspects of care with almost 60 % of patients receiving a standard of care that was considered 'less than good practice' [17]. Political involvement perhaps stimulated the necessary changes. In 2008, Professor Lord Darzi, then a labour minister, published 'High Quality for All-NHS Next Stage Review Final Report'. This report concluded that there were compelling arguments for rationalising the number of hospitals receiving patients with major trauma and the creation of specialised centres [18]. In 2010, the National Audit Office estimated that the annual lost economic output as a result of major trauma was between £3.3 billion and £3.7 billion [19]. Of the 193 hospitals that had emergency departments, the number of patients with major trauma seen each year ranged from 18 to 265 depending on geography and hospital size. Only 114 hospitals contributed data to the Trauma Audit Research network (59 %) and these showed a range of outcomes following trauma, from five unexpected survivors to eight unexpected deaths per 100 trauma patients. Even in those contributing data, the amount and quality were variable and the performance of the remaining 41 % of hospitals could not be judged. The report concluded that 450–600 lives could be saved each year in England with better organisation of trauma care. In 2010, three major trauma networks were established in London with a fourth commencing in early 2011. The London ambulance service was given the authority to bypass emergency departments and go direct to the major trauma centre, if the patient was considered to have sustained major traumatic injuries.

In 1978, the first ATLS course was tested in conjunction with the Southeast Nebraska Emergency Medical Service [20]. The course was adopted by the American College of Surgeons a year later and was conducted nationally under the College auspices in January 1980 with the first international course in 1986. Around 50,000 clinicians are trained each year on over 3000 courses in 60 countries. Similar courses have been established for pre-hospital personnel, nursing staff and allied health care professionals. Many lessons from conflict have been adopted into civilian trauma care over the last few decades. Exsanguination from extremity injury was the commonest cause of preventable death in the Vietnam conflict. Since 2005, the US military have adopted a haemorrhage control policy that includes the use of combat tourniquets with the incidence of death from extremity haemorrhage falling by over two thirds [21]. The use of tourniquets, haemostatic dressings, tranexamic acid, early use of blood and blood products have all been translated from military to civilian practice.

The strengthening of trauma care has been identified as a priority in many low and middle income countries. Trauma system development has recently been reviewed and a wide variety of heterogeneous programmes have been successful [22, 23].

What Is a Regional Trauma Network?

Regional trauma networks can be described as exclusive or inclusive. An inclusive trauma system is one which is responsible for all aspects of trauma care in a defined area, providing differing levels of service provision according to capability. The system is responsible for all aspects of care from injury to rehabilitation and including injury prevention. In contrast, an exclusive system focuses trauma care on the level 1 or major trauma centre. The principal risk of inclusive trauma systems is that the patient is wrongly triaged to a hospital that is unable to provide the full range of care required, necessitating transfer of the patient for definitive care. Inclusive systems may also dilute the volumes of trauma seen at the major centre. For exclusive systems the principal concern is over-triage of patients to the major centre, overwhelming the services there with patients who could quite appropriately be managed at a smaller facility. Studies suggest that over 80 % of patients admitted to trauma centres in the United States do not require specific trauma centre management [24]. Prevention, rehabilitation and the roles of the pre-hospital providers and smaller hospitals may receive less attention in exclusive systems.

Ideally, the design of trauma systems would be done after a comprehensive needs assessment within a region as there are dangers with both under and over-designating services. Trauma systems have often, however, been defined as much on the basis of existing services as the population density and patient needs. Studies suggest the need for one or two level 1 or 2 trauma centres per million population to achieve the appropriate concentration of severely injured patients in a limited number of specialty care facilities [25].

In the USA, trauma system development is usually the state's responsibility. Most of the systems currently employed in the USA are exclusive systems, focusing activity on the level 1 trauma centre. Many areas have not limited the number of trauma centres based on need, such that there are often competing trauma centres within a small area, while other parts of the country have no designated centres [26]. Similarly in Australia, major trauma centres are designated by regional administrative health services of State Health Departments. In 2010, the Royal Australasian College of Surgeons introduced a verification system comprising five levels [1–5] of trauma care. This was designated to assist in the analysis of care systems but has remained voluntary and states can designate level 1 trauma centres independent of the verification process. This has resulted in variations in levels of care and resource allocation [27].

In the UK, a trauma network is the name given to the collaboration between all providers commissioned to deliver trauma care in a geographical region. The network includes all providers of trauma care including pre-hospital services, trauma units (local hospitals that receive trauma admissions and due to geographical distance from the major trauma centre may be required to provide initial assessment and resuscitation of the major trauma patient), the major trauma centre and rehabilitation units. Several trauma networks, covering the south of the UK, are shown in Fig. 2.2.

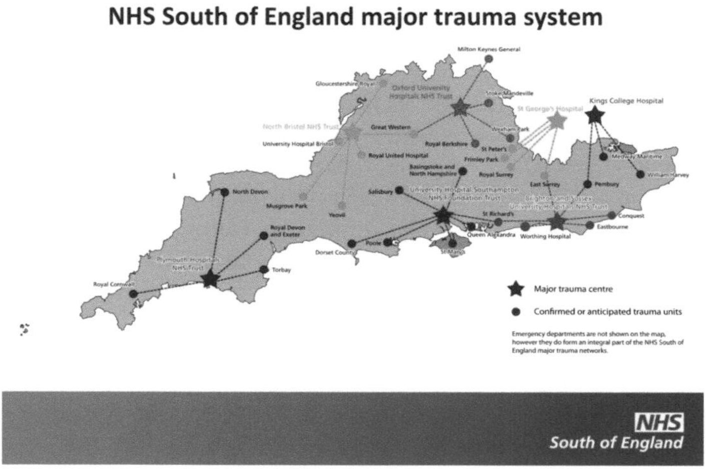

FIGURE 2.2 Trauma networks across the south of the United Kingdom showing the hub and spoke setup of Major Trauma Centres and Trauma Units (NHS South of England *with permission*)

Prior to the launch of the national trauma networks, designation criteria were established for both major trauma centres and trauma units. Not all major trauma centres achieved all of the necessary designation criteria prior to going live and indeed some centres have still not established all of the necessary requirements 3 years into the re-organisation. Some networks designated all hospitals wishing to retain trauma services as trauma units and have since un-designated those that failed to meet the necessary standards whereas other networks insisted that trauma unit status would only be granted if the hospital met the necessary standard and that there was also a geographical requirement. There are currently 12 combined adult and paediatric major trauma centres in England with a further four designated as paediatric-only and 8 adult-only major trauma centres. There are two geographical areas where major trauma services are provided by a consortium of hospitals (with specialties split over multiple sites) although a review of one of these consortia in 2015 suggested that all major trauma should be co-located to one site.

What Are the Advantages of Clustering the Care of Critically Injured Patents in Major Trauma Centres?

Trauma system performances in the USA were first evaluated by means of expert panel studies. The development of registries for trauma care has subsequently allowed comparison among trauma systems. In 2006, a systematic review of studies evaluating trauma system performance in the USA found 14 articles [28]. Of these, 8 showed improved odds of survival. Meta-analysis of all published studies found a 15 % reduction in mortality in favour of trauma systems. A review of outcomes at 18 trauma centres and 51 non-trauma centres in the USA, found a 20 % reduction in the risk of death in a trauma centre that increases to 25 % when outcome data is extended to 1 year [29]. A number of studies have shown the impact of volume of cases on outcome with suggestions that trauma centres should treat a minimum of 240 cases of severe trauma each year to maintain experience [30].

Cohorting major trauma patients at level 1 centres allows identification of low incidence error patterns. A 9 year review of admissions at a level 1 trauma centre in Seattle identified 64 of 2594 deaths (0.1 % of trauma patient admissions, 2.5 % of deaths) that had errors in their care [31]. Error patterns identified included failure to successfully intubate, secure or protect the airway, delayed operative control of haemorrhage, inadequate DVT or gastrointestinal prophylaxis, lengthy initial operations rather than damage-control surgery, over-resuscitation and complications of feeding tubes. A similar study from California found 51 preventable or potentially preventable deaths from 2081 deaths over an 8 year period with over 35,000 trauma admissions [32]. Delay in control of haemorrhage was a major cause in 13 cases. In six of these there was failure to activate the trauma team and in seven there was delay in taking the patient to the operating theatre. Two cases resulted from failure to activate a second surgical team when the first was already operating. Four cases had delay in securing an airway. In six cases, a missed injury contributed to death. The most common recurrent cause of preventable death remained human error, resulting in delays in treatment, inadequate monitoring and missed injuries.

A review of 6 years of management of severely injured (Injury Severity Score >15) patients in New South Wales, Australia found an increased odds of death for patients managed at a level 3 hospital compared to those managed at a level 1 hospital (OR 2.00; 95 % CI 1.29–3.11) [27]. 48 patients died at the level 3 hospital in the time period studied (17 %). 42 patient records were reviewed and 6 deaths were considered preventable or possibly preventable. Each death had multiple problems identified, the majority of which occurred in the prehospital phase of care or in the emergency department.

In the UK, recent data from TARN has shown a more than 60 % improvement in mortality from major trauma compared to 2008 (https://www.tarn.ac.uk/Content.aspx?c=3477). The data also indicates that the improvement has been largely in the last 3 years following the development of major trauma networks. Although very encouraging, data collection remains incomplete especially outside the major trauma centres and this improvement refers only to in-hospital mortality. The ELOTS study reported the differences in patient outcomes in London following the introduction of the London trauma networks [33]. Although national data indicated that at the time of the study nearly half of all patients sustaining major trauma were managed entirely outside the MTC, only cases that were admitted directly to the MTC or were transferred to the MTC were studied. 321 cases were reviewed and a higher quality of care was noted when compared with the NCEPOD study of 2007. In the study, 69 % of patients were felt to have received a 'good standard of care' compared to 48 % in the NCEPOD study. Greatest benefit was noted in the reduction in organisational deficits. Significant differences remained in the standard of care received by patients who were initially managed in trauma units compared to the major trauma centres. Eight percent of patients in the MTC were considered to have room for improvement in at least one aspect of management compared to 1 in 3 patients at the trauma units.

The number of cases of paediatric major trauma each year are relatively small. It is not clear whether children should be treated at dedicated paediatric major trauma centres or within adult centres with paediatric experience [34].

How Do We Assess the Quality and Performance of Trauma Systems?

The outcome for patients sustaining major trauma will depend on three factors: the severity of injury, patient specific factors such as age and co-morbidities and trauma system performance. There are a variety of scoring systems for the severity of the injury sustained [35]. The Abbreviated Injury Scale (AIS) lists over 200 injuries based on anatomy. Patients with multiple injuries are scored by adding together the squares of the three highest AIS scores in three regions of the body, to give an Injury Severity Score (ISS). An ISS greater than 15 is defined as major trauma, 9–14 as moderate trauma and ≤8 as minor trauma. The Revised Trauma Score (RTS) assesses the physiological response to trauma. By convention, the first measurements when the patient arrives at hospital are used. These can obviously be influenced by pre-hospital practice and if the patient is intubated, the RTS cannot be measured. Overall measures of the probability of survival have been derived by combining anatomical and physiological scores: TRISS includes the RTS, ISS, the age of the patient and whether the injury was blunt or penetrating. This methodology is now being superseded by better outcome prediction models.

To assess the performance of inclusive trauma systems, simple measures of in-patient outcome such as mortality rates are insufficient and an approach that uses an extended number of metrics is advisable, as shown in Fig. 2.3.

A review in 2011 found only one international trauma registry that routinely collected morbidity outcome measures for both adults and children [36]. Deaths from trauma may occur before the hospital or following the acute hospital episode. A 7 year nationwide study in Sweden found 1112 hospital injury deaths with 17,703 pre-hospital deaths [8]. Pre-hospital deaths were more likely in males (73 %) whereas hospital deaths were evenly distributed. Nearly three quarters of pre-hospital deaths occurred in patients less than 64 years of age. A smaller study in Miami-Dade County found 512 trauma deaths that were not transported to hospital [37]. 80 % of deaths were male, mostly resulting from neurotrauma and haemorrhage. In this study, more than 1 in 5 cases had potentially survivable injuries. The effects of trauma may continue long-after the acute episode. A follow-up study of trauma patients in Washington State found excess post-injury mortality at 3 years of 10 % above age and sex-adjusted norms [38]. In the elderly, one study of patients with traumatic brain injury found that post-discharge mortality was 3.5

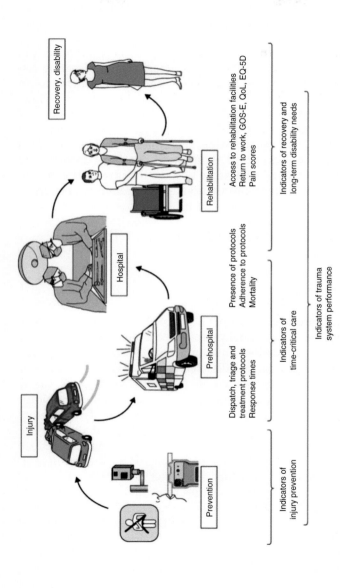

FIGURE 2.3 The injured patient's journey and measures to assess trauma system performance (From Gruen et al. [48], with permission)

times greater than that of the general population with half of the deaths occurring within 6 months of discharge [39]. Extending the period for outcome measurement also allows the impact of morbidity to be studied. In-hospital data does not take into account the improvements made following discharge from the acute admission. The cost-effectiveness of care can also only be assessed following longer-term follow-up. Hospital costs are only a fraction of the lifetime costs for patients who are left unable to work and require long-term care. Effective system-wide monitoring can be achieved through the linkage of databases containing information about pre-hospital care, acute hospital management, rehabilitation care, coroner information and economic assessments.

What Are the Ongoing Issues in Trauma Critical Care?

Prevention

Many approaches have been adopted worldwide to reduce the burden of potentially preventable injury. These include legislation, education, environmental changes such as road design and emergency disaster preparation that reduce or eliminate the risks or increase protective factors [40]. In the USA, there has been a dramatic fall in the numbers of motor vehicle related deaths due to a combination of road safety measures, safer cars and changes in driver behaviours. The correct use of lap-shoulder belts and car airbags can reduce fatalities for occupants of vehicles by >60 %. The use of seatbelts in the USA was reported as 83 % in 2008, whereas in China their use by drivers varies from 30 to 66 %, with <10 % of front-seat passengers wearing seatbelts. In the USA, concern has been expressed regarding the increasing numbers of elderly drivers and the finding that as drivers age, the risk of a fatal accident increase in a non-linear fashion [40]. By 2030 it is estimated that drivers over 65 years will account for 25 % of drivers involved in fatal car accidents. Prevention of road traffic crashes and injuries in the elderly requires a variety of approaches including car design, roadway design and person specific measures including trying to identify who should stop driving due to an unacceptable risk of crashing.

Motorcyclists are nearly forty times more likely to die in a road traffic accident than car occupants [41]. Motorcycle helmets have been shown to reduce the risk of death by >40 % but reports from low and middle income countries show that helmets are underused. Restrictions on the size of engine that learner drivers can ride have resulted in a 25 % reduction in casualties among young motorcyclists in the UK [42].

In low and middle income countries, child pedestrians comprise 30–40 % of all road traffic deaths [41]. Risk factors for child pedestrian injury include male gender, younger age, low income families, high traffic volumes and high vehicle speed. The probability of pedestrian death from road crashes increases significantly with increasing speed. Introduction of 20 mph zones in the U.K. has resulted in >40 % reduction in road casualties with the percentage reduction greatest for younger children [43].

In 2004, around 1.6 million people died worldwide due to violence, the vast majority, around 1.5 million, in low and middle income countries [41]. The highest rates are found in young males between 15 and 29 years where a history of early aggression, low IQ, substance misuse and exposure to media violence are individual risk factors. Low socioeconomic class, academic failure, gang membership, high crime areas with easy access to firearms are additional risk factors. Tackling these issues clearly requires multi-focused prevention strategies.

Unintentional falls are major public health issues for the elderly. Over 400,000 people die from falls each year and in 2002, they were the second highest cause of unintentional deaths after road traffic accidents. Over three quarters of fall related deaths occur in low and middle income countries. Many studies have identified that exercise, vitamin D supplementation, cataract surgery and review and withdrawal of psychotropic medication can be effective in reducing falls [41].

In 2012, drowning was the cause of an estimated 372,000 deaths [44]. The vast majority of deaths are in low and middle income countries. Drowning in children under 1 year occurs predominantly in bathtubs or buckets where lack of supervision is the main factor. Fifty percent of cases occurring in the 1–4 age group in higher income countries are in swimming pools where lack of barriers is a factor. In low and middle income countries, most drowning in 1–4 years is in natural bodies of water. Simple measures to separate children from bodies of water and teaching water safety can have significant impacts.

Rehabilitation and Outcomes

The Victorian State Trauma Registry collects detailed follow-up information regarding patient outcomes following major trauma [45]. At 24 months post-injury, the factors that influenced whether a major trauma patient experienced a good recovery differed for adult and paediatric patients. For paediatric patients, the most important factor influencing functional outcome was the type of injury sustained, with patients experiencing chest and abdominal injuries experiencing the highest probability of recovery, followed by those with isolated head injuries and children who experienced only orthopaedic injuries. Socioeconomic and demographic factors were not important predictors of functional outcome in children. In contrast, pre-existing disability, socioeconomic status, age, pre-existing conditions, compensation status and the types of injuries sustained all influenced whether an adult major trauma patient experienced a good functional recovery at 24 months. The probability of experiencing a good recovery was highest for patients who experienced injuries to the chest and/or abdomen only and lowest for patients with spinal cord injury or orthopaedic injuries only. Increasing age, the presence of pre-existing medical, mental health, drug or alcohol conditions reduced the probability of a good functional outcome. At 24 months post-injury, the probability of returning to work ranged from 38 % for spinal cord injury patients to 79 % for major trauma patients who experienced injuries to the chest and/or abdomen only. Women were less likely than males to return to work at 24 months, and the probability of return to work decreased by 5–10 % with each decade of increasing age. The probability of return to work was 33–50 % lower for patients with pre-existing mental health, drug or alcohol conditions, or severe pre-existing medical conditions, respectively. Education below university level reduced the probability of return to work. The RESTORE study aims to provide an overview of patient outcomes for over 2500 adult and paediatric major trauma patients in the 5 years following injury to help guide provision of rehabilitation services [46].

In the UK the availability of rehabilitation services for patients sustaining multiple injuries varies widely and has been described as lacking co-ordination [19]. Services have often developed on the basis of local geography and expertise rather than on population demand with the actual needs of patients not being systematically appraisal. Many of the spinal injuries and burns centres are located on the sites of military hospitals from the 2nd World War rather than linked to major trauma centres. Experience from Headley Court, the military rehabilitation centre, has shown the benefits of having most forms of rehabilitation services on one site to enable holistic delivery of care to all patients with emphasis on vocational outcomes [47]. In low and middle income countries, there is an immense burden of disability related to extremity injuries and relatively simple interventions and rehabilitation may provide significant benefit.

References

1. World Health Organization. Injuries and violence: the facts. Geneva: WHO; 2010.
2. World Health Organization. The global burden of disease 2004. Geneva: WHO; 2008.

3. Hashmi A, Ibrahim-Zada I, Rhee P, et al. Predictors of mortality in geriatric trauma patients: a systematic review and meta-analysis. J Trauma Acute Care Surg. 2014;76:894–901.
4. World Health Organization. WHO global report on falls prevention in older age. Geneva: WHO; 2007.
5. Masud T, Morris RO. Epidemiology of falls. Age Ageing. 2001;30:3–7.
6. Department of Health and Human Services. Special focus report – elderly major trauma patients. Department of Health: Victoria, Australia 2013 (available at http://docs2.health.vic.gov.au/docs/doc/Special-Focus-Report--Elderly-Major-Trauma-Patients).
7. National Highway Traffic Safety Administration. Traffic safety facts 1999: older population. Publication no. DOT HS 809 091. Washington DC: NHTSA; 2000.
8. Gedeborg R, Chen L-H, Thiblin I, et al. Prehospital injury deaths – strengthening the case for prevention: nationwide cohort study. J Trauma. 2012;72:765–72.
9. Kopits E, Cropper M. Traffic fatalities and economic growth (policy research working paper no 3035). Washington DC: The World Bank; 2003. http://documents.worldbank.org/curated/en/2003/04/2329628/traffic-fatalities-economic-growth.
10. Peden M, Scurfield R, Sleet D, et al. World report on road traffic injury prevention. Geneva: WHO; 2004.
11. National Committee on Trauma and Committee on Shock. Accidental death and disability: the neglected disease of modern society. Washington DC: National Academies Press; 1966.
12. American College of Surgeons. Optimal hospital resources for care of the seriously injured. Bull Am Coll Surg. 1976;61:15–22.
13. Rainer TH, de Villiers-Smit P. Trauma systems and emergency medicine. Emerg Med. 2003;15:11–7.
14. NSW Institute of Trauma and Injury Management. The NSW trauma registry profile of serious to critical injuries. Sydney: NSW Institute of Trauma and Injury Management; 2007. p. 1–83.
15. Response to the Australian Commission for the safety and quality in health care on the 'Australian Safety and Quality goals for health care – consultation paper.' Australian Trauma Quality Improvement Program. 2012 (http://www.safetyandquality.gov.au/wp-content/uploads/2012/01/National-Goals-consultation-Submission-53-National-Trauma-Research-Institute-10-Feb-2012.pdf).
16. Anderson ID, Woodford M, de Dombal FT, Irving M. Retrospective study of 1000 deaths from injury in England and Wales. BMJ. 1988;296:1305–8.

17. Findlay G, Martin IC, Carter S, et al. Trauma; who cares? A report of the National Confidential Enquiry into Patient Outcome and Death 2007. London; 2007. p. 1–149.
18. Darzi A. High quality care for all, NHS next stage review final report. London: Department of Health; 2008. p. 1–92.
19. Morse A, Fisher A, Ross C, et al. Major trauma care in England. London: National Audit Office; 2010. p. 1–41.
20. American College of Surgeons. Advanced trauma life support. 9th ed. Chicago: American College of Surgeons; 2012.
21. Eastridge BJ, Mabry RL, Seguin P, et al. Death on the battle-field (2001–2011): implications for the future of combat casualty care. J Trauma Acute Care Surg. 2012;73(6 Suppl 5):S431–7.
22. Henry JA, Reingold AL. Prehospital trauma systems reduce mortality in developing countries: a systematic review and meta-analysis. J Trauma Acute Care Surg. 2012;73:261–8.
23. Callese TE, Richards CT, Shaw P, et al. Trauma system development in low- and middle-income countries: a review. J Surg Res. 2015;193:300–7.
24. Moore EE. Trauma systems, trauma centres and trauma surgeons: opportunities in managed competition. J Trauma. 1995;39:1–11.
25. MacKenzie EJ, Hoyt DB, Sacra JC, et al. National inventory of hospital trauma centres. JAMA. 2003;289:1515–22.
26. Blackwell T, Kellam JF, Thomason M. Trauma care systems in the United States. Injury. 2003;34:735–9.
27. Curtis K, Chong S, Mitchell R, et al. Outcomes of severely injured adult trauma patients in an Australian health Service: does trauma centre level make a difference? World J Surg. 2011;35:2332–40.
28. Celso B, Tepas J, Langland-Orban B, et al. A systematic review and meta-analysis comparing outcome of severely injured patients treated in trauma centres following the establishment of trauma systems. J Trauma. 2006;60:371–8.
29. MacKenzie EJ, Rivara FP, Jurkovich GJ, et al. A national evaluation of the effect of trauma-centre care on mortality. N Engl J Med. 2006;354:366–78.
30. Chiara O, Cimbanassi S. Organised trauma care: does volume matter and do trauma centres save lives? Curr Opin Crit Care. 2003;9:510–4.
31. Gruen RL, Jurkovich GJ, McIntyre LK, et al. Patterns of errors contributing to trauma mortality. Lessons learned from 2594 deaths. Ann Surg. 2006;244:371–80.

32. Teixeira PGR, Inaba K, Hadjizacharia P, et al. Preventable of potentially preventable mortality at a mature trauma centre. J Trauma. 2007;63:1338–47.

33. Cole E, Lecky F, West A, et al. The impact of a pan-regional inclusive trauma system on quality of care. Ann Surg. 2016; 264(1):188–94.

34. NHS Clinical Advisory Group. Management of children with major trauma. London: National Health Service; 2011. p. 1–22.

35. Lecky F, Woodford M, Edwards A, et al. Trauma scoring systems and databases. Br J Anaesth. 2014;113:286–94.

36. Sleat GK, Ardolino AM, Willett KM. Outcome measures in major trauma care: a review of current international trauma registry practice. Emerg Med J. 2011;28:1008–12.

37. Davis JS, Satahoo SS, Butler FK, et al. An analysis of prehospital deaths: who can we save? J Trauma Acute Care Surg. 2014;77:213–8.

38. Davidson GH, Hamlat CA, Rivara FP, et al. Long-term survival of adult trauma patients. JAMA. 2011;305:1001–7.

39. Peck KA, Calvo RY, Sise CB, et al. Death after discharge: predictors of mortality in older brain-injured patients. J Trauma Acute Care Surg. 2014;77:978–83.

40. Binder S. Injuries among older adults: the challenge of optimising safety and minimizing unintended consequences. Inj Prev. 2002;8(Suppl IV):iv2–4.

41. Curry P, Ramaiah R, Vavilala MS. Current trends and update on injury prevention. Int J Crit Illn Inj Sci. 2011;1:57–65.

42. Broughton J. The effect on motorcycling of the 1981 Transport Act. Crowthorne: Transport and Road Research Laboratory; 1987.

43. Grundy C, Steinbach R, Edwards P, et al. Effect of 20mph traffic zones on road injuries in London, 1986–2006: controlled interrupted time series analysis. BMJ. 2009;339:b4469.

44. World Health Organisation. Global report on drowning: preventing a leading killer. 2014. WHO Geneva (http://www.who.int/violence_injury_prevention/publications/drowning_global_report/en/).

45. Victorian State Trauma System. Victorian state trauma registry summary report 1 July 2013 – 30 June 2014. http://docs2.health.vic.gov.au/docs/doc/4E2375A167894BBDCA257E770001219C/$FILE/1501013_DHHS%20State%20trauma%20registry%20annual%20report%2013-14%20WEB.pdf.

46. Gabbe BJ, Braaf S, Fitzgerald M, et al. RESTORE: recovery after serious trauma outcomes, resource use and patient experiences study protocol. Inj Prev 2014. doi:10.1136/injuryprev-2014-041336. [Epub ahead of print].
47. Ladlow P, Phillip R, Etherington J, et al. Functional and mental health status of UK military amputees post-rehabilitation. Arch Phys Med Rehabil. 2015. pii: S0003-9993(15)00648-6. doi:10.1016/j.apmr.2015.07.016. [Epub ahead of print].
48. Gruen RL, Gabbe BJ, Stelfox HT, Cameron PA. Indicators of the quality of trauma care and the performance of trauma systems. Br J Surg. 2012;99 Suppl 1:97–104.

Chapter 3
Pre-hospital Management of the Critically Injured Patient

Paul S.C. Rees

Abstract Pre hospital management of critically injured patients is challenging but the application of a framework for key decisions can aid management in stressful austere environments. The field is continually evolving and evidence emerging for the use of novel therapies such as Resuscitative Balloon Occlusion of the Aorta (REBOA) for uncompressible lower body haemorrhage. Patients with traumatic cardiac arrest pose a particular challenge but the application of a management framework that includes that early use of focussed echocardiography and aggressive volume resuscitation can produce unexpected survivors from what had previously been considered a universally fatal condition. Resuscitative thoracotomy has been widely adopted by military and civilian healthcare providers and has a role in selected patients. The nature of the pre-hospital retrieval

P.S.C. Rees, MD, FRCP, DipIMC
School of Medicine, University of St Andrews, North Haugh,
St Andrews KY16 9TF, UK
e-mail: cardiacexpert@nhs.net

S.D. Hutchings (ed.), *Trauma and Combat Critical Care in Clinical Practice*, In Clinical Practice,
DOI 10.1007/978-3-319-28758-4_3,

service is of importance and there is evidence that specialist physician delivered care improves outcomes. One such service, the UK military Medical Emergency Response Team (MERT), is described in detail.

Keywords   Pre-hospital care • Major trauma • Exsanguinating haemorrhage • Resuscitative balloon occlusion of the aorta • Resuscitative thoracotomy • Pre-hospital trauma systems • Medical emergency response team • Military • Conflict

Part One: Key Clinical Questions in Pre-hospital Trauma Critical Care

What Are the Key Initial Decisions and Interventions in the Management of the Critically Injured Patient Pre-hospital?

The management of severely injured, critically ill patients imposes considerable challenges on clinical teams and a structured approach that covers rapid diagnosis and management is essential. These issues are magnified in the austere and rapidly changing pre-hospital environment. One suggested pathway, outlining the key questions and decisions that need to be made at each step during the pre-hospital management of critically injured patients, is shown in Fig. 3.1. Many of the concepts covered in this diagram are expanded upon later in this chapter or in other sections of this book.

Should Drug-Assisted Intubation Be Provided Pre-hospital?

Effective management of the airway is critical, and the ability to provide a definitive airway by means of drug-assisted endotracheal intubation is a key requirement in the pre-hospital care of critically injured patients. In the largest

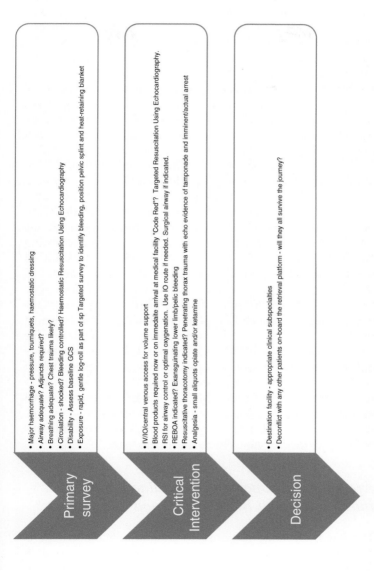

Primary survey
- Major haemorrhage - pressure, tourniquets, haemostatic dressing
- Airway adequate? Adjuncts required?
- Breathing adequate? Chest trauma likely?
- Circulation - shocked? Bleeding controlled? Haemostatic Resuscitation Using Echocardiography
- Disability - Assess baseline GCS
- Exposure - rapid, gentle log-roll as part of sp Targeted survey to identify bleeding, position pelvic splint and heat-retaining blanket

Critical Intervention
- IV/IO/central venous access for volume support
- Blood products required now or on immediate arrival at medical facility "Code Red"? Targeted Resuscitation Using Echocardiography.
- RSI for airway control or optimal oxygenation. Use IO route if needed. Surgical airway if indicated.
- REBOA indicated? Exsanguinating lower limb/pelvic bleeding
- Resuscitative thoracotomy indicated? Penetrating thorax trauma with echo evidence of tamponade and imminent/actual arrest
- Analgesia - small aliquots opiate and/or ketamine

Decision
- Destination facility - appropriate clinical subspecialties
- Deconflict with any other patients on-board the retrieval platform - will they all survive the journey?

FIGURE 3.1 Key decisions and interventions in the pre-hospital management of critically injured patients

reported series of pre-hospital physician endotracheal intubation, involving over 29,000 patients treated by London's Air Ambulance, over 7000 underwent physician-led advanced airway management. The intubation success rate was 99.3 %, with no significant difference between base specialty of the intubating physician. In the few cases where failure occurred, the rescue strategy employed was immediately successful. By comparison, in a prospective case series of 429 patients treated during 324 UK physician-led Medical Emergency Response Team (MERT) missions in Afghanistan, (48 % with blast injuries, 25 % gunshot wounds), the most common physician intervention was rapid sequence induction (RSI) of anaesthesia for airway control, performed in 45 % [1]. Usually, administration of anaesthetic agents is performed via intravenous access, but this can be difficult to achieve in the more austere and mobile military retrieval platform. In this setting, intraosseous (IO) administration has been used for achieving RSI with good results – in the setting of the critically ill exsanguinating military polytrauma patient the usual UK MERT procedure was for bilateral humeral IO devices to be used for blood product administration, inserted by the prepositioned flight nurse and flight paramedic respectively, whilst the flight physician gained access with a sternal IO device for administration of medications including RSI drugs. Previously only documented in case reports, a prospective observational study of 34 trauma patients undergoing IO drug administration for RSI (29 in-flight on MERT, 5 in-hospital) confirms a very high first-pass intubation rate in the hands of an experienced physician [2]. The data concerning drug-assisted intubation provided by non-physicians is less clear.

Are There Advantages to Providing Pre-hospital Intervention with Blood and Blood Components?

The haemodynamic response to traumatic haemorrhage is complex and has only recently been properly delineated. A transient, adaptive hypotensive state seems to exist, and previously supported interventions which interfere with this (such as rapid volume expansion) may, paradoxically, lead to increased mortality [3]. The exception to this appears to be early but judicious pre-hospital intervention with blood products, which may attenuate the coagulopathy seen with haemorrhagic shock [4]. Animal models of complex traumatic haemorrhagic shock also suggest a reduction in the systemic inflammatory response, and an improvement in markers of tissue perfusion associated with the early use of blood products during resuscitation [5]. Aggressive blood product delivery, coupled with contemporary critical care, has been shown to reverse the metabolic derangements seen with severe haemorrhage. However, large volumes of blood product (~27 units red cells and plasma), administered alongside surgical haemorrhage are required to achieve this [6]. In the pre-hospital phase, a more measured "holding pattern" approach seems more logical, using targeted resuscitation with the initial aim of maintaining essential organ perfusion. The rationale and techniques for such targeted resuscitation are outlined in Chaps. 5 and 6. As yet the use of pre-hospital blood products has yet to be tested in a prospective randomised study and the results of the upcoming RePHILL study (EUDRACT ID 2015-001401-13) are awaited with interest. Even where not actually delivering blood products pre-hospital, the retrieval team has a role in the identification of patients where the immediate availability of blood products after arrival in hospital may be beneficial, pre-alerting the receiving facility to allow them to prepare in advance for a potential massive transfusion [7]. If the retrieval phase is prolonged, the use of focussed echocardiography to guide volume resuscitation, including blood components, may be of benefit, as outlined in Chap. 6.

Is There a Novel Pre-hospital Solution to Incompressible Exsanguinating Haemorrhage?

Resuscitative Endovascular Balloon Occlusion of the Aorta (REBOA) provides a rapid and effective method of achieving "proximal control" of exsanguinating haemorrhage, avoiding the requirement to deliver resuscitative thoracotomy and provide sustained manual aortic compression [8]. Accessed via a 6–9 F sheath in the femoral artery, usually inserted under ultrasound guidance, a standard angioplasty guide wire is passed into the aorta. Over this, a suitable balloon catheter is advanced into the distal aorta, at which point the balloon is inflated with saline solution to achieve haemostasis, as shown in Fig. 3.2. This therapy has been well studied in animal models, and has been used to achieve stabilisation in patients presenting with pelvic trauma, prior to retrieval to specialist centres with pelvic surgery and interventional radiology facilities. Further case series have been described in American and Japanese major trauma centres [9–11]. Intravascular balloon positioning is usually provided inhospital, by means of fluoroscopy, not available in the pre-hospital setting. Novel systems are being developed that allow fluoroscopy-free balloon placement [12], and London's Air Ambulance has been the first in the world to successfully deploy this therapy in the pre-hospital setting.

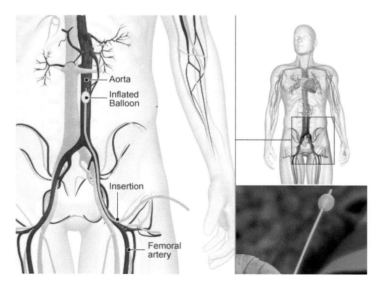

FIGURE 3.2 Resuscitative Balloon Occlusion of the Aorta (REBOA) – schematic showing placement and deployed balloon

In an analysis of 174 deaths due to exsanguinating trauma in a military setting, with a mean pre-hospital time of 61 min, 66 occurred en-route to hospital, and 29 after arrival in the receiving facility. From injury analysis, 1 in 5 patients had a focus of haemorrhage in the abdomen or around the abdomino-pelvic junction that could have been potentially treated with REBOA [13]. Similar analyses have confirmed potential utility (though less frequent) within civilian major trauma centres, and in systems with long travel times to definitive care [14, 15]. REBOA is not without its complications, and there is a well-described syndrome of metabolic consequences of aortic balloon occlusion, mostly driven by ischaemia of both lower limbs [16]. However, haemorrhage control is effective, and future modification of the equipment has the potential to optimise REBOA, including allowing isolation of one iliac artery when a unilateral injury exists and possibly providing more proximal occlusion to control abdominal and thoracic bleeding [8, 17]. A robust training programme will be required to allow operators to deliver this potentially life-saving elegant endovascular haemorrhage control solution [18].

What Are the Key Initial Decisions and Interventions in the Management of Traumatic Cardiac Arrest in the Pre- hospital Setting?

Traumatic Cardiac Arrest (TCA) has historically been considered an un-survivable condition. This was certainly supported by evidence from civilian cohorts which showed a survival rate of around 3 % for both blunt and penetrating injuries associated with a loss of cardiac output [19]. However, more recent data from contemporary military practice suggests that with effective early intervention the chance of survival may be much higher, up to 24 % in one series [20]. This increased efficacy may be due to more timely intervention, including prompt surgical control of incompressible haemorrhage and aggressive pre-hospital interventions.

A key early question is whether the patient has a true cardiac arrest or an ultra low cardiac output state. Focussed echocardiography is the most effective way of making this assessment and may show a hyper-dynamic heart with cavity collapse, indicative of extreme hypovolaemia. Ultrasound also enables an immediate diagnosis of two other potentially treatable causes of TCA, tension pneumothorax and cardiac tamponade. Both these conditions can be effectively treated in the pre-hospital setting.

Aggressive volume resuscitation, probably with blood products, will invariably be required in this scenario as discussed elsewhere in this chapter and more completely in Chaps. 5 and 6. There has been some debate regarding the effectiveness of chest compressions in the context of TCA. Whilst it is certainly true that such treatment is perhaps the single most important aspect of management of non traumatic cardiac arrest it does not follow that it is equally efficacious in a patient with critical hypovoalemia or obstructive cardiac output impairment. A recent review article written by military clinicians suggested that if chest compressions were performed then they should be prioritised below more proven treatments such as volume resuscitation and thoracostomy [21].

Resuscitative thoracotomy is a specific intervention which can be considered in the context of TCA and is discussed in more detail in the following section.

Figure 3.3 shows a suggested pathway of decision making and treatment for patients with TCA.

Is Pre-hospital Resuscitative Thoracotomy Effective?

Pre-hospital resuscitative thoracotomy (RT), delivered within a physician-led, highly organised trauma resuscitation service can yield good results [22]. A retrospective analysis of 15 years of the London's air ambulance service identified 71 patients who underwent this therapy, of whom

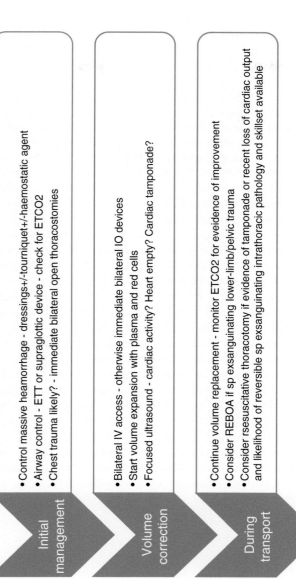

FIGURE 3.3 Key decision and intervention points in the management of traumatic cardiac arrest

13 survived (18 %). Of the survivors, 11 had a good neurological outcome, and 2 had significant neurological deficits. All the survivors had cardiac tamponade, remediable by immediate pericardotomy and evacuation of clot and blood [23]. RT can also be an effective treatment following cardiac arrest from ballistic military trauma. In a retrospective cohort study using UK Joint Theatre Trauma Registry (JTTR) data between 2006 and 2011, 65 cases who underwent this therapy were analysed, of whom 14 survived. Of the 10 who suffered traumatic cardiac arrest in the field, there were no survivors. 29 suffered a cardiac arrest during the retrieval phase, of whom 3 survived. 20 arrested within the emergency department, of whom 11 survived. Injury severity scores were the same across all the groups, and the provision of rapid thoracotomy seems the most important determinant of survival (6 min from arrest in survivors vs 18 min in those who died) [24]. Additionally, physiological stabilisation en-route and avoidance of the development of loss of cardiac output might also be able to modify outcomes in this critically injured group. However, although pre-hospital resuscitative thoracotomy has been successful in highly developed civilian trauma retrieval services, it is acknowledged that it is a difficulty therapy to deliver in the context of a military setting, and especially in the back of a helicopter during the retrieval phase. Severe intrathoracic injuries are likely to be encountered which may not be amenable to single-operator delivered therapies, with major arterial and pulmonary hilar injuries a major source of mortality in this setting, particularly in association with severe head injury [25, 26]. Immediate handheld ultrasound might also aid in patient selection by promptly identifying the pathology most likely to be reversible – cardiac tamponade.

Part Two: Pre- hospital Trauma Care Systems

What's the Best Model for Primary Trauma Retrieval in a Civilian Pre-hospital System?

The majority of emergency medical services (EMS) systems rely on provision of an emergency medical technician (EMT) or paramedic response for the bulk of incidents. In some countries, an enhanced level of care may be available from specialist paramedic practitioners, flight paramedics with additional training such as critical care paramedics, specialist nurses or a physician with critical care skills. The requirement for intervention and stabilisation in the pre-hospital phase varies according to injury type and a balance exists between optimising physiology at the scene, with meaningful inputs, offset against a potential delay in transferring the patient to definitive care. The addition of a physician allows delivery, to the scene, of therapies usually only available within the hospital, by a provider formally trained and skilled in their delivery. Key interventions at the scene may facilitate transfer direct to a specialist facility, for example allowing the delivery of patients with severe traumatic brain injury direct to an acute neurosurgical receiving facility, or allow bypass of smaller hospitals in favour of a designated multispecialty major trauma centre.

In a large North American study of long-distance rural aeromedical EMS retrievals, around 30 % of the transfers were due to major trauma. Of these, 11 % required a major intervention to achieve stabilisation prior to or during transportation. Another 42 % required a minor intervention from the flight crew, and the remainder needed no additional therapies during transport. The attendance of the aeromedical crew and its therapeutic interventions was assessed as being

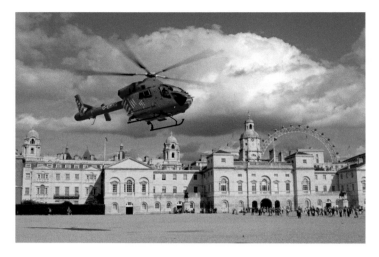

FIGURE 3.4 London HEMS McDonell Douglas MD 902 Explorer landing in central London

essential for survival in 27 % of cases, of therapeutic benefit in 55 % and non-contributory in 18 % [27]. Blunt trauma predominates in the civilian setting, and in a multicentre study of physician-led helicopter retrieval in Europe, 61 % of activations were to victims of road traffic collisions, and 30 % to incidents in the home, during sport or leisure activities. The study also highlights that, although physicians spent more time delivering therapies in the pre-hospital phase, there was an overall reduction in 30 day mortality compared with patients who received only EMS delivered care. Similarly, a further mortality reduction was noted where patients were delivered direct to a multispecialty university hospital, supporting the notion that, to optimally manage these patients, an organised regional system needs to exist, coupling a top-level pre-hospital care provider with a regional receiving system for complex cases (Figs. 3.4 and 3.5).

London's Air Ambulance is the highest volume and most established advanced pre-hospital system in the UK, delivering a team comprising a senior physician capable of

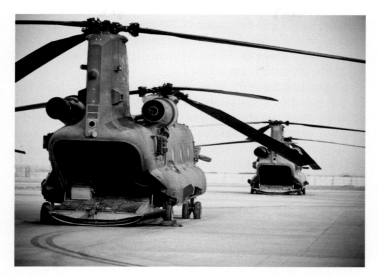

FIGURE 3.5 The cavernous interior of "Tricky 73" – Camp Bastion's duty Medical Emergency Response Team CH-47 helicopter, arguably the world's most advanced airborne trauma retrieval service. ©MoD

advanced pre-hospital trauma critical care plus a senior paramedic. The team can deploy by road or air, depending on the travel times to the incident.

What Challenges Exist When Preparing for Forward Medical Evacuation of Seriously Injured Patients from the Battlefield?

Patients with injuries sustained during military operations present a very difficult set of circumstances which require special arrangements to save life, when compared with conventional civilian trauma. Patients are often multiple in number, with multiple, complex injury patterns. Pre-hospital timelines may be long – one retrospective review of the pre-hospital timelines for 456 seriously injured UK military casualties (192 gunshot wounds, 233 blast/fragmentation injuries) in Afghanistan demonstrated that the median time from injury to handover in the emergency department was 99 min for the most critical cases [28].

Evacuation from the battlefield is now primarily achieved by the use of aviation assets. Helicopters have been routinely used by the military to transport casualties from near the point of wounding to surgical facilities since the second year of the Korean conflict [29]. With the deployment of the larger Bell UH-1 "Huey" helicopter to Vietnam in the early 1960s, there was sufficient space within the platform to perform medical interventions en-route, although these are now considered basic by today's standards. Arguably, the evolution of military pre-hospital retrieval reached its apogee with the creation of the Medical Emergency Response Team (MERT) by the UK Defence Medical Services in the Afghanistan conflict (2001–2014).

Access to the patient may be delayed by poor weather, or tactical factors such as an ongoing firefight. There may be no time in which to assess the patients before moving to definitive treatment, as the tactical situation may dictate that the transport asset being used, whether air, sea or land, may well have to move immediately after the patients are loaded, to maintain the safety of that platform and its occupants. Critical interventions such as drug-assisted intubation often have to be carried out whilst on the move, with restricted light, suboptimal communication between team members, in cramped conditions, at extremes of temperature and whilst manoeuvring tactically, if not actually under enemy attack.

What Is the Optimal Team for Providing pre Hospital Care to Critically Injured Patients in the Military Setting?

From the available published military datasets, the main emerging theme is that severely injured patients benefit from early intervention by the most skilled available care provider.

A US study, using the JTTR database of combat injuries in Afghanistan compared outcomes in patients who received pre-hospital care from an emergency medical technician (EMT) helicopter system with those treated by critical care trained flight paramedics (CCFP). They found a 48 h mortality of 15 % in the EMT group, compared with 8 % in the CCFP cohort. After correcting for potentially confounding variables, there was still a 66 % lower risk of death in the CCFP-treated cohort, supporting the basic tenet of providing the highest skill mix possible when dealing with complex multisystem trauma patients [30].

Although prospective randomised trial data in this area is lacking due to operational constraints, there is clear evidence of benefit from the provision of physician-delivered care during the retrieval phase following battlefield injury. Formal evidence on which to base the design of an optimal system is sparse, although a literature review in 2007 does identify one randomised controlled trial confirming benefit from physician-led care, as well as several cohort studies analysing the benefit of specific interventions. There is an association between the deployment of a physician with critical care skills and improved survival in victims of major trauma, identifying emergency intubation, ventilation and intercostal drainage as key interventions likely to result in improved clinical outcomes, particularly where long transfer distances exist [31].

A registry study looking at US and UK casualties evacuated to a trauma facility in Afghanistan between 2008 and 2012 confirms that for most injuries with low injury severity scores, medic-led retrieval is effective. However, in the group of patients with an Injury Severity Score (ISS) of 16–50, mortality was reduced from 18.2 to 12.2 % where a physician-led advanced medical retrieval system was used, as was time to reach the operating theatre in those with an ISS of 51–75 [32]. Similarly, in a study of 865 patients comparing pre-hospital shock index (heart rate/systolic blood pressure) with admission values, marked differences were found, attributable to the capabilities of the forward aeromedical evacuation platform deployed. Four-hundred and seventy-eight were treated by the physician-led UK MERT, 291 by USAF PEDRO (paramedic-led) and 96 by US Army DUSTOFF (EMT) crews, and these were compared across three injury severity score groups. In the lowest severity group, an improvement was seen across all retrieval platforms. In the middle group (ISS 10–25), both MERT and PEDRO achieved an improvement in SI on admission, with a sustained improvement only in the MERT cohort. This improvement was also seen in the top ISS group (ISS 26 and above) in the MERT group, whereas a trend to deterioration was seen in the PEDRO group. These data suggest that the use of a forward aeromedical evacuation platform with a greater clinical capability is associated with haemodynamic improvement in the most critically injured casualties [33].

Do These Advanced Systems Improve Survival Following Battlefield Trauma?

In a study looking at mortality resulting from 14,252 individual injuries occurring in 2,792 UK battlefield trauma patients from 2003 through to 2012, using the New Injury Severity Score (NISS), a marked improvement was seen across the study period. The NISS associated with a 50 % chance of survival was 32 in 2003, rising each successive year to 60 in 2012 (Fig. 3.6). Put simply, more patients were surviving despite having more severe injuries, attributable to advances in trauma care systems; with physician-led retrieval, advanced resuscitation en-route and direct delivery to a pre-alerted multispecialty consultant team being key components [34]. The hard lessons learned from years of delivery of tactical evacuation and advanced retrieval

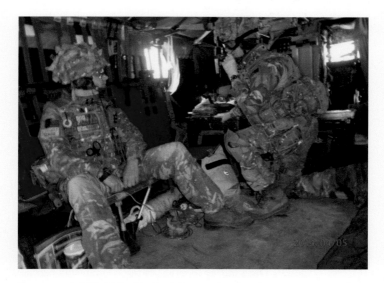

FIGURE 3.6 UK MERT physician and critical care nurse prepare equipment to receive a casualty with penetrating head injury caused by a gunshot wound. Standard personal equipment is augmented by the addition of extra survival and escape equipment for missions into hostile territory – this can be seen on the kneeling clincian's body armour. Additionally, a pouch containing the equipment required to perform emeregncy resuscitative thoracotomy is carried in a leg-pouch, to ensure ready access. The ability to achieve controlled ventilation by means of RSI, and the physicain's authority to divert the mission to a unit with neurosurgery on-site proved valuable in this case (With kind permission of ©Paul Rees)

systems in the military setting should be harnessed and tailored to optimise existing civilian services, using an evidence–based, data-driven improvement programme to improve outcomes [35] (Fig. 3.7).

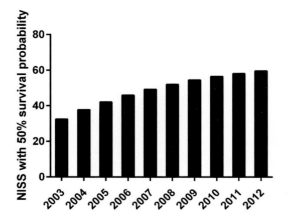

FIGURE 3.7 New Injury Severity Score (NISS) associated with 50 % chance of survival following injury. Data applies to casualties treated by the UK DMS during a period of the Afghanistan conflict (2003–2014) and shows the improvement in survival rates associated with the development of the trauma service

References

1. Calderbank P, Woolley T, Mercer S, Schrager J, Kazel M, Bree S, et al. Doctor on board? What is the optimal skill-mix in military pre-hospital care? Emerg Med J. 2011;28(10):882–3.
2. Barnard EB, Moy RJ, Kehoe AD, Bebarta VS, Smith JE. Rapid sequence induction of anaesthesia via the intraosseous route: a prospective observational study. Emerg Med J. 2015;32(6): 449–52.
3. Kirkman E, Watts S. Haemodynamic changes in trauma. Br J Anaesth. 2014;113(2):266–75.
4. Watts S, Nordmann G, Brohi K, Midwinter M, Woolley T, Gwyther R, et al. Evaluation of Prehospital Blood Products to Attenuate Acute Coagulopathy of Trauma in a Model of Severe Injury and Shock in Anesthetized Pigs. Shock. 2015;44 Suppl 1:138–48.
5. Doran CM, Doran CA, Woolley T, Carter A, Male K, Midwinter MJ, et al. Targeted resuscitation improves coagulation and outcome. J Trauma Acute Care Surg. 2012;72(4):835–43.

6. Morrison JJ, Ross JD, Poon H, Midwinter MJ, Jansen JO. Intra-operative correction of acidosis, coagulopathy and hypothermia in combat casualties with severe haemorrhagic shock. Anaesthesia. 2013;68(8):846–50.

7. Weaver AE, Hunter-Dunn C, Lyon RM, Lockey D, Krogh CL. The effectiveness of a 'Code Red' transfusion request policy initiated by pre-hospital physicians. Injury. 2016;47(1):3–6.

8. Morrison JJ, Ross JD, Houston R, Watson JD, Sokol KK, Rasmussen TE. Use of resuscitative endovascular balloon occlusion of the aorta in a highly lethal model of noncompressible torso hemorrhage. Shock. 2014;41(2):130–7.

9. Saito N, Matsumoto H, Yagi T, Hara Y, Hayashida K, Motomura T, et al. Evaluation of the safety and feasibility of resuscitative endovascular balloon occlusion of the aorta. J Trauma Acute Care Surg. 2015;78(5):897–903.

10. Norii T, Crandall C, Terasaka Y. Survival of severe blunt trauma patients treated with resuscitative endovascular balloon occlusion of the aorta compared with propensity score-adjusted untreated patients. J Trauma Acute Care Surg. 2015;78(4): 721–8.

11. Brenner ML, Moore LJ, DuBose JJ, Tyson GH, McNutt MK, Albarado RP, et al. A clinical series of resuscitative endovascular balloon occlusion of the aorta for hemorrhage control and resuscitation. J Trauma Acute Care Surg. 2013;75(3):506–11.

12. Chaudery M, Clark J, Morrison JJ, Wilson MH, Bew D, Darzi A. Can contrast-enhanced ultrasonography improve Zone III REBOA placement for prehospital care? J Trauma Acute Care Surg. 2016;80(1):89–94.

13. Morrison JJ, Ross JD, Rasmussen TE, Midwinter MJ, Jansen JO. Resuscitative endovascular balloon occlusion of the aorta: a gap analysis of severely injured UK combat casualties. Shock. 2014;41(5):388–93.

14. Barnard EB, Morrison JJ, Madureira RM, Lendrum R, Fragoso-Iniguez M, Edwards A, et al. Resuscitative endovascular balloon occlusion of the aorta (REBOA): a population based gap analysis of trauma patients in England and Wales. Emerg Med J. 2015;32(12):926–32.

15. Morrison JJ, Lendrum RA, Jansen JO. Resuscitative endovascular balloon occlusion of the aorta (REBOA): a bridge to definitive haemorrhage control for trauma patients in Scotland? Surgeon. 2014;12(3):119–20.

16. Markov NP, Percival TJ, Morrison JJ, Ross JD, Scott DJ, Spencer JR, et al. Physiologic tolerance of descending thoracic aortic balloon occlusion in a swine model of hemorrhagic shock. Surgery. 2013;153(6):848–56.

17. Morrison JJ, Rasmussen TE. Noncompressible torso hemorrhage: a review with contemporary definitions and management strategies. Surg Clin North Am. 2012;92(4):843–58, vii.

18. Brenner M, Hoehn M, Pasley J, Dubose J, Stein D, Scalea T. Basic endovascular skills for trauma course: bridging the gap between endovascular techniques and the acute care surgeon. J Trauma Acute Care Surg. 2014;77(2):286–91.

19. Soar J, Perkins GD, Abbas G, et al. European Resuscitation Council Guidelines for Resuscitation 2010 Section 8. Cardiac arrest in special circumstances: Electrolyte abnormalities, poisoning, drowning, accidental hypothermia, hyperthermia, asthma, anaphylaxis, cardiac surgery, trauma, pregnancy, electrocution. Resuscitation. 2010;81:1400–33.

20. Russell RJ, Hodgetts TJ, McLeod J, et al. The role of trauma scoring in developing trauma clinical governance in the Defence Medical Services. Philos Trans R Soc B. 2011;366:171–91.

21. Smith JE, Le Clerc S, Hunt PAF. Challenging the dogma of traumatic cardiac arrest management: a military perspective. Emerg Med J. 2015;32(12):955–60.

22. Coats TJ, Keogh S, Clark H, Neal M. Prehospital resuscitative thoracotomy for cardiac arrest after penetrating trauma: rationale and case series. J Trauma. 2001;50(4):670–3.

23. Davies GE, Lockey DJ. Thirteen survivors of prehospital thoracotomy for penetrating trauma: a prehospital physician-performed resuscitation procedure that can yield good results. J Trauma. 2011;70(5):E75–8.

24. Morrison JJ, Poon H, Rasmussen TE, Khan MA, Midwinter MJ, Blackbourne LH, et al. Resuscitative thoracotomy following wartime injury. J Trauma Acute Care Surg. 2013;74(3):825–9.

25. Morrison JJ, Mellor A, Midwinter M, Mahoney PF, Clasper JC. Is pre-hospital thoracotomy necessary in the military environment? Injury. 2011;42(5):469–73.

26. Morrison JJ, Stannard A, Rasmussen TE, Jansen JO, Tai NR, Midwinter MJ. Injury pattern and mortality of noncompressible torso hemorrhage in UK combat casualties. J Trauma Acute Care Surg. 2013;75(2 Suppl 2):S263–8.

27. Fallon MJ, Copass M. Southeast Alaska to Seattle emergency medical air transports: demographics, stabilization, and outcomes. Ann Emerg Med. 1990;19(8):914–21.

28. McLeod J, Hodgetts T, Mahoney P. Combat "Category A" calls: evaluating the prehospital timelines in a military trauma system. J R Army Med Corps. 2007;153(4):266–8.

29. Olson Jr CM, Bailey J, Mabry R, Rush S, Morrison JJ, Kuncir EJ. Forward aeromedical evacuation: a brief history, lessons learned from the Global War on Terror, and the way forward for US policy. J Trauma Acute Care Surg. 2013;75(2 Suppl 2): S130–6.

30. Mabry RL, Apodaca A, Penrod J, Orman JA, Gerhardt RT, Dorlac WC. Impact of critical care-trained flight paramedics on casualty survival during helicopter evacuation in the current war in Afghanistan. J Trauma Acute Care Surg. 2012;73(2 Suppl 1):S32–7.

31. Davis PR, Rickards AC, Ollerton JE. Determining the composition and benefit of the pre-hospital medical response team in the conflict setting. J R Army Med Corps. 2007;153(4):269–73.

32. Morrison JJ, Oh J, DuBose JJ, O'Reilly DJ, Russell RJ, Blackbourne LH, et al. En-route care capability from point of injury impacts mortality after severe wartime injury. Ann Surg. 2013;257(2):330–4.

33. Apodaca AN, Morrison JJ, Spott MA, Lira JJ, Bailey J, Eastridge BJ, et al. Improvements in the hemodynamic stability of combat casualties during en route care. Shock. 2013;40(1):5–10.

34. Penn-Barwell JG, Roberts SA, Midwinter MJ, Bishop JR. Improved survival in UK combat casualties from Iraq and Afghanistan: 2003–2012. J Trauma Acute Care Surg. 2015;78(5): 1014–20.

35. Bailey JA, Morrison JJ, Rasmussen TE. Military trauma system in Afghanistan: lessons for civil systems? Curr Opin Crit Care. 2013;19(6):569–77.

Chapter 4
The Trauma Team and Initial Management of the Critically Injured Patient

Simon J. Mercer

Abstract   Recent conflicts in Afghanistan and Iraq have driven the development and refinement of the trauma team based approach to complex injury. This has arguably contributed to the remarkable outcomes seen, with many casualties recovering from seemingly unsurvivable injuries. Many concepts developed by the military have subsequently been adopted by civilian healthcare providers. Human factors and non-technical skills play a vital role in the initial management of the critically injured patient and can be taught and practiced alongside more traditional clinical skills. The

S.J. Mercer
Honorary Senior Lecturer, Postgraduate School of Medicine,
University of Liverpool, Lecturer in Military Anaesthesia
Education, National Institute of Academic Anaesthesia,
Liverpool, UK

Consultant Trauma and Emergency Anaesthetist, Deputy College
Tutor, Aintree University Hospitals NHS Foundation Trust,
Liverpool, UK
e-mail: simonjmercer@hotmail.com

S.D. Hutchings (ed.), *Trauma and Combat Critical Care
in Clinical Practice*, In Clinical Practice,
DOI 10.1007/978-3-319-28758-4_4,
© Crown Copyright 2016

trauma team leader performs a vital role within the trauma team, assimilating and communicating information and taking decisions at certain key points. These decision points can be predicted in advance and include whether to perform early CT imaging and early surgical intervention for control of exsanguinating haemorrhage. Effective communication underpins all of the work of the trauma team and should be conducted in a standardized fashion in order to reduce error.

Keywords Trauma teams • Major trauma centers • Military trauma • Human factors • Damage control resuscitation

Introduction

This chapter will describe the initial management of the critically injured patient conducted by the receiving trauma team. Recent conflicts in Afghanistan and Iraq have allowed the development and refinement of the processes used to treat severe traumatic injury and as a consequence many patients are leaving hospital after sustaining injuries that were previously considered unsurvivable [1, 2]. Many of these processes and concepts, developed by the UK Defence Medical Services (UK DMS) over the last decade, have now been adopted by the UK National Health Service [1, 3] particularly in the area of human factors [4].

What Are Human Factors and Why Are They Important in Trauma Care?

Much of the success of the trauma team in recent military conflicts has been attributed to excellent human factors [5] with rehearsal in pre-deployment training [6] and refinement on operations. Human factors has been defined as '*Enhancing clinical performance through an understanding of the effects of teamwork, tasks, equipment, workspace, culture and organisation on human behaviour and abilities and application of that knowledge in clinical settings'* [7]. There has been research into human factors for anaesthetists [8], surgeons [9] and scrub practitioners [10] and much of this work can be directly translated into clinical practice. Another definition of human factors is *'the cognitive, social, and personal resource skills that complement technical skills, and contribute to safe and efficient task performance'* [11] with key aspects including situational awareness, teamwork, leadership, followership, communication and decision making.

The Anaesthetists Non-Technical Skills Framework [ANTS] [12] is shown in Table 4.1 and consists of categories and elements all of which are highly relevant to trauma scenarios. This framework was developed by observation of the behaviors of anaesthetists in the operating theatre environment and is broken down into four separate behavior categories, namely: task management, team working, situational awareness and decision-making. Although a framework for trauma has not yet been developed there is certainly much

TABLE 4.1 Anaesthetists non-technical skills (ANTS)

Category	Element
Task management	Planning and preparing management
	Prioritizing
	Providing and maintaining standards
	Identifying and utilizing resources
Team working	Coordinating activities with team members working
	Exchanging information
	Using authority and assertiveness
	Assessing capabilities
	Supporting others
Situational awareness	Gathering information awareness
	Recognizing and understanding
	Anticipating
Decision making	Identifying options
	Balancing risks and selecting options
	Re-evaluating

overlap that can be transferred to the trauma team. *Task management* describes how the team prepares to receive a patient. The *team working* elements dictate the process of the primary survey, gathering information to ensure that the team leader has the opportunity to maintain *situational awareness* and not miss the subtle signs of a severely injured patient with rapidly changing physiology. Robust *decision making* is essential to ensure that the patient receives the right intervention at the right time by the right person. The ANTS framework is often used for training by the UK DMS.

Why Is a Trauma Team Needed?

The Report 'Trauma Who Cares' [13] highlighted deficiencies in the provision of trauma care in the UK. The model trauma team is a resource rich unit of individuals with specific skills and competencies required to stabilise a casualty and then make rapid decisions about further management. By providing a dedicated trauma team seriously injured patients will not only receive effective early stabilistation but, crucially, the correct decisions will be made regarding their ongoing management after initial resuscitation is complete.

What Does a Trauma Team Consist Of?

Salas describes a team as being '*a distinguishable set of two or more people who interact dynamically, interdependently, and adaptively towards a common and valued goal, who have each been assigned specific roles or functions to perform, and who have a limited life-span membership*' [13]. Since their inception, UK major trauma centers have made a significant investment in staffing the trauma team. Personnel involved are listed in Table 4.2 and a typical military trauma team is shown in Fig. 4.1.

This is a senior team which facilitates early decision making and prompt institution of appropriate treatment. It is common for the trauma team leader to be a consultant

TABLE 4.2 A typical trauma team from a UK Major Trauma Centre

Personnel	Role
Trauma team leader (consultant)	To lead the trauma team Co-ordination of tasks Ultimate responsibility for the patient
Emergency doctors (ST trainee)	Primary survey
Anaesthetist (ST5+)	Airway management
ODP	To support the anaesthetist
General surgeon	To assist in timely diagnosis for chest and abdominal injuries To insert a chest drain if required
Orthopaedic surgeon	To assist in timely diagnosis for injuries involving fractured pelvis and long bones.
Scribe	To make an accurate record of events on the trauma pathway
Nurse 1	To assist as part of the trauma team
Nurse 2	To run the rapid infuser
HCA	To assist the team
Runner	To collect blood products

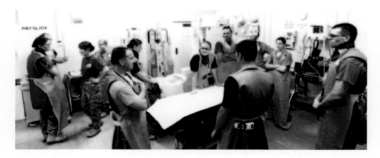

FIGURE 4.1 Trauma team assembled prior to patient arrival at the UK Role 3 Hospital, Camp Bastion, Afghanistan (Dr Mark de Rond with permission)

usually, but not always, in Emergency Medicine. UK Major Trauma Centres undergo regular peer review where the competencies of the trauma team leader are assessed. Training should include courses focusing on a team based approach, such as the European Trauma Course (www.european-trauma.com), alongside regular training using 'in situ simulation' in their own department.

What Process Activates the Trauma Team?

The trauma team is a resource rich unit and as such draws on experience from all parts of an acute hospital. It is clear that the activation criteria must be robust to ensure that this valuable resource is not wasted. Many centers have adapted the activation criteria previously used in the UK Role 3 hospital in Afghanistan [14] shown in Table 4.3. This is tailored to the mechanism of injury and the anatomy and physiology of the casualty. The decision to activate the trauma team is made using the information from the pre-hospital system with a typical activation being about 20 min prior to the arrival of the casualty. Local policy will dictate whether other elements, such as a massive transfusion protocol, also need to be activated prior to the arrival of the patient.

Why Does the Trauma Team Need to Be Assembled Prior to a Casualty Arriving?

A period of preparation is very important for the trauma team. The team is introduced by name and role and competencies confirmed. The team leader then briefs the team and conveys their mental model (an idea of what might happen during the trauma call based on the information given and their prior experience). Contingency planning is also discussed, for example dealing with a difficult airway. Some Major Trauma Centers have the provision for providing

TABLE 4.3 Trauma team activation criteria at the UK Role 3 Hospital, Camp Bastion, Afghanistan

Mechanism of injury or history

Penetrating trauma	Gunshot or shrapnel wound
	Blast injury (Landmine/Improvised Explosive Device/Grenade)
	Stab wound
Blunt trauma	Motor vehicle crash with ejection
	Motorcyclist or pedestrian hit by vehicle >30 km/h
	Fall > 5 m
	Fatality in the same vehicle
	Entrapment and/or crush injury
	Inter-hospital trauma transfer meeting

Anatomy and physiology of casualty

Anatomy	Injury to two or more body regions
	Fracture of two or more long bones
	Spinal cord injury
	Amputation of a limb
	Penetrating injury to head, neck, torso, or proximal limb Burns >15 % BSA in adults or >10 % in children or airway burns
	Airway obstruction
Physiology	Systolic blood pressure <90 mmHg or pulse >120 beats/min (adults)
	Respiratory rate <10 or >30 per minute (adults)
	$SpO_2 < 90 \%$
	Depressed level of consciousness or fitting
	Deterioration in the emergency department
	Age > 70 years
	Pregnancy >24 weeks with torso injury

blood and blood products in the form of a 'shock pack' to be issued prior to the patient arriving (often termed a Code Red) A shock pack might consist of four units of packed red blood cells, four units of fresh frozen plasma with the option of further 'shock packs' to contain platelets. Once the team has assembled then they must remain in the trauma bay until the trauma team leader dismisses them.

What Is the Role of the Trauma Team Leader?

A leader is '*a person whose ideas and actions influence the thought and the behaviour of others*' [11]. Whilst leading the team, the trauma team leader (TTL) must look to be able to influence, inspire and direct actions in order to attain a desired objective, namely to rapidly assess and stabilise a patient and make a decision regarding their next location of treatment. In addition to the leadership aspect of the TTL there is an element of management required as situations are analysed, goals set, activities co-ordinated and the team directed.

The TTL is directing the team and as such is required to adopt a position which maintains a hands off approach to the management of the patient. This allows them to maintain situational awareness, defined as '*the perception of the elements in the environment within a volume of time and space, the comprehension of their meaning and the projection of their status in the near future*' [15]. Standing at the end of the trauma trolley ensures that the TTL is not drawn into a technical task and so maintains an overall picture of an often rapidly changing situation. It is also essential that this picture be regularly relayed to the team in the form of a 'sit-rep' or update [16]. Situational awareness has three stages, as outlined in Fig. 4.2. The TTL is responsible for ensuring that these stages are followed in order to minimise errors.

Once the team is assembled, the TTL briefs the trauma team based on the information from the pre-hospital alert and outlines what could potentially happen during the trauma call.

The TTL is required to co-ordinate information from the primary survey, initial investigations (radiology and blood tests) and make a decision on the next stage of the patients care. Communication is vital and the TTL must ensure that there is control and calm in the trauma bay. The TTL is ultimately responsible for the casualty until handed over to another senior doctor in theatre or critical care. They are also responsible for the completion of any patient documentation.

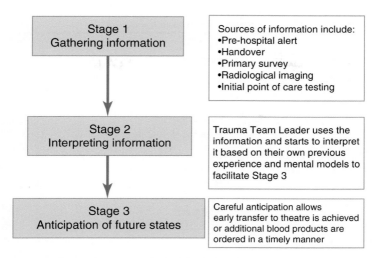

FIGURE 4.2 The three stages of situational awareness in a trauma setting

How Should the Handover of the Patient Be Conducted?

It is important that all members of the trauma team listen to the handover of the patient from the pre-hospital team and it should ideally be done in silence. Situational awareness will be impaired without a proper handover. A structured format is important in order to ensure that essential information is conveyed. The AT-MIST acronym, used by the UK Defence Medical Services, is outlined in Table 4.4 with an example.

What Are the Initial Actions of the Trauma Team?

There has been a recent shift in the conduct of the primary survey. Traditionally, one individual would systematically review and treat problems in a 'vertical' hierarchical approach, starting with control of the (A)*irway* then moving on to assessment of (B)*reathing* etc. This has been replaced by a

TABLE 4.4 AT-MIST format for trauma handover

A	Age	25 years
T	Time of injury	1830
M	Mechanism of injury	Pedestrian V Car
I	Injuries sustained	Head injury Possible pelvic injury
S	Signs and symptoms	Oxygen saturation (SaO_2) 92 % Respiratory rate 32, Heart rate 130, No radial pulse, Agitated, GCS 11/15
T	Treatment given	Oxygen 15 L, 16G cannula inserted in left ante-cubital fossa

'horizontal' approach in which multiple members of the trauma team simultaneously assess and treat (*A*)*irway*, (*B*)*reathing* and (*C*)*irculatory* abnormalities [17]. Experience during recent operations has lead military healthcare providers to adopt an approach that also emphasizes early control of <c>*atastrophic haemorrhage*, leading to a <c>ABC paradigm [1, 3, 18]. The following tasks must be considered during the primary survey which has been likened to a 'Formula One' pit stop.

- Primary survey <c>ABC
- Checking of tourniquet and pelvic binder positioning
- Administer oxygen
- Cervical spine immobilisation
- Additional vascular access
- Blood samples taken for
  - Full Blood Count
  - Thrombolestometry (e.g., RoTEM®)

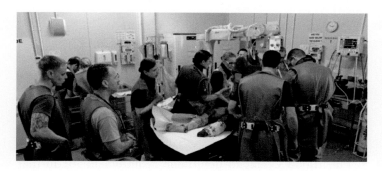

FIGURE 4.3 Military trauma team conducting a 'horizontal' primary survey in the UK Role 3 Hospital, Camp Bastion, Afghanistan (Dr Mark de Rond with permission)

- – Venous blood gas
- – Group and Save
- Focused assessment with sonography for trauma scan (FAST)
- Focused ultrasound to exclude pneumothorax and assess intravascular volume status
- Chest and pelvis X-Rays
- Commencement of haemostatic resuscitation, via a rapid infuser if required
- Rapid sequence induction if required
- Consideration of drugs, for example:
  - – Antibiotics
  - – Tranexamic Acid (15 mg/kg)
  - – Tetanus
  - – Analgesia
  - – Calcium Chloride

A military trauma team conducting a primary survey is shown in Fig. 4.3.

What Investigations Are Carried Out in the Trauma Bay and How Do They Help the Decision Making Process?

The initial investigations will add to the information from the handover and primary survey and guide the trauma team leaders decision-making. These include the following:

- Full Blood Count to determine requirement for further transfusion of pack red cells and platelets
- Venous Gas [pH, base deficit, lactate, K^+, ionized Ca^{2+}]. When serial measurements are taken then the base deficit and lactate concentration allows guidance on the success of resuscitation [4, 19]. Ionized potassium may rise and ionized calcium fall during massive transfusion and these must be promptly corrected
- Rotational thromboelastometry (e.g., RoTEM®) is a 'point of care' test of coagulation [5, 20]. Up to 25 % of major trauma patients have acute coagulopathy of trauma shock [6, 21]; thromboelastometry can guide the effective use of blood component therapy, providing information much faster than lab based methods
- Group and Save
- Blood glucose
- Chest X-Ray may indicate gross chest trauma and signs such as fractured ribs and massive haemo or pneumothorax
- Pelvic X-Ray may show gross disruption of the pelvis
- Focused assessment with sonography for trauma scan (FAST) may indicate if there is free fluid in the abdomen
- Chest ultrasound examination may reveal a pneumothorax
- Focused echocardiography may be helpful in determining intra vascular volume status as well as evidence of cardiac injury

What Is Damage Control Resuscitation?

Damage Control Resuscitation (DCR) is defined as '*a systemic approach to major trauma combining the <c>ABC paradigm with a series of clinical techniques from point of wounding to definitive treatment in order to minimize blood loss, maximize tissue oxygenation and optimize outcome* [7, 22]'. The elements of DCR have been described as permissive hypotension, haemostatic resuscitation and damage control surgery (DCS) [8, 19]. Permissive hypotension is when the administration of fluid is restricted, accepting a limited period of sub-optimal end-organ perfusion until haemorrhage is controlled [9, 19]. Haemostatic resuscitation is the administration of blood and blood products when required instead of using filler fluids such as crystalloid.

Damage Control Surgery (DCS) describes a process where the completeness of initial surgical repair is sacrificed in order to curtail initial operating times and mitigate the combined physiological insults of trauma and surgery [11, 23]. This process is described in more detail in Chap. 13. The linkage of DCR to DCS requires an effective team approach between surgeons and anaesthetists/intensivists which tests many elements of the human factors equation described earlier in this chapter [12, 24].

What Are the Initial Critical Decision Points in the Management of a Complex Trauma Patient?

Once handover has taken place and whilst the primary survey is being completed in a horizontal fashion [12, 17], the TTL must focus on the first critical decision point, the initial destination of the patient as shown in Fig. 4.4. Options are:

- *Transfer to CT for imaging and possible radiological intervention*

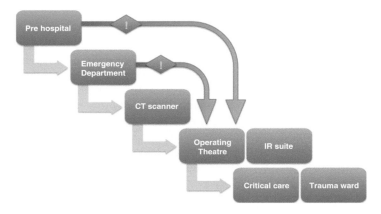

FIGURE 4.4 Trauma patient pathway, *red diamonds* indicate the key initial decision points

- This is the most common pathway for major trauma patients and allows:

    (a) Rapid identification of life-threatening injuries such as sites of active bleeding.

    (b) Identification or exclusion of head or spinal injury. This will later facilitate clearing of the cervical spine.

    (c) The prompt and accurate triage of patients to the operating theatre for thoracic, abdominal (or both) surgeries or the angiography suite for endovascular haemorrhage control.

- Reporting of the CT should ideally be performed immediately by a senior radiologist and occur in the presence of the key decision makers (TTL and senior operating surgeons) as shown in Fig. 4.5 [13, 25].
- *Immediate transfer to theatre for surgical haemostasis*
- This will occur exceptionally prior to imaging but is sometimes necessary for control of exsanguinating haemorrhage, particularly from penetrating torso trauma. In the UK Role 3 Hospital in Afghanistan this process was described as 'right turn resuscitation' due to the layout of the facility and consisted of a process of by-passing the emergency department altogether and immediately entering the operating theatre [14, 26].

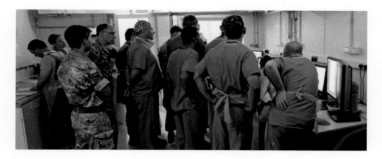

FIGURE 4.5 Reporting of the CT at the UK Role 3 Hospital, Camp Bastion, Afghanistan (Dr Mark de Rond with permission)

- *Remaining in the trauma bay for a fixed period of time*
- The rationale for this could include the administration of further blood products in an attempt to achieve more physiological stability prior to transfer. Often, however, ongoing resuscitation, including the administration of a massive transfusion protocol occurs concurrently with imaging. This requires a high level of command and control by the TTL.
- *Early transfer to Critical Care*
- This may occur if a patient arrives from another hospital where they underwent axial imaging and do not require any immediate surgical interventions.
- *Early transfer to ward based care*

- Generally the case only for patients who have been over-triaged to the Major Trauma Centre and who do not require any further imaging or treatment.

How Should Communication Occur Within the Trauma Team?

The TTL is aided by other senior members of the trauma team in ensuring that decisions are made in a timely manner. The UK DMS introduced the concept of 'The Trauma WHO' into deployed clinical practice [2, 15–17]. The original WHO Checklist was introduced worldwide to reduce error and improve patient safety during surgery [27] but the rapidity of events in trauma requires an abbreviated, yet safe, method of completing this process. The four stages are:

1. The Command Huddle
2. SNAP Brief
3. Sit-Reps
4. Debrief

1. The Command Huddle

This occurs in the resuscitation bay, is 'consultant delivered', and co-ordinated by the trauma team leader as shown in Fig. 4.6. This experienced group are able to quickly determine the next stages of the patient pathway and the interventions required. The key players in the command huddle include:

- Trauma Team Leader
- Consultant General Surgeon
- Consultant Orthopaedic Surgeon
- Consultant Anaesthetist

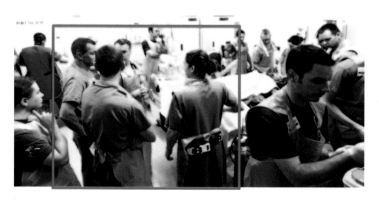

FIGURE 4.6 An example of a command huddle approach to communication during a trauma call at the UK Role 3 Hospital, Camp Bastion Afghanistan. Senior surgical specialists consult with the trauma team leader whilst patient resuscitation continues (Dr Mark de Rond with permssion)

- Deployed Medical Director (essentially the senior clinician of a deployed military treatment facility)

2. The SNAP brief

   This occurs prior to the start of any surgery and in a time critical situation this 'snap' briefing should be kept to a minimum.

   - The surgeon should give the clinical & imaging findings and state the surgical plan
   - The anaesthetist will state the blood given so far, rate of infusion and coagulopathy and any other clinical problems that have been recognised or are evolving

3. Sit-Reps

   This should only occur when there is new information to pass between the teams and a usual guide is every 10–30 min.

   The anaesthetist states:

   - The time since the start and the duration of the procedure
   - Blood products given
   - Rate of infusion of blood products
   - Blood gases, coagulopathy (ROTEM®) and temperature
   - Any developing problems

      The surgeon will state:

- Surgical phase (for example vascular control, resuscitative/therapeutic packing etc.)
- New developing problems/findings
- Future intentions

   A suggested acronym for the Sit-Rep is:

- **T**: **T**ime
- **B**: **B**lood (units given so far & rate of transfusion) & **B**lood gases
- **C**: **C**lotting & **C**old (i.e., temp)
- **S**: **S**urgical progress or discussions on new surgical plan

4.Debrief

Following the safe transfer of the patient to the critical care unit, the team sit down and discuss elements of the patient pathway that went well and those that need to be improved. This is an ideal opportunity to identify any latent errors (errors in the system) and immediately implement strategies to prevent them. It also allows for identification of further training needs for members of the team and if further support is required for team members based on their recent experience.

References

1. Mercer SJ, Tarmey NT, Woolley T, Wood P, Mahoney PF. Haemorrhage and coagulopathy in the defence medical services. Anaesthesia. 2012;68:49–60.
2. Arul GS, Pugh H, Mercer SJ, Midwinter MJ. Human factors in decision making in major trauma in Camp Bastion, Afghanistan. Ann Surg. 2015;97:262–8.
3. McCullough AL, Haycock JC, Forward DP, Moran II CG. Major trauma networks in England. Br J Anaesth. 2014;113:202–6.
4. Mercer S, Park C, Tarmey NT. Human factors in trauma. BJA Educ. 2015. http://dx.doi.org/10.1093/bjaceaccp/mku043.
5. Mercer S, Arul GS, Pugh HEJ. Performance improvement through best practice team management: human factors in complex trauma. J R Army Med Corps. 2014;160:105–8.
6. Mercer SJ, Whittle C, Siggers B, Frazer RS. Simulation, human factors and defence anaesthesia. J R Army Med Corps. 2010;156:365–9.
7. Catchpole K. Towards a working definition of human factors in healthcare. 2011. Available at: www.chfg.org/news-blog/towards-a-working-definition-of-human-factors-in-healthcare. (Accessed on 17 Sept 2015).
8. Fletcher G. Anaesthetists' non-technical skills (ANTS): evaluation of a behavioural marker system. Br J Anaesth. 2003;90:580–8.
9. Yule S, Flin R, Paterson-Brown S, Maran N. Non-technical skills for surgeons in the operating room: a review of the literature. Surgery. 2006;139:140–9.

10. Mitchell L, Flin R. Non-technical skills of the operating theatre scrub nurse: literature review. J Adv Nurs. 2008;63:15–24.
11. Flin R, O'Connor P, Crichton M. Safety at the sharp end: a guide to non-technical skills. Aldershot: Ashgate; 2008.
12. Flin R, Patey R, Glavin R, Maran N. Anaesthetists' non-technical skills. Br J Anaesth. 2010;105:38–44.
13. National Confidential Enquiry into Patient Outcome and Death. Trauma who cares? 2007. (Available at http://www.ncepod.org.uk/2007report2/Downloads/SIP_summary.pdf).
14. Ministry of Defence. Clinical guidelines for operations. Joint Service Publication 999. Change 3, September 2012. Available at: https://www.gov.uk/government/uploads/system/uploads/attachment_data/file/79106/20121204-8-AVB-CGO_Online_2012.pdf.
15. Endsley MR. Toward a theory of situation awareness in dynamic systems. Human Factors J Human Factors Ergon Soc. 1995;37:32–64.
16. Arul GS, Pugh H, Mercer SJ, Midwinter MJ. Optimising communication in the damage control resuscitation-damage control surgery sequence in major trauma management. J R Army Med Corps. 2012;158:82–4.
17. Smith J, Russell R, Horne S. Critical decision-making and timelines in the emergency department. J R Army Med Corps. 2011;157:273.
18. Hodgetts TJ. ABC to ABC: redefining the military trauma paradigm. Emerg Med J. 2006;23:745–6.
19. Jansen JO, Thomas R, Loudon MA, Brooks A. Damage control resuscitation for patients with major trauma. Br Med J. 2009;338:1778–8.
20. Keene DD, Nordmann GR, Woolley T. Rotational thromboelastometry-guided trauma resuscitation. Curr Opin Crit Care. 2013;19:605–12.
21. Brohi K, Singh J, Heron M, Coats T. Acute traumatic coagulopathy. J Trauma Inj Infect Crit Care. 2003;54:1127–30.
22. Hodgetts TJ, Mahoney PF, Kirkman E. Damage control resuscitation. J R Army Med Corps. 2007;153:299–300.
23. Midwinter M. Damage control surgery in the era of damage control resuscitation. J R Army Med Corps. 2009;155:323–5.
24. Midwinter MJ, Woolley T. Resuscitation and coagulation in the severely injured trauma patient. Philos Trans R Soc B Biol Sci. 2010;366:192–203.

25. Chakraverty S, Zealley I, Kessel D. Damage control radiology in the severely injured patient: what the anaesthetist needs to know. Br J Anaesth. 2014;113:250–7.
26. Tai N, Russell R. Right turn resuscitation: frequently asked questions. J R Army Med Corps. 2011;157:S310.
27. Sewell M, Adebibe M, Jayakumar P, Jowett C, Kong K, Vemulapalli K, et al. Use of the WHO surgical safety checklist in trauma and orthopaedic patients. Int Orthop (SICOT). 2010;35:897–901.

Chapter 5
Haemodynamic Resuscitation Following Traumatic Haemorrhagic Shock: An Overview

William R.O. Davies and Sam D. Hutchings

Abstract   Resuscitation of patients with trauma associated shock has evolved over the last 60 years, in part driven by developments during military conflict. An empirical high volume crystalloid based approach has been replaced by more targeted early use of blood products. There is some evidence that the use of pre-defined goal directed resuscitation can improve outcome in trauma shock but this should be tempered by the recent experience of the failure of such a strategy in patients with severe sepsis. An individualized, targeted strategy may represent a more optimal approach but firm evidence is lacking. Although trauma resuscitation is still dominated by a pressure centric paradigm, targets that reflect

W.R.O. Davies, MBChB, MRCP, FRCA, FFICM (✉)
Intensive Care, Royal Sussex County Hospital,
Brighton BN2 5BE, UK
e-mail: will.ro.davies@gmail.com

S.D. Hutchings, MRCS, FRCA, FFICM, DICM, DipIMC
Department of Critical Care, Kings College Hospital,
Denmark Hill, London SE5 9RS, UK

S.D. Hutchings (ed.), *Trauma and Combat Critical Care*   83
in Clinical Practice, In Clinical Practice,
DOI 10.1007/978-3-319-28758-4_5,

flow and perfusion may be more sensitive end points of resuscitation. An overall strategy that concentrates on global flow, alongside tissue perfusion is suggested. Such a strategy needs to be tailored to the environment and the endpoints of resuscitation will necessarily change as the patient progresses through the trauma care pathway.

Keywords Traumatic hemorrhagic shock • Blood products • Goal directed therapy • Individualized resuscitation • Pressure targeted resuscitation • Tissue perfusion • Haemodynamic monitoring • Focused echocardiography

How Has the Approach to Trauma Resuscitation Evolved

Discovering the optimal approach to shock resuscitation has been a central concern of clinicians and physiologists for many decades. Fluid therapy has long been considered the cornerstone of resuscitation practice, however defining which fluids, when, and to what targets, has created fierce debate.

Fluid resuscitation during World War II and the Korean conflict was comprised of colloid solutions and banked whole blood; the strategy emphasised the need for restoration of circulatory blood volume. However, there was also a recognition of the potential negative consequences of aggressive fluid resuscitation prior to definitive haemorrhage control. With this approach early survival improved in comparison to previous conflicts. However, many of these early survivors later died from acute renal failure [1]. In the 1960s the physiological animal models developed by Shires and others influenced a shift towards isotonic crystalloid solutions [2]. Their experimental data suggested that, in Traumatic Haemorrhagic Shock (THS), extracellular fluid was redistributed into both the intravascular and intracellular spaces. It was therefore concluded that optimal resuscitation required a large volume of crystalloid fluid to correct this extracellular deficit. This approach to resuscitation was practiced during the Vietnam conflict and coincided with a reduction in the incidence of acute renal failure but the emergence of 'shock lung' or 'Da Nang lung', later described as adult respiratory distress syndrome. This newly described pathology raised concerns over the potential iatrogenic consequences of a high volume crystalloid based resuscitation strategy. However, this same crystalloid based approach was adopted by the Advanced Trauma Life Support (ATLS) teaching on shock resuscitation, which advocated early infusion of two litres of Ringer's Lactate for shocked trauma patients. Whilst this approach may restore intravascular volume and improve oxygen delivery in patients with controlled haemorrhage, animal models demonstrated that, in uncontrolled haemorrhage, this approach was counterproductive. These studies from the 1980s and 1990s showed that although small volumes of fluid were required to avoid haemodynamic collapse, attempts to normalise blood pressure values consistently led to increased total blood loss and reduced survival [3]. Following recognition of these concerns 'hypotensive' or limited volume resuscitation was advocated, most notably following the landmark trial by Bickell et al. in 1994 [4]. Adoption of this approach has significantly reduced the quantity and rate of initial fluid administration in trauma patients, with greater emphasis on rapid diagnostics and definitive haemorrhage control. Current ATLS and military trauma care guidelines reflect this approach, with shocked patients receiving low volume resuscitation to specific endpoints prior to definitive haemorrhage control. The last two decades have witnessed further developments in resuscitation strategy, with a greater emphasis on damage control principles, haemostatic resuscitation, and identifying more sensitive resuscitation end-points.

Is 'Goal Directed Resuscitation' Appropriate for Patients with THS?

In the 1980s Shoemaker and others hypothesised that optimal resuscitation required the achievement of 'supranormal' oxygen delivery goals in order to meet the raised metabolic demands of the surgical stress response [5]. Early trials of this strategy in trauma patients reported fewer organ failures and shorter hospital stays, particularly when the targeted DO2 values were attained within 24 h of injury [6, 7]. However, targeting 'supranormal' DO2 was also demonstrated to be futile or harmful once patients had established critical illness [8, 9]. A prospective randomized study of unselected ICU patients reported an increase in mortality when fluids and inotropes were targeted to defined 'supranormal' DO2 [9]. Subsequently, investigators demonstrated that in major trauma patients admitted to an ICU, targeting more modest DO2 targets during the first 24 h led to a reduced incidence of intra-abdominal hypertension, abdominal compartment syndrome, MOF and death [10]. This strategy was also associated with less crystalloid volume loading and fewer blood transfusions in the first 24 h [10, 11]. Following a seminal study by Rivers and colleagues [12], which showed a substantial benefit in the application of Early Goal Directed Therapy (EGDT) in septic patients, a multitude of critical care societies and organisations endorsed and advocated a similar approach. However, concern about the physiological basis of the applied treatments, which were predominantly central venous pressure and central venous oxygen saturation targets achieved through fluid therapy, inotropic support and blood transfusion, prompted three large international trials designed to replicate the original single centre protocol [13–15]. These trials either showed no difference or a deleterious effect from the application of EGDT. The publication of these trials has led many in the critical care community to question the basis of a 'one size fits all' approach to therapy and, as a consequence, there is increasing research interest in so called 'individualised resuscitation'.

Is Blood Pressure an Appropriate Resuscitation Target for Patients with THS ?

The definition, detection and reversal of all forms of shock has been based predominantly upon pressure centric models of blood flow, with targets typically expressed in terms of systolic blood pressure (SBP). However, studies have indicated that the ATLS classifications of hypovolaemic shock do not accurately reflect clinical reality, with SBP changes not occurring to the degree suggested [16, 17]. Pragmatically, SBP is used as a surrogate for bulk blood flow due to ease of measurement. However, it should be appreciated that SBP correlates poorly with cardiac output (CO), oxygen delivery and tissue perfusion. Pressure is a function of flow and resistance and therefore a state of high systemic vascular resistance (SVR) will maintain a normal range for SBP despite significantly reduced blood flow. Furthermore, regional flows can vary significantly due to marked changes in local vascular resistance, whilst global systemic pressures remain within normal limits. The most established definition of shock, SBP < 90 mmHg, has been shown to be a late marker, correlating poorly with injury severity, and lacking sensitivity and specificity for predicting patient outcomes [18, 19]. Despite these limitations, SBP remains a major component of trauma triage guidelines.

The adaptive response to hypovolaemia increases sympathetic outflow and vascular tone, increasing SVR and maintaining perfusion pressure to vital organs at the expense of less vital tissues. In this context, global flow remains decreased and the shock state persists despite normalisation of vital signs. This occult hypoperfusion (OH) is a state of 'compensated' shock, defined as an elevated blood lactate level in the absence of clinical signs of shock. Following resuscitation, it has been demonstrated that up to 80 % of normotensive trauma patients with adequate urine output remain in a state of OH [20]. Early identification and correction of OH directly impacts on patient survival and morbidity [21]. Conversely, there is a strong association between failing to meet metabolic demands and mortality as shown in Fig. 5.1.

In summary there is a post-traumatic therapeutic window within which individualised, quantitative, flow targeted resuscitation may influence the outcome of severely injured trauma patients.

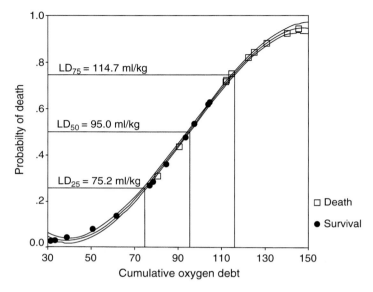

FIGURE 5.1 Probability of death as function of oxygen debt (O2D) in a pig model of haemorrhagic shock. Points plotted along the regression line and its 95 % confidence limits represent the values of cumulative O2D at 60 min of haemorrhage for survivors (*marked with circles*) and non-survivors (*marked with squares*) (Reproduced from Rixen [24])

What Is the Relationship Between Global Blood Flow, Regional Blood Flow and Tissue Perfusion Following THS?

Trauma, shock and ischaemia-reperfusion initiate an acute inflammatory response. The release of inflammatory mediators, combined with shedding of the endothelial glycocalyx layer, results in increased capillary permeability and potential microcirculatory dysfunction. In this situation apparently normal systemic haemodynamics may not translate into normal perfusion in all tissues. Local vascular resistance in specific tissue beds influences local perfusion patterns. Our current understanding of microcirculatory mechanics is limited; however, it is clear that an adequate circulating volume is a prerequisite for adequate tissue perfusion, and thus maintaining a normal circulating volume remains a priority. The ultimate aim of resuscitation is to restore effective tissue perfusion and to normalise cellular metabolism. Although the first key step in resuscitation is optimisation of global flow, strategies should also consider ways to optimise regional perfusion and microcirculatory blood flow.

How Should the Approach to Resuscitation of the Critically Injured Patient Be Adapted to the Environment?

Trauma patients, almost by definition, present in challenging environments, which can be remote from traditional healthcare provision and sometimes even frankly dangerous. The strategy for haemodynamic optimization of THS must therefore take the environment into account. The remainder of this section describes four distinct locations in which trauma patients will be managed as they move from the point of injury to the critical care unit and outlines an appropriate strategy for each phase of treatment that corresponds to this location. An overview of these phases is shown in Table 5.1. The specifics of management, including a discussion of the various haemodynamic monitoring devices, can be found in Chap. 6.

Pre-hospital Resuscitation

Treatment priorities in the pre-hospital phase are haemorrhage control, avoiding further physiological deterioration and rapid safe transport to definitive care. The 'platinum 10 minutes' concept emphasises the need for early and effective haemorrhage control (i.e. direct pressure, arterial tourniquets) and reversal of obstructive causes of shock (e.g. tension pneumothorax). Patients with ongoing bleeding from non-compressible haemorrhage require rapid transport to a

TABLE 5.1 Phases of trauma shock resuscitation

Phase	Timeframe	Clinical setting	Treatment priorities	Resuscitation targets	Monitoring options
Salvage	Seconds – minutes "Platinum 10 minutes"	Pre-hospital	Immediate life saving interventions Haemorrhage control Prevent cardiovascular collapse Transfer	Clinical: pulses, mentation	Fingertips – pulses 'eyeball' – global visual assessment of patient condition
Optimisation	Minutes – hours "Golden hour"	Pre-hospital ED OR	Limit depth and duration of shock Increase oxygen delivery Optimise cardiac output Repay oxygen debt Achieve homeostasis	Clinical: heart rate, pulse pressure, MAP Preload: SVV/ SPV/PPV Biochemical: BD, lactate	NIBP/IABP ETCO2 ABG ROTEM® ODM/fTTE/NICOM

Stabilization	Hours – days "Silver day"	OR ICU	Targeted therapies to avoid fluid overload/excess Maintain homeostasis (with particular attention to pH, temperature and coagulation)	Clinical: heart rate, pulse pressure, MAP Preload: SVV/SPV/PPV Biochemical: BD, lactate Oxygen Delivery (DO2)	Flow monitoring Invasive cardiac output ABG ROTEM®
De-escalation	Days – weeks	ICU	Normalisation of fluid balance Weaning from organ support Avoiding iatrogenic insults	Clinical: heart rate, pulse pressure, MAP Biochemical: BD, lactate	Focused on clinical assessment Remove invasive lines

Adapted from Vincent [25]

THS Traumatic haemorrhage shock, *ED* Emergency department, *OR* Operating room, *ICU* Intensive care unit, *NIBP* Non-invasive blood pressure, *IABP* Invasive arterial blood pressure, *ABG* Arterial blood gases, *ROTEM* Rotational thromboelastometry, *ETCO2* End-tidal carbon dioxide, *ODM* Oesophageal doppler monitor, *NICOM* Non-invasive cardiac output monitor, *BD* Base deficit, *MAP* Mean arterial pressure, *fTTE* Focus transthoracic echocardiography, *SVV* Stroke volume variation, *SPV* systolic pressure variation, *PPV* pulse pressure variation

trauma center for haemorrhage control by surgical or radiological interventions, or actions to provide this in the pre-hospital environment, e.g. aortic balloon occlusion. During this early 'salvage' phase, the goal of resuscitation is to prevent circulatory arrest and achieve a minimum vital organ perfusion pressure.

Clinical end-points for titrating fluid therapy must be pragmatic and easily identifiable, e.g. palpable pulses or mentation. In the pre-hospital setting it may be difficult to exclude non-compressible haemorrhage, therefore consensus opinion supports a 'no fluid' or low volume (250 ml fluid bolus) approach. Guidelines recommend that in adults with blunt trauma, no fluid be administered in the pre-hospital phase if a radial pulse is present. In penetrating trauma, a palpable central pulse is the chosen resuscitation end-point. However, it should be noted that there is a poor correlation between the presence, or absence, of pulses and the actual SBP [22].

In austere and remote environments the pre-hospital phase of care may run into many hours or days. In scenarios involving prolonged evacuation timelines there comes a point where permissive hypoperfusion no longer confers a survival advantage. In these settings, treatment of hypovolaemia and reversal of oxygen debt may become a more appropriate strategy. Animal studies conducted by the UK Ministry of Defence have demonstrated that withholding fluid resuscitation for more than 1 h following complex traumatic injury is associated with a decreased chance of survival; this has lead to the suggestion of a so called "Novel Hybrid" model of resuscitation [23].

Resource limitation often dictates that the clinician rely on clinical end-points for resuscitation, however this leaves open the spectre of occult hypoperfusion. If resources permit more sophisticated haemodynamic monitoring may have a place, especially when pre-hospital time lines are predicted to be extended. Pre-hospital monitoring systems should be light, robust, and easily deployable. Ideal devices should also be capable of air transportation, unaffected by vibration artifact, and have reliable independent power supplies. Bulky processing and display units make many current systems impractical. However, in prolonged retrieval scenarios the use of non-invasive systems such as focused transthoracic echocardiography (fTTE), bioreactance derived cardiac output monitoring and supra-sternal Doppler may offer a useful additional level of monitoring. Recent experience has demonstrated that the use of non-invasive monitoring and point-of-care testing (e.g. coagulation, blood gas analysis) are feasible for aeromedical evacuation services.

Resuscitation in the Emergency Department

In the emergency department it is reasonable to continue hypovolaemic resuscitation for a short period, whilst the clinical assessment is completed and haemorrhage control measures are optimized. In the actively exsanguinating patient, it is appropriate to sacrifice perfusion for coagulation and haemorrhage control. Once the injury pattern is fully defined the focus should be on rapid decision making that expedites definitive haemorrhage control. It is critical that actively bleeding patients are transferred to an area where definitive haemorrhage control can occur early, rather than delaying the process in pursuit of further diagnostics. In some circumstances this may require the patient to bypass the emergency department and proceed directly to the operating room. Prior to achieving haemorrhage control, resuscitation targets should remain clinical, e.g., palpable pulses and mentation, and fluids should only be administer to prevent haemodynamic collapse.

Formal goal directed therapy in the actively exsanguinating patient is neither appropriate nor achievable. Clinical evidence suggests that if differing pressure targets are set prior to haemorrhage control, the actual mean arterial pressures achieved are very similar, despite differences in resuscitation strategy. Furthermore, following a strategy aimed at a lower pressure target has been associated with significantly decreased transfusion requirements and postoperative coagulopathy, in the absence of increased morbidity or mortality.

Resuscitation targets should be adjusted to improve tissue perfusion if there is no identifiable surgically or angiographically correctable bleeding point. In this group, resuscitation should move to an 'optimisation' phase, where the goal is to increase global oxygen delivery (DO2) and reverse tissue ischaemia. There is a narrow window of opportunity here, where aggressive and targeted resuscitation may offset impending morbidity. Haemostatic resuscitation to SBP, pulse pressure and HR will begin to address gross hypovolaemia, whilst measurement of lactate and base deficit will quantify the severity of the shock state. Early adoption of flow monitoring should be considered at this point, as should the measurement of dynamic indices of coagulation. fTTE examination provides a non-invasive means of rapidly identifying the type(s) of shock present in trauma patients and is also an invaluable way of rapidly assessing intra vascular volume status. An oesophageal Doppler probe can be quickly inserted into the intubated patient and flow based monitoring used to guide early resuscitation.

Resuscitation in the Operating Room/ Interventional Radiology Suite

Patients who are taken to the operating room or interventional radiology suite for damage control surgery or embolisation should receive resuscitation in line with the principles of damage control resuscitation. A hypovolaemic approach should continue until definitive haemorrhage control is declared. Effective team dynamics and clear communication are crucial in aiding the appropriate direction of resuscitation efforts. Once haemorrhage control is confirmed the team should utilise invasive lines and cardiac output monitoring to titrate blood products, pharmacotherapy and respiratory support to biochemical, coagulation and haemodynamic parameters. The therapeutic goal is now complete reversal of shock. Haemodynamic targets should move beyond a pressure centric paradigm and focus on preload and afterload optimisation.

High-risk trauma patients in the operating room or interventional radiology suite should have an arterial line inserted. Display of an arterial pressure waveform provides the clinician with the ability to make crude 'eyeball' estimates of preload (systolic pressure variation), contractility (change in pressure/change in time) and afterload (diastolic and pulse pressures) when formal CO monitoring is not available. Haemodynamic responses to titrated opiate sympatholysis provide useful information regarding the degree of sympathetic tone and relative hypovolaemia. These patients may benefit from flow monitoring to guide damage control resuscitation and optimise volume status. In this context an oesophageal Doppler probe, pulse contour derived cardiac output monitors or even a pulmonary artery catheter will provide improved accuracy. Ideally these systems will remain in situ once the patient is transferred to the ICU, allowing seamless continuity of resuscitation.

In the resource-limited environment, resuscitation efforts should be targeted to an integration of clinical end-points such as urine output, capillary refill time, core-peripheral temperature gradients, as well as pulses, HR and SBP. In this environment, where blood products are often scarce, point of care devices which estimate haemoglobin concentration can help guide perioperative transfusion practice.

Resuscitation in the Intensive Care Unit

Following the intraoperative phase of damage control surgery/resuscitation, management priorities change as critical illness becomes more established. Resuscitation strategies are directed at restoring organ function after the combined insults of hypovolaemia, hypoperfusion, surgery and the associated inflammatory response. An early priority is to ensure an adequate preload in the face of an evolving relative hypovolaemia secondary to inflammation related vasodilatation. The degree of vasoplegia will relate to the severity of shock and subsequent reperfusion injury. This manifests clinically as warm peripheries, a falling blood pressure and if uncorrected, signs of impaired end organ perfusion. It should be borne in mind that ongoing overt blood loss from areas of debrided tissue is common and this will be more pronounced in patients who remain coagulopathic. The priorities in the early care of these ICU patients are to correct hypothermia, coagulopathy and acidaemia, monitor for ongoing bleeding, and continuously optimise intra vascular volume.

Resuscitation should be individualised and utilise blood gas analysis, thromboelastography and flow monitoring. This 'optimisation' phase may continue for the first 24 h following injury, while metabolic debts are repaid and homeostasis is restored. This is a critically important time, dubbed the 'Silver Day', within which quantitative flow targeted resuscitation can influence clinical outcomes. Close attention must be paid to deterioration requiring return to the operating room or interventional radiology suite, as well as to detecting and reversing occult hypoperfusion. In resource-poor settings, the clinician may not have the benefit of advanced monitoring, however close attention to fluid balance, temperature, analgesia, and clinical markers of end organ perfusion will allow a pragmatic approach to a challenging scenario.

Once homeostasis has been restored, the resuscitation strategy should move toward a 'stabilisation' phase, where the aim is to prevent organ dysfunction. The focus here is on preventing complications from iatrogenic interstitial oedema secondary to fluid therapy. Following this phase, care should then begin to focus on 'de-escalation', where organ support is weaned and intrinsic function is restored. Attention should be paid to normalising total body water and salt content. Fluid restrictive, natriuretic, and diuretic strategies may be appropriate in some patients at this point.

What Are the Unanswered Questions in Trauma Resuscitation?

Compared to other disease states, such as severe sepsis, the pathological mechanisms underpinning the response to complex severe trauma remain relatively understudied. The consequences of 15 years of combat operations have pushed the frontiers of trauma research, particularly in relation to trauma associated coagulopathy, but there remain many unanswered questions as to the best resuscitation strategy following complex traumatic haemorrhage. Some of the areas of ongoing interest to clinical academics, including those working within the research divisions of the UK and allied militaries are shown in Table 5.2.

TABLE 5.2 Ongoing research questions in trauma shock resuscitation

Question	Potential avenues/speculation
If early goal-directed therapies improve outcome, when is early enough?	Started within first 6 h from injury?
At what stage from point of wounding does shock need to be fully reversed to prevent secondary morbidity?	12–24 h?
What is the upper limit of a period of permissive hypotension/ hypoperfusion?	60–90 min in animal models (HypoResus trial, Clinical trials. gov NCT01411852- awaiting publication)
What other patient factors influence the duration of tolerable hypoperfusion?	Co-existing brain injury, age, comorbid hypertension/vascular disease, genomics?
What are the relationships between shock, inflammation, coagulation, immune function and multi-organ dysfunction	Complex. Multiple ongoing projects including the Inflammation and Host Response to Injury group (www.gluegrant.org), ACIT Trial (UK CRN ID 537), MICROSHOCK study (Clinical trials.gov NCT02111109)
How can we ensure that optimised global flow is translated into optimised tissue perfusion?	By measuring microcirculatory flow parameters, lactate clearance and base deficit? Point of care perfusion measurement is a real possibility in the next 5 years

References

1. Butler F. Fluid resuscitation in tactical combat casualty care: brief history and current status. J Trauma. 2011;70(5):s11–2.
2. Shires T. Fluid therapy in hemorrhagic shock. Arch Surg. 1964;88:688–93.
3. Fouche Y. Changing paradigms in surgical resuscitation. Crit Care Med. 2010;38:S411–20.
4. Bickell W. Immediate versus delayed fluid resuscitation for hypotensive patients with penetrating torso injuries. N Engl J Med. 1994;331:1105–9.
5. Shoemaker W. Prospective trial of supranormal values of survivors as therapeutic goals in high-risk surgical patients. Chest. 1988;94:1176–86.
6. Fleming A. Prospective trial of supranormal values as goals of resuscitation in severe trauma. Arch Surg. 1992;127(10):1175–9.
7. Bishop MH. Prospective randomized trial of survivor values of cardiac index, oxygen delivery, and oxygen consumption as resuscitation endpoints in severe trauma. J Trauma. 1995;38:780–7.
8. Gattinoni L. A trial of goal-oriented hemodynamic therapy in critically ill patients. N Engl J Med. 1995;333:1025–32.
9. Hayes M. Elevation of systemic oxygen delivery in the treatment of critically ill patients. N Engl J Med. 1994;330:1717–22.
10. Balogh Z. Supranormal trauma resuscitation causes more cases of abdominal compartment syndrome. Arch Surg. 2003;138:637–43.
11. McKinley B. Normal vs supranormal oxygen delivery goals in shock resuscitation: the response is the same. J Trauma. 2002;53:825–32.
12. Rivers E. Early goal-directed therapy in the treatment of severe sepsis and septic chock. N Engl J Med. 2001;345:1368–77.
13. Investigators PCESS. A randomized trial of protocol-based care for early septic shock. N Engl J Med. 2014;370:1683–93.
14. Investigators ARISE. Goal-directed resuscitation for patients with early septic shock. N Engl J Med. 2014;371:1496–506.
15. Mouncey P. Trial of early, goal-directed resuscitation for septic shock. N Engl J Med. 2015;372:1301–11.
16. Mutschler M. A critical reappraisal of the ATLS classification of hypovolaemic shock: does it really reflect clinical reality? Resuscitation. 2013;84:309–13.

17. Guly H. Vital signs and estimated blood loss in patients with major trauma: testing the validity of the ATLS classification of hypovolaemic shock. Resuscitation. 2011;82:556–9.
18. Parks J. Systemic hypotension is a late marker of shock after trauma: a validation study of advanced trauma life support principles in a large national sample. Am J Surg. 2006;192:727–31.
19. Newgard C. A critical assessment of the out-of-hospital trauma triage guidelines for physiologic abnormality. J Trauma. 2010;68(2):452–62.
20. Scalea T. Resuscitation of multiple trauma and head injury: role of crystalloid fluids and inotropes. Crit Care Med. 1994;22:1610–5.
21. Blow O. The golden hour and the silver day: detection and correction of occult hypoperfusion within 24 hours improves outcome from major trauma. J Trauma. 1999;47:964–9.
22. Deakin CD, Low JL. Accuracy of the advanced trauma life support guidelines for predicting systolic blood pressure using carotid, femoral, and radial pulses: observational study. BMJ. 2000;321(7262):673–4.
23. Kirkman E, Watts S, Cooper G. Blast injury research models. Philos Trans R Soc Lond B Biol Sci. 2011;366(1562):144–59.
24. Rixen D. Bench-to-bedside review: oxygen debt and its metabolic correlates as quantifiers of the severity of hemorrhagic and post-traumatic shock. Crit Care. 2005;9:441–53.
25. Vincent JL. Circulatory shock. N Engl J Med. 2013;369:1726–34.

Chapter 6
Haemodynamic Optimisation of the Critically Injured Patient

William R.O. Davies and Sam D. Hutchings

Abstract Haemodynamic optimisation of the shocked, bleeding trauma patient requires a systematic approach. The initial focus should be on haemorrhage control but must move quickly to assessment and targeted treatment of the shock state. Optimisation of global volume status can be challenging but there are a multitude of devices available to assist clinicians. Focused echocardiography can be performed at all stages of the trauma care pathway and allows for exclusion of restrictive cardiac impairment as well as assessment of cardiac contractility and optimisation of volume status. After ensuring adequate

W.R.O. Davies, MBChB, MRCP, FRCA, FFICM (✉)
Intensive Care, Royal Sussex County Hospital, Eastern Road,
Brighton BN2 5BE, UK
e-mail: will.ro.davies@gmail.com

S.D. Hutchings, MRCS, FRCA, FFICM, DICM, DipIMC
Department of Critical Care, Kings College Hospital,
Denmark Hill, London SE5 9RS, UK

S.D. Hutchings (ed.), *Trauma and Combat Critical Care in Clinical Practice*, In Clinical Practice,
DOI 10.1007/978-3-319-28758-4_6,

intravascular volume, clinicians must focus on improving tissue perfusion and reversing the shock state as quickly as possible. Serial measurement of lactate alongside central venous oxygen saturations and carbon dioxide tension provide therapeutic targets. Patients may exhibit occult microcirculatory hypo-perfusion despite normal macro circulatory values and new monitoring tools, such as point of care videomicroscopy may help to identify these patients who require individually targeted therapy. The 'optimal' blood pressure during and following trauma resuscitation remains unclear and there is probably wide inter-individual variation.

Keywords Haemorrhagic shock • Major trauma • Resuscitation • Blood pressure • Cardiac output • Haemodynamic monitoring • Focused echocardiography • Lactate • Perfusion • Microcirculation

Introduction

In Chap. 5 we discussed how trauma shock resuscitation has evolved in the modern era and outlined the kinds of haemodynamic optimisation that should be considered at each stage of the trauma pathway, from point of injury through to the intensive care unit. In this chapter we will discuss how clinicians can implement this strategy using existing monitoring tools, as well as exploring how new technology may change the existing paradigm of trauma shock resuscitation.

Achieving optimal resuscitation requires individualised, timely, goal-directed titration of therapies to sensitive endpoints. This 'quantitative resuscitation' consists of a structured approach to haemodynamic optimisation, utilising intravascular volume expansion and possibly vasoactive drugs to achieve explicit goals, which should be tailored to the individual rather than applied across an entire

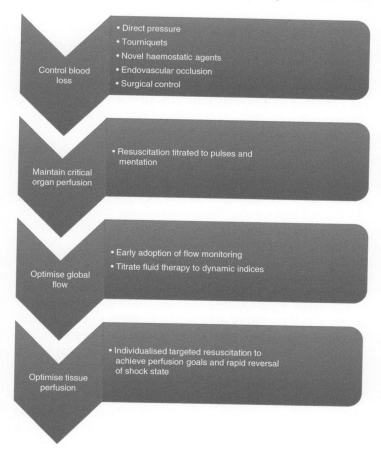

FIGURE 6.1 Suggested process for haemodynamic optimisation of the shocked trauma patient

population of patients. A suggested step-wise approach that moves from maintenance of critical organ blood flow through optimization of global preload and hence to ensuring ongoing adequacy of tissue perfusion is shown in Fig. 6.1

Part One: Assessment and Optimisation of Cardiac Output and Global Blood Flow

How Should Global Flow and Cardiac Output Be Optimized During Trauma Shock Resuscitation?

In early traumatic hemorrhagic shock (THS) the deficit in global flow is usually secondary to acute intravascular volume loss and fluid administration is the obvious therapeutic strategy. In some trauma scenarios an obstructive reduction in cardiac output, caused by a tension pneumothorax or cardiac tamponade, may be present. These conditions need to be excluded early during resuscitation and again if patients demonstrate new haemodynamic instability. Point of care ultrasound is the most reliable method of diagnosing these conditions.

Empirical fluid challenges assume that the patient's left ventricle (LV) is functioning on the ascending portion of the Frank-Starling curve and has a 'recruitable' cardiac output (CO). Once the LV is functioning near the 'flat' part of this curve, fluid loading has less effect on CO and only serves to increase interstitial oedema. Increasing evidence suggests that excessive fluid resuscitation is associated with worse outcomes [1], therefore resuscitation requires the administration of an optimal amount of fluid, and no more. In fact, some clinicians would suggest that once a patient has become a non responder to fluid then they have already received too much volume.

Predicting fluid responsiveness and intravascular volume status in critically ill patients can be challenging. The standard definition of volume responsiveness is a >15 % increase in CO in response to volume expansion [2]. Although the volume of the fluid bolus has not been standardised, between 250 and 500 mL, administered over a period of 20–30 min, is most commonly used [3]. The passive leg raise (PLR) technique provides an alternative to the fluid challenge by utilising a reversible 'auto-transfusion' mechanism. The technique involves lifting the legs passively from the horizontal position by 30–45° inducing a gravitational transfer of blood from the lower limbs toward the intra-thoracic compartment. A sustained, 15 s, increase in cardiac output 30 s after PLR predicts fluid responsiveness. This PLR assessment can allow an assessment of 'fluid tolerance', whilst avoiding iatrogenic insults from unnecessary fluid challenges.

Traditional static haemodynamic parameters, such as central venous pressure (CVP), have been shown to be poor predictors of volume responsiveness except in patients with relatively obvious hypovolemia [4]. In mechanically ventilated patients pulse contour analysis can produce more sensitive dynamic indices of volume responsiveness, e.g., pulse pressure variation (PPV), systolic pressure variation (SPV) and stroke volume variation (SVV). However, these techniques require relatively large tidal volumes (≥ 8 ml/kg). In addition patients should have no spontaneous breathing effort and be free of major arrhythmia and right ventricular dysfunction.

Suggested haemodynamic resuscitation endpoints are shown in Table 6.1.

It should be emphasised that not all patients who are volume responsive require fluid. The healthy LV has a physiological reserve that will allow continued SV increases in response to increasing preload. Clinicians must integrate all the available information regarding global, organ and tissue flow, prior to administering volume. Some researchers are beginning to suggest that patients with objectively adequate tissue perfusion, measured for example by using SDF videomicroscopy, do not benefit from fluid administration, even if they are classically 'volume responsive' [5]. This approach merits further investigation, but at present the existing technology is not sufficiently adapted for routine clinical use.

A suggested approach to the optimisation of intra vascular volume during trauma shock resuscitation, adapted

Table 6.1 Possible resuscitation targets based on global flow/intravascular volume parameters

End point (device)	Measures	Advantages	Disadvantages	Therapeutic target
CVP PCWP (CVC, PAC)	Pressure within the venous system as a marker for intravascular volume	Continuous monitoring	Pressure not volumetric and affected by cardiovascular compliance. Very poor correlation with volume status when used as a static parameter	Sustained CVP/PCWP rise of >2–3 cmH$_2$O following a fluid challenge
GEDVI (PiCCO)	Global end diastolic volume (preload)	Well correlated with preload. Not influenced by mode of ventilation	Requires repeat thermodilution and dedicated monitoring device. Reference values derived from healthy volunteers	680–800 ml/m^2
SVV PPV SPV (Pulse contour devices, arterial line)	Intravascular volume status variation with ventilation	Continuous monitoring, Well correlated with volume status in selected patients	Requires arterial cannula. Inaccurate in patients with variable or low tidal volumes. SPV not well correlated with intravascular volume unless significant hypovolaemia	<15 %

IVC collapsibilty (fTTE)	Intravascular volume status variation with ventilation	Non invasive, Well correlated with preload in selected patients	Single snap-shot, cannot be used for continuous monitoring, Training and experience required to acquire images Unclear thresholds especially in spontaneously breathing patients	<20 % (in mechanically ventilated patients) <40 % variability (spontaneously breathing patients)
VTi variability (fTTE, Suprasternal Doppler, Carotid Doppler)	Intravascular volume status variation with ventilation	Non invasive, Well correlated with preload in selected patients	Single snap-shot, cannot be used for continuous monitoring, Training and experience required to acquire images Inaccurate in patients with variable or low tidal volumes	<15 %

CVP central venous pressure, *PCWP* pulmonary capillary wedge pressure, *GEDVI* global diastolic volume index, *SVV* stroke volume variation, *PPV* pulse pressure variation, *SPV* systolic pressure variation, *fTTE* focused transthoracic echocardiography, *VTi* velocity time integer, *IVC* inferior vena cava, *PiCCO* pulse contour cardiac output

from the process used by the Defence Medical Services of the United Kingdom (UK DMS) is shown in Fig. 6.2.

Which Tools Are Available to Aid Clinicians in Optimising Global Flow During Trauma Shock Resuscitation?

Devices that monitor global flow or volume provide haemodynamic information that helps guide resuscitation. Correct interpretation of the data, combined with appropriate and goal-directed interventions form a vital part of shock resuscitation. The decision to use flow monitoring and which device to deploy will depend on the clinical environment and phase of resuscitation as discussed in Chap. 5.

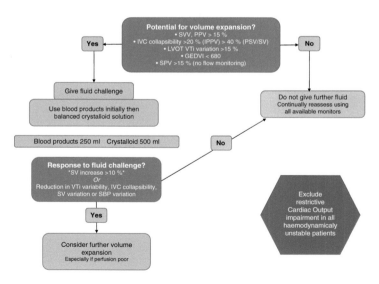

FIGURE 6.2 Suggested process for optimising global flow and intravascular volume during trauma shock resuscitation based on UK DMS critical care guidelines

Focused Transthoracic Echocardiography (fTTE)

Recent years have seen an upsurge of interest and enthusiasm for the use of echocardiography to answer focused questions relating to the haemodynamic management of critically ill patients. In many ways focused transthoracic echocardiography is the ideal monitor for optimizing volume status in critically injured patients. Modern devices are compact and portable, enabling use throughout the trauma care pathway. The technique is non-invasive and rapid, lacking the requirement for device insertion and calibration associated with many other monitoring systems. Competency in fTTE is increasingly becoming a standard part of many training programs for acute care clinicians and can also be delivered by non-medically trained personal [6]. The UK DMS have adopted fTTE as the preferred technique for assessing volume status in critically injured patients on deployed military operations (Fig. 6.3).

Using focused echo to determine volume status is achieved using two techniques: (i) determination of inferior vena cava (IVC) collapsibility and (ii) assessment of left ventricular outflow tract (LVOT) Doppler Velocity Time Integral (VTi) variability. During normal respiration the reduction in intra-thoracic pressure is transmitted to the IVC and causes a reduction in the calibre of the vessel, the degree of collapse being related to the intravascular volume. The reverse effect occurs during mechanical positive pressure ventilation, although the magnitude of change is less. Precise data is lacking but as a general rule IVC collapse of up to 40 % during spontaneous breathing and up to 20 % during intermittent positive pressure ventilation (IPPV) is taken to be within physiological norms. Values over these limits are suggestive of hypovolaemia [7]. Figure 6.4 shows an example of IVC variability.

Changes in preload occurring as a result of intra-thoracic pressure differences during respiration can cause variation in the ejected stroke volume. The degree of variation is related to the tidal volume and intravascular volume status. Doppler

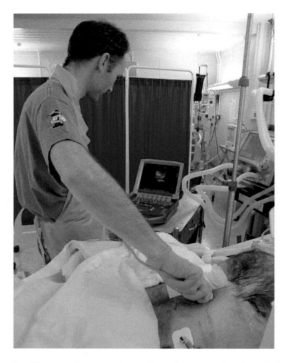

FIGURE 6.3 Focussed trans thoracic echo examination being performed by one of the authors on the ICU of the UK Role 3 hospital at Camp Bastion, Afghanistan

measurement of the VTi of blood flow through the LVOT provides an accurate measure of stroke volume. Variation in LVOT VTi of more than 15 % is suggestive of hypovolaemia in a patient receiving mandatory ventilation with a fixed tidal volume [8] (Fig. 6.5).

Because the VTi is directly proportional to the stroke volume it can also be used as an absolute value when assessing the impact of fluid administration i.e., a rise in VTi of more than 10 % following a fluid challenge is a good indicator of volume responsiveness and has the advantage of being non invasive.

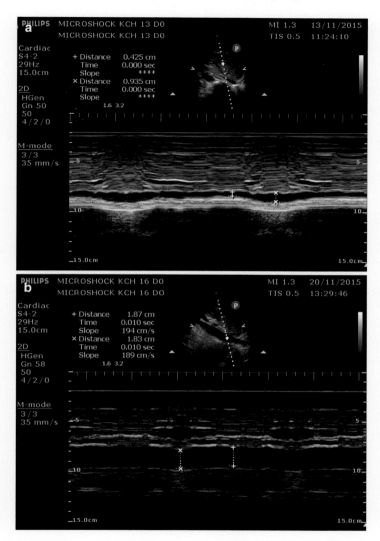

FIGURE 6.4 M- Mode view of the IVC in two patients following traumatic injury, both of whom are intubated and ventilated. (**a**) Shows a small calibre IVC with a 55 % increase in diameter during inspiration, indicative of significant hypovolaemia. (**b**) Shows a larger IVC with no variation across the respiratory cycle, indicating a potentially full venous circulation

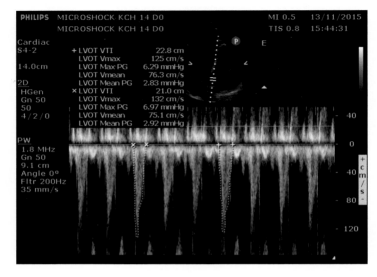

FIGURE 6.5 Pulse wave Doppler image obtained from the LVOT of a ventilated patient. The VTi has been measured and there is minimal change across the respiratory cycle, suggesting the absence of hypovolaemia

Pulmonary Artery Catheter

Bolus thermodilution utilising the pulmonary artery catheter (PAC) is still often described as the clinical gold standard method for measuring CO, even though it is now rarely used in clinical practice. The main disadvantages of the PAC are that it is maximally invasive, carries the risk of severe complications, and requires a skilled technician to correctly position the catheter. The PAC also provides predominantly pressure based indices which may not be as accurate as volumetric indices, particularly where vascular compliance is abnormal. Broad consensus is now not in favour of routine use of the PAC in the management of shock states and they are generally reserved for cardiogenic shock, particularly when an accurate real time assessment of pulmonary artery pressure is required.

Devices That Use Pulse-Contour Analysis

Stroke volume and cardiac output can be calculated from the arterial pressure waveform if the arterial compliance and resistance are known. Commercial pulse-contour analysers use pressure volume conversion algorithms to derive volumetric indices. These systems can be divided into two main categories:

- Systems requiring indicator dilution CO measurement to calibrate the pulse contour, e.g., lithium dilution & thermodilution:

  The **LiDCO** monitor (Lithium Dilution Cardiac Output, LiDCO Systems, Cambridge UK) combines pulse contour analysis with lithium indicator dilution for continuous SV monitoring. The 'nominal SV' is adjusted to an 'actual SV' using a patient-specific calibration factor which is derived from a lithium indicator dilution CO measurement. The LiDCO system does not require central venous cannulation and the lithium doses used do not exert pharmacologically relevant effects. Recalibration is required after acute haemodynamic changes and after any intervention that alters vascular impedance [9].

  The **PiCCO** monitor (Pulse Contour Continuous Cardiac Output, Pulsion, Munich, Germany) combines pulse contour analysis with transpulmonary thermodilution CO measurement. This system requires both central venous and central arterial catheterisation (femoral or brachial). The SV is calculated from the area under the systolic portion of the arterial waveform. Arterial compliance and resistance are derived from the diastolic decay curve. The PiCCO uses transpulmonary thermodilution CO measurement for algorithm calibration, and the thermodilution curve can be used to measure the global end-diastolic volume (GEDV) and extravascular lung water. The calibration is considered to remain accurate for several hours, however it is advisable to recalibrate after periods of haemodynamic instability or following significant fluid shifts. The contour-based algorithm is dependent upon the shape of the arterial waveform and is therefore sensitive to damping [9].

- Systems requiring patient biometrics for arterial impedance estimation:

  The **FloTrac** system (Edwards Lifesciences, Irvine, CA, USA) is operator independent and only requires peripheral arterial catheterisation. The basic principle of the system is the linear relationship between pulse pressure and SV. This system estimates vascular compliance from patient biometric values and vascular tone from waveform characteristics.

  The **LiDCO rapid** system (LiDCO Systems, Cambridge, UK) uses the pulse pressure algorithm validated in the original LiDCO system and applies it to an uncalibrated arterial waveform analysis. This system uses a nomogram to estimate the patient specific aortic compliance and the algorithm estimates stroke volume from the arterial pressure waveform.

Calculation of CO and SV by arterial pressure waveform analysis is influenced by several confounding factors, including acute changes in vascular tone, e.g., secondary to vasoactive drugs and acute fluid shifts. When compared with thermodilution CO and Doppler based monitoring, these uncalibrated systems are poor at tracking changes in SV and can produce unreliable estimates of CO, particularly in haemodynamically unstable patients. It is also important to appreciate the influence of the site of the arterial catheter when interpreting data from pulse contour analysis. Significant differences have been described between peripheral and central sites in a variety of clinical scenarios [10]. Essentially, in haemodynamically unstable patients with rapidly changing intravascular volume and tone, it is unreasonable to expect uncalibrated systems using peripheral arteries to accurately reflect the true state of the circulatory system.

Devices That Use Doppler Assessment of Blood Flow

The **Oesophageal Doppler** monitor (CardioQ-ODM, Deltex Medical, Chichester, UK) measures blood velocity in the descending thoracic aorta by means of a Doppler transducer placed at the tip of a minimally invasive flexible probe (Fig. 6.6). The probe is inserted to the mid oesophagus where small adjustments to position and gain are required to obtain an optimal Doppler signal. This signal produces a velocity time integer (VTi) measurement that is factored into an algorithm to produce SV and CO. The algorithm incorporates a nomogram to estimate aortic cross sectional area and derive total left ventricular stroke volume.

There is a steep but rapid learning curve to obtaining optimal Doppler signals and the probe may require frequent adjustments of position to ensure beam alignment with aortic flow. Visual display of the signal waveform provides useful feedback when optimising beam alignment and focus. Despite its limitations, the UK National Institute for Health and Care Excellence has endorsed the use of the ODM for goal-directed fluid therapy in high-risk surgical patients. In the setting of trauma resuscitation, optimisation of SV using the ODM has been associated with a decrease in blood lactate levels, a lower incidence of infectious complications, and reduced ICU and hospital length of stay [11].

The **USCOM** device (USCOM Ltd, Sydney, Australia) uses a small hand-held probe that is placed in the suprasternal notch, directing a Doppler ultrasound beam toward the ascending aorta (Fig. 6.7). As with the ODM, VTi measurements are factored into nomogram based algorithms to produce SV and CO. The accuracy of the system relies on obtaining an optimal flow signal, which is dependent on operator ability and patient factors. Studies comparing USCOM measurements of CO with those obtained by standard thermodilution techniques have shown mixed results [12]. A major advantage of the USCOM is its small size and portability. However, the handheld probe makes it impractical for continuous monitoring.

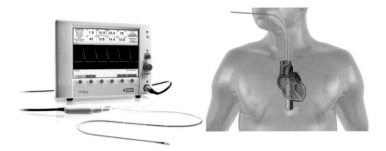

FIGURE 6.6 Oesophageal Doppler Monitor (With permission Deltex Medical)

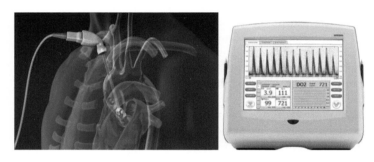

FIGURE 6.7 USCOM supra-sternal Doppler cardiac output monitoring system (With permission USCOM)

Devices That Use Thoracic Bioreactance

The thorax can be considered as an electrical circuit containing a resistor and a capacitor, which together produce the thoracic impedance. Pulsatile ejection of blood from the heart modifies the values of resistance and compliance, leading to instantaneous changes in the amplitude and phase of the impedance. The **NICOM** system (Cheetah Medical, Portland, USA) measures the bioreactance or the phase shift in voltage across the thorax. It consists of a high-frequency sine wave generator and 4 dual-electrode contacts that are placed onto the surface of the chest wall. The NICOM signal processing unit determines the relative phase shift between the input and output signals, producing a value that allows calculation of SV. The NICOM demonstrates acceptable accuracy, precision, and responsiveness when compared with echocardiographic measurements of cardiac output [13]. In the elective surgical population NICOM performs similarly to the ODM in guiding goal directed fluid therapy although some question the clinically acceptable limits of agreement between the two devices [14]. The NICOM is completely non-invasive, simple to configure and requires no repositioning once attached.

Devices That Use Plethysmographic Waveform Analysis

Several devices exist that attempt to provide a non invasive continuous estimate of arterial pressure using a finger cuff occlusion technique. The ClearSight device (Edwards Lifsciences, Irvine, California USA) uses a high speed oscillating cuff placed around the wrist to produce a constant volume of blood within the finger. The resulting arterial waveform is then reconstructed into a brachial trace using an algorithm. Cardiac output is calculated by integration of this waveform. Although easy to apply and use, these devices have poor accuracy when compared to more invasive systems and also function poorly during low flow states, making them unsuitable for shock resuscitation.

Features of plethysmography, derived from a routine pulse oximetry waveform, are associated with changes in blood volume. Pre hospital respiration induced variation in plethysmography has been investigated for its association with major hypovolemia in trauma patients [15]. In isolation this technique had poor predictive power, but when combined with five basic vital signs (HR, respiratory rate, SpO2, SBP, and diastolic blood pressure) the plethysmography waveform metrics have reasonable power for predicting the presence of major haemorrhage. The automated analysis and integration of vital signs, including the plethysmography variability, has potential utility as a non-invasive means of detecting hypovolemia in the actively bleeding trauma patient.

Part Two: Assessment and Optimisation of End Organ Perfusion

How Should Tissue Perfusion Be Assessed in the Critically Injured Patient?

Ensuring the adequacy of tissue perfusion is the ultimate goal of trauma shock resuscitation. However, assessment of tissue perfusion is challenging and there are fewer methods available than exist for optimizing global flow. Many of these methods are also highly subjective. A summary of the methods for assessing tissue perfusion are shown in Table 6.2.

Clinical Measures

Examination of the cutaneous, renal and neurological systems can yield useful clinical signs of tissue hypoperfusion. Cold and clammy skin, with vasoconstriction and cyanosis is suggestive of tissue hypoperfusion. In low CO states, capillary refill time is prolonged and significant peripheral central temperature gradients are evident. Compared with patients with warm extremities, those with cool extremities following initial resuscitation appear to have a higher degree of late organ dysfunction [16]. However, vasoconstrictive responses to cold and pain can act as confounders, particularly in the pre-hospital environment.

Urine output (UOP) provides a crude marker of renal perfusion but can be falsely reassuring in the context of high sympathetic tone and relative hypertension. Furthermore, there exists a time lag between the perfusion of the renal parenchyma and the appearance of urine and hence UOP does not provide a 'real-time' estimate of the adequacy of

TABLE 6.2 Possible resuscitation targets based on perfusion parameters

End point	Measures	Advantages	Disadvantages	Therapeutic target
Base deficit	Tissue perfusion	Routinely measured Sensitive marker of shock	Predictive ability diminishes over duration of ICU admission Confounded by other acid base variables (e.g., hyperchloraemia)	< -2 mmol/l
Lactate clearance	Tissue perfusion	Routinely measured Sensitive marker of shock	Can be influenced by non perfusion factors (e.g., alcohol, adrenergic agonists)	20 % reduction over 2 h during resuscitation
SvO2/ScvO2	Whole body oxygen supply and demand	Rapidly changes with therapy Sensitive marker of oxygen extraction	Requires CVC Masks flow heterogeneity and local shunting	>70 %

(continued)

Table 6.2 (continued)

End point	Measures	Advantages	Disadvantages	Therapeutic target
ScvCO2 – SaCO2 (CO2 gap)	Ratio of CO2 production to removal	Rapidly changes with therapy Sensitive marker of tissue perfusion	Requires CVC	<6 mmHg (0.8 kPa)
StO2 (e.g., NIRS)	Tissue oxygen tension	Non-invasive	Limited availability of equipment Lack of data regarding optimal target Confounded by peripheral vasoconstriction	>65 %
SDF (e.g., Cytocam)	Microcirculatory flow and vessel density	Minimally invasive May be used as point of care test when validated	Specialist equipment and offline analysis currently required	Global MFI >2.5

Urine output	Renal perfusion (surrogate)	Simple bedside assessment	Time lag Multiple confounding factors e.g., hypertension, ADH	>0.5 ml/kg/h
Conscious level	Brain perfusion (surrogate)	Simple bedside assessment	Subjective, lack of precision Inter observer variation Confounded by sedation/analgesia	GCS 15
Skin temperature	Soft tissue perfusion (surrogate)	Simple bedside assessment	Confounding factors e.g., environmental cold Subjective, lack of precision Inter observer variation	Lack of peripheral – central temperature gradient

SvO2 mixed venous O2 saturation, *ScvO2* central venous O2 saturation, *ScvCO2* central venous CO2 tension, *SaCO2* arterial CO2 tension, *StO2* tissue oxygen saturation, *NIRS* near infra red spectroscopy, *SDF* side stream darkfield videomicroscopy, *MFI* Microcirculatory Flow Index, *GCS* Glasgow Coma Score, *CVC* central venous catheter

renal perfusion. In addition, the endocrine response to the 'stress' of trauma, haemorrhage and surgery produces an increase in anti diuretic hormone levels and therefore an appropriate oliguria which adds a further confounder.

The neurologic response to reduced cerebral perfusion pressure manifests clinically as an altered mental state, which typically includes obtundation, disorientation, and confusion. However, the cerebral perfusion pressure is typically well preserved when perfusion to less vital organs may be grossly reduced. Furthermore, a multitude of confounders can affect the patients mental state, including prescription and illicit drugs and direct brain trauma. These factors make mental state a poor discriminator of whole body perfusion.

Lactate Measurement

The pathophysiology of lactate production, clearance, and kinetics are complex, however hyperlactataemia is associated with reduced DO2 and tissue hypoperfusion. Lactate levels are influenced by the adequacy of the macrocirculation, microcirculation and mitochondrial function. Persistent hyperlactataemia for >12 h following ICU admission is strongly associated with subsequent infectious complications, ICU length of stay, MOF and death [17]. Goal-directed fluid therapy in trauma patients has been shown to improve lactate clearance, reduce infectious complications, and reduced hospital and ICU length of stay [11].

The time to clear lactate from the blood and the absolute lactate level are both suitable resuscitation endpoints. Although changes in serum lactate occur more slowly than changes in cardiac output, the lactate level should decrease over a period of time with effective resuscitative therapy. There remains some debate over the optimal target for lactate clearance as shown in Table 6.3. However, targeting a decrease of at least 20 % in the blood lactate level over a 2 h period appears to be associated with reduced in-hospital

TABLE 6.3 Evidence for resuscitation goals based on lactate levels

Author (year) (Ref.)	Evidence	Clinical setting
Abramson et al. (1993) [30]	All survivors normalised lactate by 24 h from ICU admission	Trauma
Jones et al. (2010) [31]	Initial lactate clearance of 10 % over 2 h is as effect as using ScvO2 in targeted resuscitation	Sepsis
Jansen et al. (2010) [32]	Targeting a 20 % reduction in plasma lactate over 2 h is associated with reduced in-hospital mortality	Critical Illness (ICU patients)
Odom et al. (2013) [33]	Both initial lactate and lactate clearance at 6 h independently predict death in trauma patients	Trauma

mortality. Handheld point-of-care devices now exist for pre-hospital, emergency department, or ICU determinations of lactate and base deficit.

Base Deficit

The initial base deficit (BD) in patients with traumatic haemorrhagic shock is a sensitive measure of both the degree and the duration of inadequate tissue perfusion. BD has also been shown to correlate with transfusion requirements, severity of coagulopathy, rates of organ failure and all cause mortality in the general trauma population [18, 19]. When the probability of death is analysed as a function of BD, a critical threshold exists above a BD of 6.0 mmol/l. At this point an exponential rise in probability of death begins. Failure to reduce BD between hospital and ICU admission strongly predicts poor outcome. It is therefore suggested that serial BD be used as an index of the effectiveness of early resuscitation. However, it has also been shown that the predictive ability of BD diminishes over the course of the ICU stay and is inferior when compared to lactate clearance. This reduction in predictive ability may be influenced by the infusion of unbalanced crystalloids during resuscitation.

Venous Oxygen Saturation

The relationship between global oxygen supply and demand can be used to infer the adequacy of tissue perfusion [20]. In health, global oxygen extraction is approximately 25 % and therefore normal venous oxygen saturation (SvO2) is approximately 75 %. SvO2 is typically decreased in patients with low flow states or anaemia, when increased oxygen extraction occurs to maintain normal aerobic metabolism. Clinically, SvO2 measurements can only be taken from mixed venous blood via a PAC but the central venous oxygen saturation (ScvO2) measured via a central venous catheter is a convenient surrogate. Under normal conditions ScvO2 is slightly less than SvO2, but in critically ill patients it is often greater. ScvO2 values <70 % have been used to identify patients with compromised DO2. However, in pathological shock states ScvO2 can elevated by microvascular shunting or mitochondrial dysfunction and can therefore give a false impression of the adequacy of tissue perfusion and cellular oxygen delivery.

CO2 Gap

The difference between CO_2 tension in the arterial and central venous blood, the 'CO2 gap', is reflective of the ability of the body to remove CO_2 from the tissues and is therefore dependent on cardiac output and the state of the local microcirculation. Unlike, ScvO2, the CO2 gap it is not influenced by haemoglobin concentration or saturation and may be a more sensitive marker of supply and demand. Studies have suggested that a CO2 gap of >6 mmHg (0.8 kPa) is inversely correlated with cardiac output and is also associated with a reduced lactate clearance [21]. The CO2 gap also appears to correlate well with the state of the microcirculation, as visualised using SDF imaging [22]. As it is easy to measure, once central venous access is secured, it seems reasonable to adopt as a marker of perfusion and resuscitation success.

Near Infrared Spectroscopy

Using a technique that relies on the differential light absorption characteristics of oxygenated and deoxygenated haemoglobin, near infra-red spectroscopy (NIRS) can provide information on tissue oxygen saturation (StO2). The technique is completely non-invasive, using gel pads applied to the skin surface over the tissue to be assessed. The technique necessarily involves averaging the signal across quite a large area and can therefore underestimate heterogeneity or microcirculatory shunting. In addition the raw value may not be particularly effective at discriminating between areas of above and below average perfusion; the trend in values in response to time or treatment may be of more utility. The response of the NIRS signal to tourniquet induced vascular occlusion and release can provide a useful marker of microcirculatory performance but this technique has limited utility in clinical practice [23]. One clinical study has suggested that baseline NIRS readings at presentation to hospital can predict the development of organ failure in trauma patients, but the results barely reached significance and need to be confirmed [24].

Sublingual Videomicroscopy

It is possible to assess tissue perfusion through direct visualisation of small vessels at various sites throughout the body. Historically this required the use of large microscopes and tissue dyes, so called intra-vital microscopy, and was therefore mainly limited to experimental work in small animal models. The development of handheld microscopes, such as the Braedius Cytocam, shown in Fig. 6.8 has revolutionised this area of research [25]. The latest generation devices use a Sidestream Dark Field (SDF) technique which involves illuminating the edges of the examined field with visible green light in a 530 nm wavelength from a circular array of diodes. This light illuminates the target tissue from the edges, whilst the field itself is excluded from external light. Haemoglobin (both oxygenated and deoxygenated) absorbs the green light and thus appears black. Thus perfused blood vessels appear as black lines on a white/greyscale background. Lighter gaps within blood vessels are caused by plasma or by leucocytes, shown in Fig. 6.9. The sublingual microvascular bed is commonly used as it is easy to access in both intubated and non-intubated patients. It also probably represents an essential central circulatory bed and hence flow impairments here are likely to be particularly concerning to clinicians. Producing qualitative data from SDF

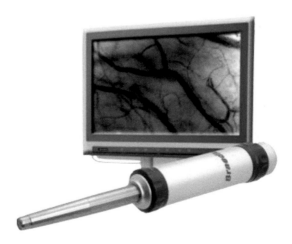

FIGURE 6.8 The Cytocam IDF Videomicroscope (Image courtesy of Braedius Medical)

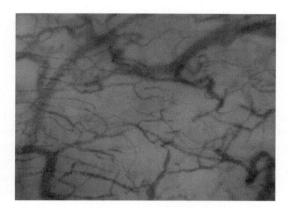

FIGURE 6.9 Microcirculation image obtained from a critically injured patient. Individual erythrocytes can be visualised within capillaries

images currently requires editing and processing into discrete sequences followed by off-line analysis which generates data on vessel density and flow. At its most basic this analysis can be entirely manual, consisting of a subjective assessment of flow using a qualitative scale. More commonly, semi-automated software is used to assist in the process, but a significant amount of user interaction is still required and each ten second video sequence can take up to thirty minutes to process, even with an experienced analyst. Given the widespread heterogeneity seen within the microcirculation during shock states it is important to obtain a large number of video sequences, ideally five, at each time point being examined, thus increasing the amount of video sequences that need to be analysed. This prolonged off-line analysis has, thus far, limited the use of this technique to research rather than as a clinical point-of-care perfusion test. However, with some experience it is possible to make a quicker subjective analysis of flow at the bedside and this opens up the possibility of using this technique clinically. A current multi-centre UK study is exploring whether acute changes in microcirculatory perfusion can be identified at a very early stage in the trauma care pathway using this technique; (MICROSHOCK study, Clinical Trials.gov: NCT02111109).

How Can Tissue Perfusion Be Optimised?

In most patients admitted to critical care following traumatic haemorrhagic shock (THS), supplemental oxygen and the optimisation of preload are the only therapies required to ensure appropriate organ perfusion. However, some trauma patients may suffer myocardial depression and/or alterations in vascular resistance that influence DO2 and tissue perfusion. If these conditions are not detected or optimised the duration of shock may be prolonged. A structured approach, such as shown in Fig. 6.10, that ensures optimization of preload in tandem with assessing the adequacy of perfusion should be adopted.

Patients who do not meet perfusion goals should have myocardial dysfunction excluded, ideally using echocardiography. Patients with myocardial depression may require

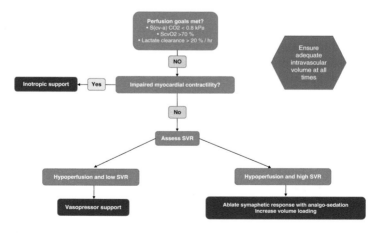

FIGURE 6.10 Suggested process for optimising perfusion during trauma shock resuscitation based on UK DMS critical care guidelines

inotropic support, but the utility of inotropes in this setting is unclear and is not currently supported by an evidence base. Of more importance is the degree of vasoconstriction, which is probably the leading cause of poor tissue perfusion following traumatic injury. There appears to be a wide variation between patients in this regard and identifying those individuals who demonstrate an exaggerated vasoconstrictor response could help titrate therapy. Unfortunately, no monitoring devices in current clinical use can accurately assess tissue perfusion in real time. In the near future point of care SDF videomicroscopy may prove a useful tool in identify those patients with excessive vasoconstriction, potentially providing a new therapeutic target.

Is There a Role for Vasopressor Therapy in THS?

In the context of early THS patients have hugely elevated levels of circulating catecholamines and consequently vascular resistance is greatly increased. This adaptive response continues up until a point of catastrophic cardiovascular decompensation. Use of exogenous vasoconstrictive agents may prolong the shock state by inhibiting subsequent tissue resuscitation, preventing the 'washout' of metabolic acids and endogenous anticoagulants. Supplementary vasopressors in this early phase are contrary to the doctrine of damage control resuscitation and some consider them relatively contraindicated. This position is supported by data suggesting an increase in mortality when vasopressors are used in the first 12–24 h of haemorrhagic shock [26]. Paradoxically, there is evidence from animal models suggesting that exogenous vasopressors can improve right heart filling through the constriction of venous capacitance vessels [27]. Investigators using a rat model of THS demonstrated that early application of vasopressin significantly prolonged the period of hypotensive resuscitation tolerated by shocked animals [28]. Another group showed that the use of noradrenaline reduced the requirement for blood products in a mouse model of THS [29]. This has led to claims that use of supplementary vasopressors in the pre-hospital phase may be an appropriate strategy for trauma patients with active haemorrhage, especially for those with prolonged evacuation timelines. Early vasopressor therapy is also widely used in some urban pre-hospital trauma systems, without any apparent detriment to outcomes.

In the setting of prolonged haemorrhagic shock, patients can develop profound inflammatory states, become deplete in vasopressin, and develop significant vasoplegia, leading to refractory hypotension. In such a low resistance state, tissue DO2 may be inadequate to meet demands despite an adequate preload and CO. In this context, there may be a benefit to supplementing the endogenous vasoconstrictor response. It is still imperative to optimise intravascular volume prior to using vasoactive therapies.

Is There a Role for Vasodilator Therapy Following THS?

In the acute phase following traumatic injury the sympathetic neuroendocrine response is highly active, stimulated by pain, tissue injury, ischaemia and hypovolaemia. This high sympathetic tone produces a state of intense vaso- and venoconstriction. This will generally resolve with time but is also responsive to analgesia and sedation. Once haemorrhage control is achieved and hypovolaemia is being addressed, targeted therapeutic sympatholysis may improve global tissue perfusion by reducing vascular hypertonicity in parallel with volume loading. Active vasodilatation with opiates and anaesthetic agents can facilitate earlier reversal of tissue oxygen debt, leading to timely resolution of acidaemia and coagulopathy. This strategy was commonly adopted by the UK DMS during recent operations, however the evidence base for such an approach is anecdotal at best. It may well be that some patients with hyper-vasoconstriction could benefit from this approach, the key is successfully identifying this sub group.

What Is an Appropriate Blood Pressure to Ensure Tissue Perfusion?

The relationship between mean arterial pressure (MAP) and tissue perfusion is complex and non-linear. Figure 6.11 shows the relationship between microvascular perfusion and blood pressure in a large animal model of traumatic haemorrhagic shock. Note the very large spread of microvascular perfusion at very low blood pressures, demonstrating again the large individual variation in the flow/pressure relationship.

There remains a dearth of studies exploring the relationship between pressure/flow and perfusion in this setting, with the bulk of work focusing purely on the 'optimal' blood

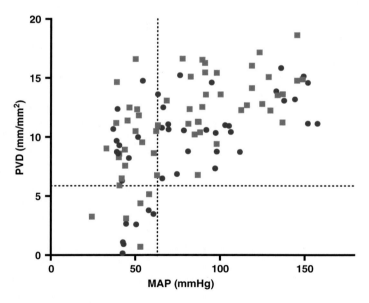

FIGURE 6.11 Data taken from a large animal model of traumatic haemorrhagic shock. Animals exhibited a wide range of microcirculatory perfusion even when markedly hypotensive (Crown copyright DSTL, with permission PVD Perfused Vessel Density; MAP Mean Arterial Pressure)

pressure target. It is however inescapable that clinicians will continue to seek guidance on blood pressure targets during resuscitation, not least because of its widespread adoption in clinical practice and ease of measurement. Individual patients and tissue beds have differing ideal perfusion pressures. A target MAP of 65 mmHg should provide adequate organ perfusion, representing approximately 80 % of normal MAP in young people; young patients generally have a compliant vasculature and are therefore likely to continue to maintain good microvascular flow rates at low pressures, as long as preload is optimised. By comparison, elderly patients with established arteriosclerosis are likely to have a more pressure dependent circulation and therefore may require a higher MAP to maintain microcirculatory perfusion.

The use of vasoactive agents for haemodynamic support should be guided by an approach that takes both arterial pressure and tissue perfusion into account. The efficacy of haemodynamic therapy should be assessed by monitoring a combination of clinical, haemodynamic and biochemical parameters. In practice, if a MAP of 65 mmHg fails to improve tissue perfusion clinicians should seek to explain why this is the case and consider using additional monitoring to optimise volume and perfusion.

When Should Inotropic Support Be Considered?

A minority of trauma patients may have myocardial dysfunction, for example following direct thoracic injury, which can lead to impaired perfusion despite an adequate filling status. Assessment of myocardial contractility should be made directly by fTTE, wherever possible. Serial assessment of cardiac biomarkers may also give an indication of the extent of myocardial injury. In the context of significant myocardial depression and delayed lactate clearance it is reasonable to commence a trial of inotropic support. There is no evidence to suggest the superiority of any particular inotropic agent in this context.

References

1. Mitchell KH, Carlbom D, Caldwell E, et al. Volume overload: prevalence, risk factors and functional outcome in survivors of septic shock. Ann Am Thorac Soc. 2015. doi:10.1513/AnnalsATS.201504-187OC.

2. Cecconi M, De Backer D, Antonelli M, et al. Consensus on circulatory shock and hemodynamic monitoring. Task force of the European Society of Intensive Care Medicine. Intensive Care Med. 2014;40:1795–815. doi:10.1007/s00134-014-3525-z.

3. Cecconi M, Hofer C, Teboul J-L, et al. Fluid challenges in intensive care: the FENICE study. Intensive Care Med. 2015;41:1529–37. doi:10.1007/s00134-015-3850-x.

4. Marik PE, Baram M, Vahid B. Does central venous pressure predict fluid responsiveness? A systematic review of the literature and the tale of seven mares. Chest. 2008;134:172–8. doi:10.1378/chest.07-2331.

5. Pranskunas A, Koopmans M, Koetsier PM, et al. Microcirculatory blood flow as a tool to select ICU patients eligible for fluid therapy. Intensive Care Med. 2013;39:612–9. doi:10.1007/s00134-012-2793-8.

6. Hutchings SD, Bisset L, Cantillon L, et al. Nurse delivered focused echocardiography to determine intravascular volume status in a deployed maritime critical care unit. Intensive Care Med Exp. 2015;3:A919. doi:10.1186/2197-425X-3-S1-A919.

7. Airapetian N, Maizel J, Alyamani O, et al.. Does inferior vena cava respiratory variability predict fluid responsiveness in spontaneously breathing patients? Crit Care. 2015;19:1–8. doi:10.1186/s13054-015-1100-9.

8. Slama M, Masson H, Teboul J-L, et al. Respiratory variations of aortic VTI: a new index of hypovolemia and fluid responsiveness. Am J Physiol Heart Circ Physiol. 2002;283:H1729–33. doi:10.1152/ajpheart.00308.2002.

9. Marik PE. Noninvasive cardiac output monitors: a state-of the-art review. J Cardiothorac Vasc Anesth. 2013;27:121–34. doi:10.1053/j.jvca.2012.03.022.

10. Takala J, Ruokonen E, Tenhunen JJ, et al. Early non-invasive cardiac output monitoring in hemodynamically unstable intensive care patients: a multi-center randomized controlled trial. Crit Care. 2011;15:R148. doi:10.1186/cc10273.

11. Chytra I, Pradl R, Bosman R, et al. Esophageal Doppler-guided fluid management decreases blood lactate levels in multiple-

trauma patients: a randomized controlled trial. Crit Care. 2007;11:R24. doi:10.1186/cc5703.

12. Thom O, Taylor DM, Wolfe RE, et al. Comparison of a suprasternal cardiac output monitor (USCOM) with the pulmonary artery catheter. Br J Anaesth. 2009;103:800–4. doi:10.1093/bja/aep296.

13. Hutchings S, Hopkins P, Campanile A. Volume assessment in critically ill patients: echocardiography, bioreactance and pulse contour thermodilution. Crit Care. 2015;19:P176. doi:10.1186/cc14256.

14. Waldron NH, Miller TE, Thacker JK, et al. A prospective comparison of a noninvasive cardiac output monitor versus esophageal Doppler monitor for goal-directed fluid therapy in colorectal surgery patients. Anesth Analg. 2014;118:966–75. doi:10.1213/ANE.0000000000000182.

15. Chen L, Reisner AT, Gribok A, Reifman J. Is respiration-induced variation in the photoplethysmogram associated with major hypovolemia in patients with acute traumatic injuries? Shock. 2010;34:455–60. doi:10.1097/SHK.0b013e3181dc07da.

16. Lima A, Jansen TC, van Bommel J, et al. The prognostic value of the subjective assessment of peripheral perfusion in critically ill patients. Crit Care Med. 2009;37:934–8. doi:10.1097/CCM.0b013e31819869db.

17. Claridge JA, Crabtree TD, Pelletier SJ, et al. Persistent occult hypoperfusion is associated with a significant increase in infection rate and mortality in major trauma patients. J Trauma Inj Infect Crit Care. 2000;48:8–14; discussion 14–5.

18. Hodgman EI, Morse BC, Dente CJ, et al. Base deficit as a marker of survival after traumatic injury: consistent across changing patient populations and resuscitation paradigms. J Trauma Acute Care Surg. 2012;72:844–51. doi:10.1097/TA.0b013e31824ef9d2.

19. Rutherford EJ, Morris JA, Reed GW, Hall KS. Base deficit stratifies mortality and determines therapy. J Trauma Inj Infect Crit Care. 1992;33:417–23.

20. Giraud R, Siegenthaler N, Gayet-Ageron A, et al. ScvO(2) as a marker to define fluid responsiveness. J Trauma. 2011;70:802–7. doi:10.1097/TA.0b013e3181e7d649.

21. Vallée F, Vallet B, Mathe O, et al. Central venous-to-arterial carbon dioxide difference: an additional target for goal-directed therapy in septic shock? Intensive Care Med. 2008;34:2218–25. doi:10.1007/s00134-008-1199-0.

22. Ospina-Tascón GA, Umaña M, Bermúdez WF, et al. Can venous-to-arterial carbon dioxide differences reflect microcirculatory

alterations in patients with septic shock? Intensive Care Med. 2015;42:1–11. doi:10.1007/s00134-015-4133-2.
23. Bezemer R, Lima A, Myers D, et al. Assessment of tissue oxygen saturation during a vascular occlusion test using near-infrared spectroscopy: the role of probe spacing and measurement site studied in healthy volunteers. Crit Care. 2009;13 Suppl 5:S4. doi:10.1186/cc8002.
24. Duret J. Skeletal muscle oxygenation in severe trauma patients during haemorrhagic shock resuscitation. Crit Care. 2015;19:141. doi:10.1186/s13054-015-0854-4.
25. Hutchings S, Watts S, Kirkman E. The Cytocam video microscope. A new method for visualising the microcirculation using Incident Dark Field technology. Clin Hemorheol Microcirc. 2015. doi:10.3233/CH-152013.
26. Sperry JL, Minei JP, Frankel HL, et al. Early use of vasopressors after injury: caution before constriction. J Trauma. 2008;64:9–14. doi:10.1097/TA.0b013e31815dd029.
27. Giraud R, Siegenthaler N, Arroyo D, Bendjelid K. Impact of epinephrine and norepinephrine on two dynamic indices in a porcine hemorrhagic shock model. J Trauma Acute Care Surg. 2014;77:564–9; quiz 650–1. doi:10.1097/TA.0000000000000409.
28. Yang G, Hu Y, Peng X, et al. Hypotensive resuscitation in combination with arginine vasopressin may prolong the hypotensive resuscitation time in uncontrolled hemorrhagic shock rats. J Trauma Acute Care Surg. 2015;78:760–6. doi:10.1097/TA.0000000000000564.
29. Harrois A, Baudry N, Huet O, et al. Norepinephrine decreases fluid requirements and blood loss while preserving intestinal villi microcirculation during fluid resuscitation of uncontrolled hemorrhagic shock in mice. Anesthesiology. 2015;122:1093–102. doi:10.1097/ALN.0000000000000639.
30. Abramson D, Scalea TM, Hitchcock R, et al. Lactate clearances and survival following injury. Time to normalize lactate is prognostic of survival. J Trauma 1993;35(4):584–9.
31. Jones AE, Shapiro NI, Trzeciak S, et al. Lactate clearance vs central venous oxygen saturation as goals of early sepsis therapy. JAMA 2010;303(8):739–46.
32. Jansen TC, van Bommel J, Schoonderbeek FJ, et al. Early lactate-guided therapy in intensive care unit patients: a multicenter, open-label, randomized controlled trial. Am J Respir Crit Care Med 2010;182:752–61.
33. Odom SR, Howell MD, Silva GS, et al. Lactate clearance as a predictor of mortality in trauma patients. J Trauma 2013; 74:999–1004.

Chapter 7
Blood Product and Fluid Therapy in the Critically Injured Patient

William R.O. Davies and Sam D. Hutchings

Abstract The logical initial resuscitation fluid following traumatic haemorrhage is blood products. However, this remains to be proven in large scale clinical trials. Haemostatic resuscitation, using targeted blood products, may have beneficial effects on vascular endothelium, including the endothelial glycocalyx. Transfusion of packed red blood cells should be targeted to a concentration of 10 g/dl in the acute setting, although this target should be reviewed in the subsequent phases of critical illness. Once the initial stabilisation phase of resuscitation has concluded, ongoing intra vascular volume replacement can be with either crystalloid or colloid solutions. There is no evidence that colloids offer beneficial effects on clinical outcomes and some association with harm.

_____

W.R.O. Davies, MBChB, MRCP, FRCA, FFICM (✉)
Intensive Care, Royal Sussex County Hospital, Eastern Road,
Brighton BN2 5BE, UK
e-mail: will.ro.davies@gmail.com

S.D. Hutchings, MRCS, FRCA, FFICM, DICM, DipIMC
Department of Critical Care, Kings College Hospital,
Denmark Hill, London SE5 9RS, UK

S.D. Hutchings (ed.), *Trauma and Combat Critical Care in Clinical Practice*, In Clinical Practice,
DOI 10.1007/978-3-319-28758-4_7,
© Crown Copyright 2016

137

Balanced salt solutions avoid the phenomena of hyperchloraemic acidosis, but there is no convincing evidence that they produce clinically superior outcomes over 0.9 % saline. Experimental synthetic haemoglobin based compounds offer many theoretical advantages but are not yet established in clinical practice.

Keywords   Fluids • Blood products • Crystalloids • Colloids • Balanced salt solutions • Normal saline • Traumatic injury • Critical illness

Which Factors Govern the Choice of Resuscitation Fluids in Shocked Patients with Traumatic Injuries?

In previous chapters we have outlined the approach to early resuscitation following haemorrhage and have emphasised targeted optimisation of intravascular volume as the initial therapeutic strategy. Bleeding patients firstly require control of haemorrhage and then transfusion with red blood cells (RBC) and blood components. Many healthcare systems, including the Defence Medical Services of the United Kingdom (UK DMS) advocate the early use of blood products in the pre hospital environment and there is evolving evidence from large animal studies that this has beneficial effects on outcomes [1]. However, these remain to be proved in a large scale clinical trial.

There is a good physiological rationale to support the early use of haemostatic resuscitation, that is resuscitation targeted to coagulation endpoints. Such an approach minimises crystalloid fluid infusion and optimises coagulation function. There is also evidence that reperfusion injury is influenced by the choice of resuscitation fluid used. In animal models, crystalloid infusions have been strongly associated with increased neutrophil activation, inflammation and increased capillary permeability. Conversely, animal data suggest that the early use of plasma can repair endothelial tight junctions, decrease para-cellular permeability, restore the endothelial glycocalyx, and increase microvascular perfusion [2]. It appears that early plasma may theoretically be the optimal resuscitation fluid for the severely injured patient, combating both the coagulopathy and endotheliopathy of trauma [3]. To this end, some pre-hospital providers now carry lyophilised plasma, which can be reconstituted and administered at point of injury. However, it must be stressed that this approach is not based on high quality evidence, and concerns around the potential immunological sequelae of plasma transfusion persist. The RePhill study (National Institute for Health Research (NIHR) Efficacy & Mechanism Evaluation Programme (EME; project number 14/152/14), which will compare pre-hospital crystalloid and blood product resuscitation is planned to commence in 2016 and may provide more answers.

Once haemostatic resuscitation is complete, trauma patients will often continue to require fluid therapy, particularly in the presence of an evolving systemic inflammatory response. Key concerns in this context are the optimal management of reperfusion once haemostasis is achieved and the point of transition from blood products to other fluids. This transition point will most likely be influenced by pragmatic decisions surrounding resource utilisation and the perceived risk-benefit profiles of differing products. A recent reappraisal of fluid therapy in critically ill patients has begun following studies demonstrating that both colloid and crystalloid fluids have potential toxicity. The selection, timing, and dosing of intravenous fluids should be evaluated carefully, with the aim of maximizing efficacy and minimizing iatrogenic toxicity.

What Is the Optimal Haemoglobin Target During Resuscitation from THS?

Systemic oxygen delivery is a function of cardiac output (CO) and the oxygen content of arterial blood (CaO_2). The main determinant of CaO_2 is the saturation of haemoglobin with oxygen. The ideal haemoglobin (Hb) concentration that balances optimal fluid flow with oxygen carrying capacity is debatable, but a figure of approximately 10 g/dl is frequently quoted. During acute resuscitation, maintaining the Hb >10 g/dL assures a safety margin in the event of occult or recurring bleeding. This acute target also correlates with a haematocrit of approximately 30 %, which is considered to be effective in maintaining platelet margination and hence supporting coagulation and haemostasis.

In trauma management, the acute transfusion of haemoglobin rich fluids generally occurs in the context of haemostatic resuscitation with blood component therapies. However, stored RBCs are relatively deplete in 2,3-diphosphoglycerate and therefore do not have the same oxygen carrying capacity as fresh whole blood. In addition, storage decreases RBC deformability and increases RBC adhesion and aggregation, impairing their transit through capillary beds. Furthermore, it is thought that stored RBCs generate bioreactive lipids, priming neutrophils and potentially contributing to the development of MOF. The storage duration of RBCs has drawn significant research attention and there is some evidence of an association between old blood transfusion and poor outcomes in trauma patients. Transfusion of older blood is independently associated with an excess of nosocomial infections, MOF and increased mortality [4]. Fresh whole blood or fresh RBCs are considered better able to increase tissue perfusion, correct coagulopathy and reverse oxygen debt. In the setting of THS, a large retrospective study has reported improved 24-h and 30-day survival for combat casualties transfused warm fresh whole blood when compared with those transfused component therapies [5]. Set against these findings are the results of the ABLE study, which showed no difference in a range of outcomes between patients who received old (22 days) vs new (6 days) RBC transfusion. However, less than 10 % of the study cohort consisted of patients with traumatic injury [6].

Once haemostasis is achieved and any oxygen debt repaid, the negative effects of transfusion may outweigh the benefits.

It is therefore reasonable to consider adopting a lower transfusion threshold once the acute phase of resuscitation is complete. The Transfusion Requirements In Critical Care (TRICC) study was a multicentre RCT that included 838 critically ill patients, of whom approximately 20 % were trauma patients. The findings of this trial suggested that a conservative transfusion trigger of <7 g/dl was as well tolerated in non ischaemic heart disease patients, as a liberal trigger of <10 g/dl [7]. One criticism of this study was that the transfused RBCs were not leucodepleted and that this may have influenced the reported outcomes. Leucodepletion has been shown to decrease the RBC storage lesion, limiting transfusion-related immunomodulation and RBC endothelial adhesion. However, in the recent TRISS trial, patients transfused leucodepleted RBCs also demonstrated no difference in 90-day mortality when a transfusion threshold of <7 g/dl was compared with <9 g/dl [8].

Some clinicians advocate tailoring transfusion for stable critically ill patients to individual patient factors, such as signs and symptoms of tissue ischemia. However, it remains to be demonstrated that a symptomatic transfusion strategy is as effective as a target haemoglobin based transfusion strategy.

Which Fluids Should Be Used During the Optimisation Phase of Shock Resuscitation?

Ongoing coagulopathy and blood loss often requires the administration of further plasma and packed cells throughout the optimisation phase of resuscitation. Cryoprecipitate and platelets may also be required to correct coagulopathy. Once the haemoglobin concentration is >10 g/dl, any coagulopathy has resolved (as indicated by normalisation of ROTEM parameters), and blood loss from drains is reducing or has stopped, a transition to an alternative fluid is required.

In a clinical setting where blood products are not available and volume resuscitation is essential, a pragmatic approach is required. Here, a major consideration is the need to balance the potential negative effects of non blood product therapy, principally dilutional coagulopathy and lack of oxygen transport capability, against the requirement to reverse shock and offset organ dysfunction. This balance requires an individualised approach led by experienced, senior clinicians. The increasing use of blood products in the pre hospital setting may help to address this issue as will the development of synthetic oxygen carrying compounds.

Which Fluids Should Be Used During the Stabilisation and De-escalation Phases of Shock Resuscitation?

When considering the relative merits of individual fluids is it important to consider the effect of fluid therapies on the development of iatrogenic interstitial oedema. There is increasing evidence that the cumulative dose of fluid administered to a patient over the duration of their ICU admission may be more important in determining outcome than the type of fluid. A large positive fluid balance in critically ill patients has been found to be independently associated with increased morbidity and mortality. This morbidity includes an increased incidence of renal dysfunction, abdominal compartment syndrome and pulmonary dysfunction [9].

Efforts to reduce cumulative fluid balance require a thorough understanding of the changing fluid requirements over time. Targeted fluid therapy is key to effective resuscitation in the early 'salvage' and 'optimisation' phases. However, once perfusion has been optimised and homeostasis has been restored, fluid requirements decrease. It is during this 'stabilisation' phase that unnecessary fluid administration contributes to cumulative fluid balance. Fluid used for drug infusions, 'maintenance' fluids, and fluid challenges in response to oliguria result in increased cumulative doses of sodium and water over time. The neuroendocrine response to the combined traumatic and surgical insults produces a physiologically appropriate oliguria. A reduction in urine output should not be used solely as a trigger or end point for fluid resuscitation, particularly in the later (>24 h) phases of resuscitation. The true maintenance fluid requirements may be unclear and the tendency is often to overestimate these volumes. There is increasing support for 'restrictive' fluid strategies to minimise cumulative fluid balance, with some evidence that these approaches are effective in reducing morbidity.

How Should Fluids Be Administered During Shock Resuscitation?

As a general principle, when practicing goal directed fluid therapy, warmed boluses of fluid should be titrated to effect. In young trauma patients the compliance of the vascular system and right ventricle is generally good and large boluses of fluid (5–10 ml/kg) are required in order to produce an appreciable effect. This effect should provide clinically significant information regarding the patient's volume status. Fluid boluses should be titrated to sensitive indices of volume responsiveness as outlined in Chap. 6.

Whilst pragmatically it is necessary for this volume to be administered over a relatively short duration, it is unclear as to what is an optimal infusion period. In the setting of trauma associated systemic inflammation, the vulnerable glycocalyx may be at risk of further shedding in response to rapid infusions of fluid. The FEAST trial raises interesting questions regarding the use of bolus resuscitation fluids in shocked patients. In the setting of febrile illness and shock in African children, mortality was increased in response to fluid boluses when compared with no fluid [10]. This occurred despite anecdotal reports of clinical improvement following fluid therapy. Clearly there is great difficulty in generalising these findings to other shock states and different clinical settings. However, it also appears certain that further research is required to better understand the optimal approach to reperfusing vascular beds following shock.

What Are the Advantages and Disadvantages of Fluids Used in Trauma Resuscitation?

The advantages and disadvantages of the various fluids used in trauma resuscitation are summarized in Table 7.1.

Crystalloid Solutions

Crystalloids are inexpensive, widely available and have an established, although unproven, role as first-line resuscitation fluids.

Hartmann's Solution/Compound Sodium Lactate

Animal studies have demonstrated superiority of Compound Sodium Lactate (CSL) over 0.9 % 'Normal' Saline (NS) as a resuscitation fluid in haemorrhagic shock. Animals resuscitated with NS require larger resuscitation volumes, become more acidaemic, and have greater reductions in their fibrinogen levels, when compared with those receiving CSL [11]. However, CSL use in shock resuscitation has been found to be particularly associated with increased neutrophil activation and cellular damage from reperfusion injury [12]. Some clinicians remain concerned over the lactate content of CSL and therefore alternative buffers such as pyruvate, acetate, gluconate, and malate have been produced. Researchers are currently investigating the potential anti-inflammatory properties of Ringer's ethyl pyruvate.

TABLE 7.1 Characteristics of fluids used for resuscitation following traumatic haemorrhagic shock

Fluid	Advantages	Disadvantages
Blood component therapy (RBC/plasma/cryoprecipitate/platelets)	Has oxygen carrying capacity Supports heamostatic resuscitation	Relatively expensive Requires 'cold-chain' logistics Potential for immunological reactions
Plasma (Fresh frozen plasma/lyophilised plasma)	Provides clotting factors May reduce endotheliopathy	Requires thawing or reconstitution from freeze-dried powder Potential for immunological sequelae
Fresh whole blood	Directly replaces what has been lost Has excellent haemostatic properties Potential survival advantage over component therapies	Requires pre-screened donor panel Logistically problematic
Sodium chloride 0.9 %	Inexpensive and widely available Fluid of choice in isolated traumatic brain injury Suggestion of increased risk of renal injury vs balanced salt solutions *not* supported by recent evidence	Potential for hyperchloraemic acidosis Acidaemia may exacerbate coagulopathy and obscure ability to track base deficit trends

(continued)

TABLE 7.1 (continued)

Fluid	Advantages	Disadvantages
Balanced salt solutions (Compound sodium lactate, Ringers acetate)	Inexpensive and widely available Associated with a decrease in the rate of major post-operative complications in abdominal surgery	Large resuscitation volumes may result in hyperlactatemia, metabolic alkalosis, and hypotonicity
Hypertonic saline	Potential for reduced tissue oedema Potentially beneficial anti-inflammatory effects. Suited to remote environments, offering a large resuscitation effect from a relatively small volume	Unestablished safety profile No evidence of clinical benefit
Human albumin solution	Has significant volume-expanding effect in early shock May provide some protection to the endothelial glycocalyx	Possibly associated with worse outcomes in traumatic brain injury Relatively expensive outside Australasia

TABLE 7.1 (continued)

Fluid	Advantages	Disadvantages
Starches	Theoretically have significant volume-expanding effect in early shock	Have coagulopathic effects Associated with increased mortality and requirement for renal support in ICU patients Withdrawn from market in most jurisdictions
Gelatins	Theoretically have significant volume-expanding effect in early shock	Have coagulopathic effects Studies suggest potential for nephrotoxicity
Haemoglobin-based oxygen carriers	Have oxygen carrying capacity Do not require 'cold-chain' logistics	Remain experimental Potential toxicity caused by NO scavenging

Sodium Chloride 0.9 %

It has been proposed that the use of 0.9 % saline (NS) in the resuscitation of the exsanguinating patient may worsen acidaemia through the development of a hyperchloraemic acidosis. This acidaemia may exacerbate coagulopathy and obscure the effect of resuscitation in terms of tracking of the base deficit. The hyperchloraemia may also cause renal vasoconstriction, decrease renal artery blood flow, and reduce glomerular filtration rate. Despite some suggestions that the use of NS is associated with a significant increase in mortality and use of renal replacement therapy in ICU patients, a large randomised controlled trial has recently shown no difference in these outcomes when NS was compared to a balanced salt solution [13]. NS remains the fluid of choice in the management of patients with traumatic brain injury, because of the requirement to maintain plasma tonicity and prevent brain swelling.

Balanced Salt Solutions

Balanced salt solutions (BSS) have been increasingly marketed in light of the potential negative outcomes associated with hyperchloraemia. Indeed, some clinicians advocate using BSS as the default choice in the initial 'salvage' and 'optimisation' phases of resuscitation. A matched-cohort observational study compared the rate of major complications in patients who received either NS or BSS for replacement of fluid losses on the day of surgery. The use of BSS was associated with a significant decrease in the rate of major complications, including a lower incidence of postoperative infection, renal-replacement therapy, and blood transfusion [14]. However, caution should be employed when infusing large resuscitation volumes as BSS may result in hyperlactatemia, metabolic alkalosis, and hypotonicity.

Hypertonic Saline

Hypertonic solutions of sodium chloride, including concentrations of 3, 5, and 7.5 %, have been proposed as resuscitation fluids. These solutions are appealing as they offer the potential for reduced water overload, reduced tissue oedema, and have potentially beneficial anti-inflammatory effects. These solutions are also suited for use in remote environments as they offer a large resuscitation effect from a relatively small and portable volume. Some hypertonic saline (HTS) solutions have also been combined with colloidal dextrans to further enhance their volume-expanding effects. However, the safety profile of HTS has not been established. Despite a sound physiological rationale, the use of HTS in patients with traumatic brain injury has not improved neurological outcome or survival. A randomised controlled trial of 229 patients with hypotension and severe traumatic brain injury who received pre-hospital resuscitation with HTS or NS had almost identical survival and neurological function 6 months after injury [15]. In addition, a subsequent RCT of pre-hospital use of hypertonic solutions was terminated early having met pre-specified futility criteria [16].

Colloid Solutions

Supporters of colloid resuscitation solutions often cite their improved volume-expanding effects when compared with crystalloids. Whilst this effect may be significant in health, in systemic inflammatory states interstitial pressures decrease and porosity increases as the endothelial glycocalyx layer becomes disrupted. Once the vascular barrier is compromised it may be that the efficacy of crystalloid becomes almost equivalent to that of colloid solutions. Evidence from RCTs demonstrates no significant difference in short-term haemodynamic end-points when comparing the two solutions, apart from transient increases in CVP and lower vasopressor requirements with hydroxyethyl starch (HES). The observed ratio of HES to crystalloid in these trials was approximately 1:1.3, which is consistent with the ratio of albumin to saline reported in the saline versus albumin fluid evaluation (SAFE) study [17].

Although most studies have suggested either no benefit or a signal of harm from the use of colloidal resuscitation in critically ill patients the CRISTAL study showed a small mortality benefit at 90 days [18]. This study should be viewed cautiously as although the numbers were large there was huge heterogeneity in terms of the type of fluid administered. In summary it is probably reasonable to suggest that colloidal based resuscitation be avoided given the lack of demonstrable benefit, higher cost and signal of harm.

Human Albumin Solution

The SAFE study compared 4 % human albumin solution with 0.9 % sodium chloride in 6,997 ICU patients and showed that albumin administration was not associated with worse outcomes. However, there was a trend towards higher mortality in the neuro-trauma subgroup that received albumin [17]. A subsequent post-hoc follow-up study of patients with traumatic brain injury who were enrolled in the SAFE study demonstrated a significant increased mortality in those patients with severe TBI who received albumin [19]. Human albumin solution should therefore be used with caution, if at all, in patients with TBI.

Starches

Starch-based colloid solutions include dextrans, hetastarch and HES. A variety of HES products have been produced with varying molecular weights and degrees of hydroxyethyl substitution. Following safety concerns, several large RCTs have sought to establish a greater understanding of the risk-benefit profile of these products. The 6S (Scandinavian Starch for Severe Sepsis/Septic Shock) trial randomly assigned patients with severe sepsis to fluid resuscitation on the ICU with either 6 % HES 130/4.2 (Tetraspan) or Ringer's acetate at a dose of up to 33 ml/kg ideal body weight per day. 798 patients were included in the modified intention-to-treat analysis. At 90 days the group receiving HES had a significantly increased risk of death and were more likely to require renal-replacement therapy [20]. The Crystalloid versus Hydroxyethyl Starch Trial (CHEST) trial randomised 7,000 ICU patients to receive either 6 % HES 130/0.4 (Voluven) in 0.9 % sodium chloride or 0.9 % sodium chloride for all fluid resuscitation until ICU discharge, death, or 90 days after randomization. In this setting, HES was associated with more adverse events and an increased requirement for renal-replacement therapy. Their was no difference in 90-day mortality between the two groups [21]. Given these safety concerns and the known coagulopathic effects of starches, there is currently no place for their use in trauma resuscitation and indeed they have been withdrawn from the market in a number of jurisdictions because of safety concerns.

Gelatins

It is currently unclear whether the results regarding the negative effects of starches can be generalised to other semi-synthetic colloids, such as gelatins. However observational data has raised similar concerns around the risk of acute kidney injury with the use of gelatin-containing solutions. The gelatins are also known to impair clotting and therefore are not the fluid of choice in trauma resuscitation.

Experimental Compounds

Military health care providers have a particular interest in the development of alternative oxygen-carrying resuscitation fluids. These fluids might act as adjuncts to resuscitation or bridging therapies until blood products are available. This might reduce some of the 'cold-chain' logistical burden on personnel tasked with providing blood-products in austere environments. Despite early enthusiasm for perflurocarbons, current research interest is focussed predominantly on haemoglobin-based oxygen carriers (HBOCs).

Haemoglobin-Based Oxygen Carriers

Early generations of HBOCs yielded positive results in animal models but met with significant safety and toxicity concerns when trialled in humans; studies reporting an increased risk of myocardial ischaemia and mortality associated with HBOCs. The potential mechanisms of toxicity were thought to be nitric oxide scavenging and free radical development associated with cell-free haemoglobin. Despite these limitations, new generations of HBOCs are under development, although none are currently licensed for clinical use [22].

References

1. Watts S, Nordmann G, Brohi K, et al. Evaluation of prehospital blood products to attenuate acute coagulopathy of trauma in a model of severe injury and shock in anesthetized pigs. Shock. 2015;44 Suppl 1:138–48. doi:10.1097/SHK.0000000000000409.
2. Torres LN, Sondeen JL, Ji L, et al. Evaluation of resuscitation fluids on endothelial glycocalyx, venular blood flow, and coagulation function after hemorrhagic shock in rats. J Trauma Acute Care Surg. 2013;75:759–66. doi:10.1097/TA.0b013e3182a92514.
3. Del Junco DJ, Holcomb JB, Fox EE, et al. Resuscitate early with plasma and platelets or balance blood products gradually: findings from the PROMMTT study. J Trauma Acute Care Surg. 2013;75:S24–30. doi:10.1097/TA.0b013e31828fa3b9.
4. Torrance HDT, Vivian ME, Brohi K, et al. Changes in gene expression following trauma are related to the age of transfused packed red blood cells. J Trauma Acute Care Surg. 2015;78:535–42. doi:10.1097/TA.0000000000000534.
5. Spinella PC, Perkins JG, Grathwohl KW, et al. Warm fresh whole blood is independently associated with improved survival for patients with combat-related traumatic injuries. J Trauma. 2009;66:S69–76. doi:10.1097/TA.0b013e31819d85fb.
6. Lacroix J, Hébert PC, Fergusson DA, et al. Age of transfused blood in critically ill adults. N Engl J Med. 2015;372:1410–8. doi:10.1056/NEJMoa1500704.
7. Hébert PC, Wells G, Blajchman MA, et al. A multicenter, randomized, controlled clinical trial of transfusion requirements in critical care. Transfusion Requirements in Critical Care Investigators, Canadian Critical Care Trials Group. N Engl J Med. 1999;340:409–17.
8. Holst LB, Haase N, Wetterslev J, et al. Lower versus higher hemoglobin threshold for transfusion in septic shock. N Engl J Med. 2014;371:1381–91. doi:10.1056/NEJMoa1406617.

9. Malbrain MLNG, Marik PE, Witters I, et al. Fluid overload, de-resuscitation, and outcomes in critically ill or injured patients: a systematic review with suggestions for clinical practice. Anaesthesiol Intensive Ther. 2014;46:361–80. doi:10.5603/AIT.2014.0060.

10. Maitland K, Kiguli S, Opoka RO, et al. Mortality after fluid bolus in African children with severe infection. N Engl J Med. 2011;364:2483–95. doi:10.1056/NEJMoa1101549.

11. Todd SR, Malinoski D, Muller PJ, Schreiber MA. Lactated Ringer's is superior to normal saline in the resuscitation of uncontrolled hemorrhagic shock. J Trauma Inj Infect Crit Care. 2007;62:636–9. doi:10.1097/TA.0b013e31802ee521.

12. Rhee P, Koustova E, Alam HB. Searching for the optimal resuscitation method: recommendations for the initial fluid resuscitation of combat casualties. J Trauma Inj Infect Crit Care. 2003;54:S52–62. doi:10.1097/01.TA.0000064507.80390.10.

13. Young P, Bailey M, Beasley R, et al. Effect of a buffered crystalloid solution vs saline on acute kidney injury among patients in the intensive care unit. JAMA. 2015;314:1701–10. doi:10.1001/jama.2015.12334.

14. Shaw AD, Bagshaw SM, Goldstein SL, et al. Major complications, mortality, and resource utilization after open abdominal surgery: 0.9% saline compared to Plasma-Lyte. Ann Surg. 2012;255:821–9. doi:10.1097/SLA.0b013e31825074f5.

15. Cooper DJ, Myles PS, McDermott FT, et al. Prehospital hypertonic saline resuscitation of patients with hypotension and severe traumatic brain injury: a randomized controlled trial. JAMA. 2004;291:1350–7. doi:10.1001/jama.291.11.1350.

16. Wade CE, Grady JJ, Kramer GC. Efficacy of hypertonic saline dextran fluid resuscitation for patients with hypotension from penetrating trauma. J Trauma Inj Infect Crit Care. 2003;54:S144–8. doi:10.1097/01.TA.0000047223.62617.AB.

17. Bernard GR, Vincent JL, Laterre PF, LaRosa SP, Dhainaut JF, Lopez-Rodriguez A, et al. Efficacy and safety of recombinant human activated protein C for severe sepsis. N Engl J Med. 2001;344(10):699–709.

18. Annane D, Siami S, Jaber S, et al. Effects of fluid resuscitation with colloids vs crystalloids on mortality in critically ill patients presenting with hypovolemic shock: the CRISTAL randomized trial. JAMA. 2013;310:1809–17. doi:10.1001/jama.2013.280502.

19. SAFE Study Investigators, Australian and New Zealand Intensive Care Society Clinical Trials Group, Australian Red

Cross Blood Service, et al. Saline or albumin for fluid resuscitation in patients with traumatic brain injury. N Engl J Med. 2007;357:874–84. doi:10.1056/NEJMoa067514.

20. Perner A, Haase N, Guttormsen AB, et al. Hydroxyethyl starch 130/0.42 versus Ringer's acetate in severe sepsis. N Engl J Med. 2012;367:124–34. doi:10.1056/NEJMoa1204242.

21. Myburgh JA, Finfer S, Bellomo R, et al. Hydroxyethyl starch or saline for fluid resuscitation in intensive care. N Engl J Med. 2012;367:1901–11. doi:10.1056/NEJMoa1209759.

22. Njoku M, St Peter D, Mackenzie CF. Haemoglobin-based oxygen carriers: indications and future applications. Br J Hosp Med (Lond). 2015;76:78–83. doi:10.12968/hmed.2015.76.2.78.

Chapter 8
Management of the Patient with Trauma Induced Coagulopathy

Sam D. Hutchings and Catherine M. Doran

Abstract Trauma induced coagulopathy (TIC) is a complex pathophysiological process and the exact mechanisms have yet to be elucidated. The primary drivers are tissue injury and hypoperfusion but contributory factors, such as acidosis, hypothermia and dilution with exogenous resuscitation fluids all play a significant part. Recognition of TIC is vital if effective management is to be instituted early and predictive scoring systems can be useful. Conventional laboratory measures of coagulation are often poor at reflecting the severity of clinical coagulopathy and viscoelastic or thromboelastographic testing, performed in the clinical environment can be of value. Specific abnormalities in the thromboelastogram

S.D. Hutchings, MRCS, FRCA, FFICM, DICM, DipIMC (✉)
Department of Critical Care, Kings College Hospital,
Denmark Hill, London SE5 9RS, UK
e-mail: sam.hutchings@kcl.ac.uk

C.M. Doran, BA, MB BCh, BAO, MD, FRCS
General Surgery, Royal Centre for Defence Medicine, Queen
Elizabeth Hospital, Mindelsohn Way, Birmingham B15 2GW, UK

S.D. Hutchings (ed.), *Trauma and Combat Critical Care in Clinical Practice*, In Clinical Practice,
DOI 10.1007/978-3-319-28758-4_8,
© Crown Copyright 2016

can help clinicians target blood component therapy more effectively and have been shown to reduce the overall use of blood products during trauma resuscitation. Treatment of TIC should be structured around an evidenced based massive transfusion protocol which should reflect local logistic realities. A plasma : PRBC ratio of 1:1 or 1:2, early use of cryoprecipitate and maintenance of a platelet count over 100 is supported by the best available evidence at the time of writing. The use of fresh whole blood and recombinant activated factor VII have been used for refractory bleeding in the context of traumatic haemorrhage, particularly by military healthcare providers.

Keywords Massive transfusion • Trauma Induced Coagulopathy • Acute Coagulopathy of Trauma Shock • Massive transfusion protocol • Plasma: PRBC ratio • Platelets • Rotational thromboelastography

Introduction

Our understanding of Trauma Induced Coagulopathy (TIC) has increased markedly over the past decade. It is now recognised that TIC is an intrinsic problem caused by tissue injury and hypoperfusion and not just a consequence of the classic triad of acidosis, dilution and hypothermia. Up to a third of critically injured patients presenting to the Emergency Department will be coagulopathic on arrival and this is independent of the time elapsed from injury or volume of pre-hospital fluid [1, 2]. TIC is associated with a higher incidence of organ failure, longer intensive care unit stay and is an independent predictor of death [3]. It has been shown that the early recognition of TIC followed by appropriate and aggressive management can correct the coagulopathy, control bleeding, reduce blood product use and improve outcomes in severely injured patients [4]. Much of the increased understanding of TIC has resulted from experience gained during military operations in Iraq and Afghanistan; the methods used by the UK Defence Medical Services (UK DMS) and others to diagnose and manage TIC have informed and driven subsequent civilian practice.

This chapter seeks to clarify the current terminology used when discussing TIC, outline the pathophysiology, discuss methods used to aid diagnosis and finally discuss current management.

Part One: Pathophysiology of Trauma Induced Coagulopathy

What Mechanisms Produce Trauma Induced Coagulopathy?

There are a multitude of terms used to describe the coagulopathy associated with traumatic injury and a casual reader could be easily confused. Essentially TIC is a result of two discrete but interrelated processes that combine to produce a clinical coagulopathy. The underlying process is the pathological changes that occur principally at the level of the vascular endothelium and which result in a disordered system of coagulation. These changes are brought about by a combination of two factors: tissue injury and systemic and microvascular hypoperfusion [5]. The combination of these two factors produces a condition known as the Acute Coagulopathy of Trauma Shock (ACoTS).

The combination of tissue trauma, inflammation and hypoperfusion alters the vascular endothelium leading to the expression of thrombomodulin. Thrombomodulin then interacts with thrombin and activates the Protein C pathway [6]. High circulating levels of activated Protein C in trauma patients on admission is correlated with increased mortality, higher transfusion requirements and rates of multi-organ failure [3].

A concurrent mechanism of ACoTS is the disruption of the endothelial gylcocalyx. Damage to the layer, in the presence of hypoperfusion, triggers the release of substances which includes syndecan-1, soluble thrombomodulin and heparin-like substances leading to auto-heparinisation [7].

Fibrinogen is a central factor in the coagulation process, responsible for haemostasis as the precursor of fibrin and integral to platelet aggregation with normal values between 2 and 4 g/L in the plasma. In the context of massive bleeding, fibrinogen is the first factor that reaches a critically low level and this is associated with a poor outcome [8]. Interestingly some investigators have suggested that correction of fibrinogen, using cryoprecipitate, may result in a plasma sparing effect, reducing the requirement for large volumes of plasma [9].

Other factors associated with traumatic injury, blood loss and subsequent resuscitation can lead to an exacerbation of this coagulopathy. Acidosis and hypothermia will materially affect the function of the proteins within the coagulation cascade and diminish the effectiveness of clot formation. Metabolic acidosis is common in trauma and a decrease in pH directly influences coagulation by inhibiting the function of the plasma proteases. When the pH is reduced from 7.4 to 7.0, the activity level of factor VIIa falls by 90 % and prothrombin activation is reduced by 70 % [10]. When examined using thromboelastometry, clot formation has been shown to decrease by 168 % at a pH 6.8 compared to a pH of 7.4 [11]. Clinically significant hypothermia (defined as a core temperature of <35 °C) is common in trauma patients; decreased motor activity, heat loss by conduction, administration of cold fluid and removal of clothing for examination all contribute to this drop. The rate of enzyme reactions involved in coagulation reduces by 10 % per °C [10].

Dilution of clotting factors during resuscitation with crystalloid or colloidal solutions, and sometimes with component blood products, can also exacerbate any coagulopathy. Analysis from the German Trauma Registry showed that coagulopathy existed in >40 % of patients who received >2 L of fluid, in >50 % with >3 L and >70 % with >4 L given early in the resuscitation phase [12].

Historically acidosis, hypothermia and dilution, classically termed the lethal triad, were assumed to be the sole causes of the coagulopathy observed following trauma. However, evolving understanding of the pathophysiological processes at work have lead to major revisions in our

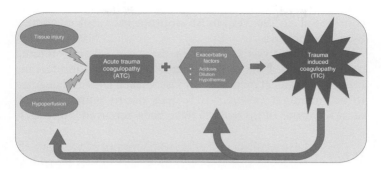

FIGURE 8.1 Overall process leading to Trauma Induced Cogulopathy (TIC). Hypoperfusion and tissue injury drive the process at the level of the vascular endothelium which is then potentially exacerbated by acidosis, hypothermia and dilution

understanding. Together the combination of ACoTS and these three external factors produce the overall condition known as Trauma Induced Coagulopathy. This coagulopathy acts to prevent haemostasis, exacerbating bleeding and thereby contributing to worsening tissue perfusion. This, along with the consequent acidosis and effects of resuscitative fluids exacerbate the existing coagulopathy, leading to further blood loss and an increasing spiral of physiological disruption. The interplay between these factors is shown in Fig. 8.1.

What Is the Significance of Hyperfibrinolysis?

Hyperfibrinolysis is the when fibrinolytic activity is greater than the rate of fibrin formation, the net result being rapid breakdown of clot integrity. The terms hyperfibrinolysis and fulminant hyperfibrinolysis are often used but have been poorly and arbitrarily defined in the literature. The measurement of fibrin/fibrinogen degradation products and D-dimers lack sensitivity and specificity as these markers are elevated in most trauma patients. Use of viscoelastic tests (further discussed in part 2 of this chapter) is currently considered to be the most appropriate tool to detect hyperfibrinolysis.

Hyperfibrinolysis is found in the most severely injured patients and is a major contributor to mortality in bleeding trauma patients. If measured by viscoelastic tests and deemed to be fulminant (where >50 % lysis occurs within 30 min) mortality rates of up to 88 % have been reported [13].

What Are the Importance of Platelets in TIC?

Platelets play a critical dual role in TIC. Firstly, they act as a haemostatic plug by aggregating at the site of vessel injury. Secondly they act as a reaction site for the proteases involved in coagulation. Platelets are activated by exposure to substances within the sub endothelial matrix and once activated undergo a number of changes that are vital to the initiation and propagation of the coagulation response. The absolute quantity of platelets (which is easy to determine) and their functional activity (which is less easy) are both critical. Additionally banked platelets have less efficacy following transfusion than native platelets (the so called "storage lesion") [14] Assessment of platelet function can utilise a number of methods, including thromboelastometry, described in more detail later in this chapter, as well as more precise laboratory based methods, such as aggregometry, which are not routinely used in clinical practice.

Part 2: Detection and Monitoring of Trauma Induced Coagulopathy

Which Patients Are at Risk of TIC?

As can be seen from a discussion of the pathophysiology the combination of massive blood loss leading to hypo-perfusion associated with extensive tissue trauma provide the conditions for the development of TIC.

Specific scoring systems have been employed to provide a prediction of the probability of a patient requiring massive transfusion. The TASH score (Trauma Associated Severe Haemorrhage) uses seven parameters, including some that are dependent on hospital investigation results, to give a score (Table 8.1). This score was validated in over 5000 patients from the German trauma registry and found to be useful in predicting coagulopathy [15].

TABLE 8.1 The TASH score

Variable	Value	Simplified points score
Haemoglobin	<7	8
	<9	6
	<10	4
	<11	3
	<12	2
Intra abdominal fluid	+ve FAST	3
Orthopaedic fractures	Clinically unstable pelvic fracture	6
	Femur fracture	3
Base excess	< −10	4
	< −6	3
	< −2	1
Systolic blood pressure	<100	4
	<120	1
Heart rate	>120	2
Sex	Male	1

A score of <8 is associated with a <5 % chance of developing TIC; 18 with a 50 % chance and over 24 an 85 % chance [15]

TABLE 8.2 The TICCS (Trauma Induced Coagulopathy Clinical Score) score

Criteria	Number of points attributed
General severity	
Critical (ED resus room)	2
Non critical (regular ED room)	0
Blood pressure	
SBP<90 mmHg (at least once)	5
SBP always >90 mmHg	0
Extent of significant injuries	
Head and neck	1
Left upper limb	1
Right upper limb	1
Left lower limb	1
Right lower limb	1
Torso	2
Abdomen	2
Pelvis	2

A cut off value of 10 is a good discriminator for those who go on to require damage control resuscitation and those with less severe injuries [16]

Early recognition is vital and a pre hospital scoring system that can be used to predict TIC has obvious advantages. The TICCS score (Table 8.2) [16] performed favourably against more complicated scoring systems, such as AIS and TASH and has the advantage that it can be used quickly in the pre hospital setting and does not require any lab based or radiological investigations.

What Are the Problems with Traditional Lab Based Methods of Coagulation?

Historically abnormalities of coagulation were diagnosed using laboratory based tests of clotting activation such as Prothrombin Time (PT) or Activated Partial Thromboplastin Time (APTT), combined with quantitative evaluation of platelets and fibrinogen. However, it is widely accepted that these *in vitro* tests only measure the initiation phase of the blood coagulation process and, as they are carried out on platelet poor centrifuged plasma samples, do not provide clinically relevant information on the dynamics and the sustainability of clot formation. A further issue is the time lag between taking samples and obtaining the results which means that clinicians are often relying on out of date information to guide the choice of blood products. In an attempt to better assess the process of coagulation *in vivo*, certain key groups of clinicians, principally those used to dealing with large blood loss, introduced viscoelastic testing into clinical practice. In centres where cardiac surgery and liver transplant are performed, use of these tests is routine and the technique is now increasingly used in the management of traumatic haemorrhage.

How Can Viscoelastic Tests Assist in the Diagnosis of TIC?

Viscoelastic tests are performed using the technique of thromboelastography (synonymous with thromboelastometry). The test is carried out by placing whole blood (from a citrated blood sample) into a receptacle into which a wire is suspended. The latter oscillates and as the clot begins to form, the change in viscosity and subsequent shear is transmitted through the wire. This change is translated into a characteristic graph known as thromboelastograph. There are two commercially

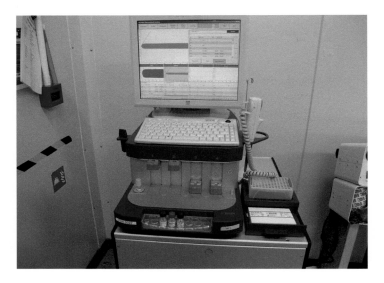

FIGURE 8.2 ROTEM device in the operating theatre at the Role 3 Hospital, Camp Bastion, Afghanistan

available machines, ROTEM® (Tem Innovations [Pentapharm] GmbH, Munich, Germany), shown in Fig. 8.2 and TEG® (Haemoscope Cooperation, Niles, IL, USA).

Several national and international guidelines recommend the use of viscoelastic testing in trauma [[4], [17]] The UK DMS were also early adopters of viscoelastic testing. In the latter stages of the conflict in Afghanistan, ROTEM® was the principal means of assessing coagulation throughout the patient pathway [18].

What Information Can Be Obtained from Thromboelastometry?

A stylized ROTEM® trace is shown in Fig. 8.3. The trace provides the following information:

Clotting time (CT) – the time in seconds from the start of the activation process to the initial clot formation when

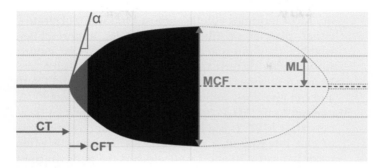

FIGURE 8.3 Stylized thromboelastometry trace demonstrating the following parameters: *CT* Clotting Time, *CFT* Clot Formation Time, *α-angle* speed of clot formation, *MCF* Maximum Clot Firmness, *ML* Maximum Lysis (Reproduced by kind permission of Tem Innovations GmbH, Germany)

the amplitude reaches 2 mm on the trace. This equates to the initiation of clotting and thrombin formation. A prolongation occurs in factor deficiency, use of anti-coagulants or in severe hypofibrinogenaemia.

Clot Formation Time (CFT) – time taken from clot initiation until a clot firmness of 20 mm is reached. This equates to fibrin polymerisation and stabilisation of the clot with platelets and Factor XIII, representing the clot formation dynamics. This time is shortened by an increase in fibrinogen and platelet function. A prolonged CFT indicates a failure for the clot to form and is also prolonged by anticoagulants such as heparin.

α-Angle – the angle between the centre line and a tangent to the curve through the 2 mm point. This demonstrates the kinetics of clot formation, i.e., the smaller the angle the weaker the clot formation. Decreased values would be expected with hypofibrinogenaemia and thrombocytopenia.

Maximum Clot Formation (MCF) – this is a measurement of the maximum firmness and is a reflection of the absolute strength of the fibrin clot equating to the maximum dynamic properties of fibrin and platelets. A reduction in the MCF indicates a deficiency of 'clottable' substrate – either platelet or fibrinogen. Platelet abnormalities, whether they are qualitative or quantitative in nature, substantially disturb the MCF. The firmness at 5 and 10 min following the CT are recorded as CA5 and CA10 and can give early indications of abnormal results.

Maximum Lysis (ML) – this is a reduction in the clot firmness after MCF. It is a function of time and reflects loss of clot integrity as a result of lysis. The lysis is often recorded as Ly 30 and Ly 60 which is the percentage of lysis that has occurred 30 and 60 min after MCF. The normal value is <15 % lysis in 60 min. This percentage increases in pathological hyperfibrinolysis.

What Are the Typical Thromboelastic Appearances of Specific Coagulation Abnormalities?

ROTEM® uses a number of channels to assist diagnostic precision, each channel producing a trace. The most commonly used channels are EXTEM, INTEM and FIBTEM. EXTEM is activated by Tissue Factor and is a broad screening test for haemostasis. INTEM activates the contact phase of haemostasis and is used when patients are heparinised. FIBTEM eliminates the platelet contribution to clot formation by inhibiting platelet function with cytochaiasin D and therefore allows for the detection of fibrinogen deficiency or fibrin polymerisation disorders. In trauma cases, where no heparin has been used, the EXTEM and FIBTEM provide sufficient information to guide haemostatic therapy.

Figure 8.4 illustrates a normal EXTEM and FIBTEM trace.

Figure 8.5 shows an example of EXTEM and FIBTEM in a patient with abnormal results. The EXTEM trace has a normal CT, meaning that the initiation phase of clotting is normal, but the prolonged CFT, decreased α-angle and decreased MCF informs the clinician there is a problem with the thrombin burst and subsequent polymerisation of the clot. The

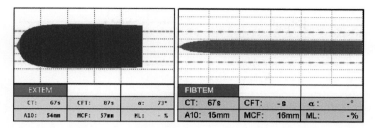

FIGURE 8.4 Normal EXTEM and FIBTEM traces. (normal EXTEM values are: CT 38–79 s; CFT 34–159 s; MCF 50–72 mm; ML <15 % in 60 min. Normal FIBTEM values are: MCF 9–25 mm)

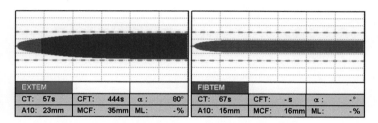

FIGURE 8.5 Platelet deficiency resulting in low MCF in EXTEM but normal fibrinogen levels as shown by normal FIBTEM trace

FIBTEM is normal, indicating normal fibrinogen levels; thus there is a platelet deficiency or functional abnormality in this patient.

Figure 8.6 shows an EXTEM trace with a normal CT, but prolonged CFT, decreased α-angle, and overall decreased MCF. From the FIBTEM trace, the MCF is significantly reduced indicating a low fibrinogen level.

Figure 8.7 shows an EXTEM trace that has a normal CT but the CFT, α-angle and MCF are reduced. In this example the ML is 100 % indicating fulminant hyperfibrinolysis. To prove this is the case, the APTEM channel beside it shows a normal trace. Here fibrinolysis has been inhibited using Aprotinin. The normal value for fibrinolysis is <15 % in 60 min, hyperfibrinolysis is indicated by a result of >15 % in

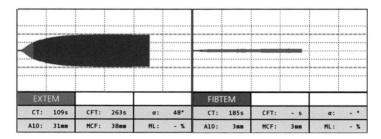

EXTEM					
CT: 109s	CFT: 263s	α: 48°			
A10: 31mm	MCF: 38mm	ML: - %			

FIBTEM					
CT: 185s	CFT: - s	α: - °			
A10: 3mm	MCF: 3mm	ML: - %			

FIGURE 8.6 Fibrinogen deficiency, as shown in FIBTEM trace, resulting in a low MCF in the EXTEM trace

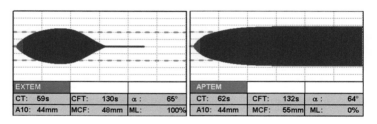

EXTEM		
CT: 59s	CFT: 130s	α: 65°
A10: 44mm	MCF: 48mm	ML: 100%

APTEM		
CT: 62s	CFT: 132s	α: 64°
A10: 44mm	MCF: 55mm	ML: 0%

FIGURE 8.7 EXTEM trace showing hyperfibrinolysis and proven by a normal APTEM when the fibrinolysis process is inhibited

60 min. Fulminant hyperfibrinolysis is when the degree of fibrinolysis is >50 % in 30 min.

Part 3: Management of Trauma Induced Coagulopathy

Once TIC has been detected clinicians must act promptly to restore the ability of the blood to clot. Overt exsanguination remains a leading cause of preventable death following traumatic injury and coagulopathy plays a prominent role in this. In addition, failure to mitigate the effects of TIC can lead to less immediately obvious effects such as exacerbation of endothelial injury with the potential for organ dysfunction.

Treatment of TIC is one of the central tenets of Damage Control Resuscitation, the process that emphasises physiological restoration over prolonged definitive operative interventions.

What Is the Effect of Resuscitation Fluids on TIC?

The choice of resuscitation fluid is the key management decision in the patient with TIC. Historically large volumes of crystalloid solutions were used, particularly in the early phases of trauma resuscitation. However, more recent practice has advocated the early use of blood products and this has obvious physiological advantages.

As detailed in the previous section point of care viscoelastic testing can help clinicians to tailor therapy, so called haemostatic resuscitation. However, in the absence of such monitoring many centres use an empirical massive transfusion protocol that lays down the pre-determined amounts of blood products that are to be given prior to the achievement of haemodynamic stability. This approach has the advantage of being easier to implement as all members of the team, including laboratory staff, are familiar with the type and amount of products to be administered. However, such an empirical approach may lead to over or under transfusion of particular blood components.

A fuller discussion of the advantages and disadvantages of various fluids used in trauma resuscitation can be found in Chap. 7. The remainder of this chapter will deal with those issues that relate to the patient with TIC and that are not covered elsewhere.

What Is the Optimal FFP/PRBC Ratio During Haemostatic Resuscitation?

The most widely debated aspect of TIC management relates to the ratio of transfused Packed Red Blood Cells (PRBC) to plasma and platelets. A large amount of retrospective cohort data, much of it derived from recent military conflicts, appeared to suggest that patients resuscitated with a high ratio of plasma to PRBC (close to 1:1) had an improved chance of survival when compared to patients treated with lower ratios (typically > 1:3) [19, 20]. However, there were considerable methodological issues with these studies, principally related to so called 'survival bias'. This phenomenon results from the fact that, for logistic reason related to the speed of delivery of plasma, patients who die early following traumatic haemorrhage will typically have received a lower plasma: PRBC ratio than survivors. Furthermore, many of these patients die from catastrophic injuries rather than as a direct result of coagulopathy leading to exsanguination.

In an attempt to control for this bias the PROMMT (PRospective Observational Multitrauma Multi cenTer) study investigators examined 905 patients who had received more than 3 units of PRBC following traumatic injury [21]. They also examined the effect of different ratios on survival, based on the time of administration. The results showed that high ratio resuscitation (close to 1:1) delivered early (within the first 6 h) appeared to be associated with a significant reduction in 30 day mortality, but that the effect was lost if higher ratios were achieved after 6 or 24 h. This makes physiological sense, it that attempting to reverse TIC late, after substantial endothelial injury has occurred is unlikely to be of benefit.

The PROMMT investigators used the data from their study to inform the design of the first multi center RCT examining plasma: PRBC ratios following traumatic haemorrhage. The PROPPR study [22] was conducted at 12 Level 1 trauma centers in North American and randomised 680 patients to receive either high ratio resuscitation (Plasma : Platelets : PRBC = 1:1:1) or low ratio resuscitation (1:1:2). The two groups were well matched with respect to injury severity and degree of coagulopathy on presentation. Although there was a significantly higher incidence of haemorrhage control in the high ratio group there was no statistical difference in either 24 h or 30 day mortality. The authors reported on a wide range of complications and sequalae, including organ dysfunction and length of critical care dependency, but again found no difference between the groups.

What do these studies tell us? It seems logical when treating haemorrhagic shock to replace the lost circulating volume with an equivalent fluid, which in this case would be whole blood. However, contemporary transfusion practice is based on the use of component blood product therapy and in this situation physiological sense would seem to suggest that replacing PRBCs, plasma and platelets in a 1:1 ratio would be logical. All the evidence prior to the PROPPR study seemed to be pointing in this direction but like so many aspects of critical care research a rational hypothesis fell foul to a well designed large RCT.

Whilst it is inescapable that patients with TIC need plasma and platelet therapy it should also be noted that there is a considerable body of evidence showing that the administration of banked frozen plasma can be associated with harm. Watson and colleagues showed a dose dependent relationship between the administration of FFP and the development of lung injury and organ failure [23]. The precise mechanism by which this occurs is unclear, although immunological modulation is likely.

In conclusion there is no strong evidence that a strategy of resuscitation based on the empirical use of FFP and platelets in a 1:1 ratio produces a benefit over a 1:2 ratio and given the potential for harm caused by excessive plasma administration such an approach should be used with caution. Many trauma centers are moving away from an empirical approach towards one targeted to point of care measures of coagulation (e.g., ROTEM®). In the absence of such technology a ratio of FFP: Platelets: PRBC of between 1:1 and 1:2 would seem to be the best approach based on the current available evidence.

How Early Should Blood Products Be Given Following Traumatic Haemorrhage?

The recognition that up to 30 % of patients were arriving in Emergency Departments following severe traumatic injury with established coagulopathy prompted some clinicians to explore the use of haemostatic resuscitation in the pre-hospital environment. Some clinician delivered pre- hospital services have been using PRBC resuscitation as an initial treatment for traumatic haemorrhage despite the logistical difficulties. However, introducing plasma into the pre hospital environment poses an even greater challenge.

Despite the enthusiasm to adopt this approach the evidence base remains minimal. A large animal study conducted by the UK Ministry of Defence explored this concept [24]. The protocol was designed to mimic a battlefield casualty who required pre-hospital treatment and evacuation and explored the differences between three possible options for pre-hospital fluid resuscitation. Twenty four pigs subjected to haemorrhage and controlled extremity injury were allowed to become shocked for a thirty minute period before receiving pre-allocated treatment with either PRBC:FFP in a 1:1 ratio, PRBCs alone, or 0.9 % saline for 60 min. After this time all animals received PRBC:FFP. The results showed that animals treated with 0.9 % saline had a significantly worse coagulopathy that only resolved towards the end of resuscitation. Animals treated with both PRBC/FFP and PRBC alone both showed significantly attenuated coagulopathy but there was no significant difference between these two groups.

The use of pre hospital blood products is about to be tested in a multi center clinical trial (RePHILL – Resuscitation with Pre-Hospital bLood products, National Institute for Health Research (NIHR) Efficacy & Mechanism Evaluation Programme EME; project number 14/152/14) which will randomise patients to receive either packed red cells and lyophilised plasma or crystalloid.

In summary the early use of blood products has numerous advantages including increasing oxygen delivery and attenuating TIC. However, logistic delivery is difficult and there is little or no evidence at present that the addition of plasma to PRBCs improves outcomes. The results of the RePhILL trial may add to our knowledge of this area and help guide future management.

What Is the Optimal Platelet Count?

As discussed in part one of this chapter, platelets play a critical role in the coagulation process. Although functional activity is important, at this time it is harder to measure than the absolute value which tends to therefore attract more interest when massive transfusion protocols are constructed. There is evidence that a lower platelet count on admission is an independent predictor of increased mortality with one study showing a 12 % reduction in mortality for every 50×10^9/L increase in platelet numbers [25]. Another cohort study used propensity scoring to examine the difference between patients receiving a low (>1:20) medium (1:2) or high (1:1) ratio of PRBC to platelets [26]. There was a significant difference in mortality between the high ratio (30 %), medium (43 %) and low ratio (48 %) groups. As discussed earlier the caveats relating to survival bias and retrospective studies are important to take into account when examining these results. However, there is a body of evidence suggesting that higher platelet counts (>100–150 $\times 10^9$/L) may confer benefit during a massive transfusion. Assessment of platelet function is more difficult but the use of thromboelastometry has obvious advantages. Anecdotally, there is often a lag between transfusion of platelets and changes to the thromboelastography trace; the platelet storage lesion may well play a role in this regard, but more research is required in this area.

Should Fibrinogen Be Given Early During Haemostatic Resuscitation?

Fibrinogen is the immediate precursor to Fibrin and is vital in clot formation. Case series and cohort studies have suggested that hypofibrinogenaemia is associated with an increased mortality following traumatic haemorrhage and uncontrolled studies that have included fibrinogen administration as part of a Massive Transfusion Protocol (MTP) have suggested that early use can improve outcomes, including mortality and reduced overall blood product requirements [27] One study [23] suggested that cryoprecipitate (a fluid containing high levels of fibrinogen) use reduced the incidence of lung injury and organ dysfunction, in direct contrast to FFP which seemed to increase the likelihood of these conditions. It is possible that this effect could result from an FFP sparing phenomena when cryoprecipitate is introduced as part of a MTP.

The current evidence base for the early use of fibrinogen supplementation is sparse and early delivery of cryoprecipitate to support a MTP is logistically challenging. However, the CRYOSTAT trial [28] which assessed the feasibility of early cryoprecipitate administration found that all of the patients allocated to early treatment with cryoprecipitate received it within the 90 min window allowed. In fact, the mean time to administration was 60 min. However, no patient received treatment within 30 min of hospital arrival highlighting the difficulties of providing treatment even within the setting of a controlled trial. Although numbers in this trial were small (n = 41) the authors commented on the apparent trend towards a lower mortality and length of critical care dependency for those patients who received early cryoprecipitate.

Further trials are urgently required in this area and the possibility of using cryoprecipitate in a plasma sparing capacity has potential. Viscoelastic tests are the ideal way of titrate the administration of fibrinogen administration. An initial treatment dose of 4 g which equates to two UK pools of cryo-precipitate was used in the CRYOSTAT study and considerably improved clot strength in ex vivo ROTEM studies.

Should Antifibrinloytics Be Given Routinely?

As discussed earlier in this chapter fibrinolysis is sometimes a component of TIC and where it occurs there is a significant increase in mortality. A number of therapeutic agents exist which can attenuate fibrinolysis such as Aprotinin (no longer in use because of safety concerns) and Tranexamic Acid (TXA). TXA was tested in a very large randomised controlled trial, CRASH 2 [29]. This study showed a reduction in both deaths from bleeding and overall mortality associated with the use of TXA. However, this unselected and heterogeneous trauma population included a large number of patients without major haemorrhage and the study did not seek to explain how TXA was able to exert its effects, which in all probability were at least partly due to reasons other than direct inhibition of fibrinolysis. Reassuringly the safety profile of TXA appeared good and there was no increased incidence of thrombosis in the treatment arm of CRASH 2. As a result of this study administration of TXA has become routine in all major trauma episodes in the UK, with 1 g given early following injury followed by a further 1 g over the next 8 h. Interestingly, CRASH 2 showed an increased mortality associated with TXA use when it was given more than 3 h after injury.

Where point of care measurement of coagulation shows evidence of hyperfibrinolysis then the decision to administer a further dose of TXA is an easy one. However more commonly thromboelastography does not show fibrinolysis, what is the correct treatment in this instance? It has been suggested that TXA has other effects on inflammation and wound healing as well as its purely antifibrinolytic effects [30]. Based on this and the fact that that TXA was given empirically in CRASH 2 to good effect and seemingly without significant harm it seems reasonable to give a further dose, even in the absence of detectable fibrinolysis.

What Is the Role of Recombinant Activated Factor VII (rFVIIa) in the Treatment of TIC?

rFVIIa or NovoSeven is licenced for use in haemophilia but has been used on multiple occasions "off label" as a treatment for refractory coagulopathy, including following traumatic injury. Its mechanism of action is two fold via both exposed tissue factor on injured endothelium and on activated platelets. Both mechanisms lead to increased activation of factors IX and X which in turn produce a burst of thrombin generation. Because of this mechanism, rFVIIa requires both sufficient numbers of activated platelets and coagulation factors (IX, X, V) to exert its effects. It is also substantially less effective in an acidic environment, losing up to 50 % efficacy at a pH of 7.0 [31]. Because it's activity is confined to areas of endothelial damage and platelet activation it theoretically should not cause a generalised hypercoagulability.

Numerous case reports, cohort studies and an RCT [32] appeared to show that rFVIIa was effective at reducing transfusion requirements following blunt trauma induced massive haemorrhage and was not associated with an increased incidence of thrombotic events. However, a larger RCT [33] evaluating rFVIIa was hindered by lower than expected mortality in both arms which meant that it is was grossly underpowered to detect a difference in the primary outcome measure. For this reason it was terminated early on grounds of futility. Again there was a reduction in the transfusion requirement in the rFVIIa arm and no discernable increase in thrombotic events.

The 2013 European guidelines on bleeding and coagulopathy [4] provide a weak recommendation to support the use of rFVIIa following traumatic haemorrhage after failure to control bleeding using a conventional MTP approach. They counsel against it's use in patients with traumatic brain injury based on case reports showing an increased mortality in this cohort. The UK DMS guideline for massive transfusion suggest that rFVIIa is only used after more than 8 units of PRBC have been transfused and in the presence of uncontrolled bleeding.

What Is the Role of Fresh Whole Blood Transfusion in the Treatment of TIC?

As noted previously, component therapy, i.e., separate administration of PRBCs, plasma and platelets is the standard approach taken to transfusion of blood products. However, in certain environments, notably austere settings and far forward military medical care the ability to transfer, store and deliver component therapy is often limited. Solutions to this problem include the use of lyophilised plasma, haemoglobin based oxygen compounds and platelets derived from local apheresis. Another solution is the use of Fresh Whole Blood (FWB), derived from a pool of pre screened volunteers who form an Emergency Donor Panel (EDP). The use of FWB is controversial. The lack of leucodepletion may heighten the potential for immunological sequalae and despite pre screening of the donor pool the interval between such screening and administration of blood opens up the potential for transfusion of undetected pathogens.

The conflicts in Iraq and Afghanistan between 2001 and 2014 saw widespread use of FWB, either as a primary resuscitation fluid in forward medical facilities or as a salvage therapy for ongoing severe coagulopathy despite the use of a conventional massive transfusion protocol. What evidence exists regarding the efficacy and safety of FWB is by necessity retrospective and uncontrolled. A US Army study [34] using propensity scoring to compare patients who had received component blood products lacking platelets with those in whom component products were augmented with FWB showed a reduction in the severity of TIC in those who received FWB. There were no obvious differences in adverse events but the sample size was too small to make accurate comparisons.

A further US Army study [35] examined data from 591 trauma casualties who had received more than 10 units of PRBC in the first 24 h after injury. Around 25 % had received FWB. Overall there was an 11 % incidence of Acute Lung Injury (ALI) in this cohort but the FWB cohort appeared slightly over represented within this group. Logistic regression analysis showed a very small increased risk of ALI associated with the use of FWB.

There is less evidence surrounding the use of FWB as a salvage therapy following uncontrolled coagulopathy in patients being managed using a conventional component therapy based MTP. Most military clinicians who served in the recent Iraq and Afghanistan conflicts will recount anecdotal incidences of the life saving role of FWB in these circumstances, often when the total amount of transfused red cells was well in excess of fifty units.

Finally, for practical and governance reasons the use of FWB is likely to remain confined to use in remote and austere environments and there is limited potential or desire to adopt the treatment into mainstream clinical practice.

What Other Complications Can Occur in a Patient Receiving a Massive Transfusion?

In addition to the direct complications associated with uncontrolled TIC there are a number of other important complications associated with massive haemorrhage and transfusion that should be monitored for and acted upon aggressively:

- Calcium: Severe hypocalcaemia can be caused by the infusion of large amounts of citrated blood products, particularly FFP. Hypocalcaemia causes failure of fibrin polymerisation as well as direct circulatory effects that may worsen perfusion. Ionised calcium levels should be checked after every six units of a massive transfusion protocol and the level kept >1.0 mmol/l by the administration of 10 ml boluses of 10 % calcium chloride

• Potassium: Hyperkalaemia can be caused by the lysis of fragile stored erythrocytes as well as direct traumatic cellular injury. It is also exacerbated by the acidosis associated with hypoperfusion. Treatment should be with prompt administration of dextrose/insulin solutions, e.g., 100 ml 20 % Dextrose with 10 units Actrapid.

• Temperature: The environment and the use of non warmed fluids can lead to rapid hypothermia following traumatic injury. The effect of hypothermia on coagulation is profound and every effort must be made to keep the core temperature above 35 °C, using fluid warming devices and convective heating systems.

• Volume overload: Modern rapid infusion devices, such as that shown in Fig. 8.8, are capable of delivering up to 750 ml of blood products every minute. Such infusion rates run the risk of causing acute circulatory overload, including the development of pulmonary oedema caused by acutely increased pulmonary hydrostatic pressure. Clinicians should be mindful of this and the use of targeted resuscitation strategies, particularly focussed ultrasound, can go some way to mitigating this risk.

Putting It All Together – What Factors Should Be Included in a Massive Transfusion Protocol (MTP)?

Trauma resuscitation is a dynamic situation with considerable potential for loss of clinical focus and control. It is therefore vital that all trauma centers who may be receiving patients with traumatic blood loss and TIC have an established protocol based approach to guide management. The recent STOP the bleeding campaign [36] aspires to reduce the incidence of death resulting from exsanguination following trauma by 20 % over 5

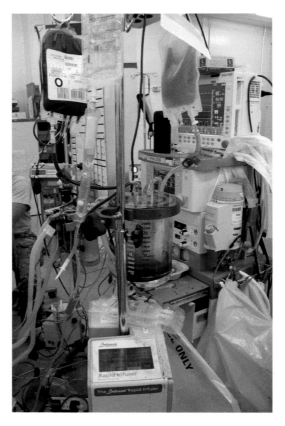

FIGURE 8.8 Belmont rapid transfusion device in use at the Role 3 Hospital, Camp Bastion, Afghanistan

years, principally through promotion and adoption of evidence based guidelines such as those produced by the multidisciplinary Task Force for Advanced Bleeding Care in Trauma [4].

The UK DMS developed a MTP based on initial experience in the Iraq conflict (2003–2009) and subsequently updated this in 2009 following experience in Afghanistan [37]. Key components of the protocol are the use of a 1:1 ratio of plasma to PRBC and early use of apheresis platelets and cryoprecipitate.

rFVIIa is reserved for cases of refractory bleeding as is the use of FWB from an emergency donor pool. UK involvement in the conflict in Afghanistan (2001–2014) and the increased incidence of blast related injuries in that conflict meant that this military MTP saw extensive use. During this period it continued to evolve, the most important element of which was the introduction of point of care viscoelastic testing to guide therapy, as described in Part 2 of this chapter.

Many civilian major trauma centers became early adopters of the "military model" MTP and in a similar fashion these were adapted over time. Nardi and colleagues describe the implementation of a MTP at two Italian trauma centers [9, 38]. This new MTP was based on point of care thromboelastography and compared with the previous protocol which used an empirical approach to blood product administration. Another significant difference was the introduction of early fibrinogen administration, in the form of cryoprecipitate. Compared to the previous protocol the authors demonstrated a significant reduction in the use of plasma with this targeted approach.

Individual MTPs must take into account the logistic factors prevailing at each individual trauma center. The Role 3 hospital at Camp Bastion was a near exclusive trauma hospital with no elective work. It was able to deliver, often in very short order, a comprehensive damage control resuscitation service that usually involved the administration of more than ten, and sometimes up to a hundred units of PRBC in the first 6 h following injury. Point of care coagulation assessment was available in the Emergency Department, Operating Theatres and Intensive Care Unit and the laboratory team was almost exclusively focused on the delivery of the MTP. Clearly, these conditions cannot be achieved at a civilian major trauma center where the focus is not exclusively on the patient with major traumatic injury. The combination of expected workload and injury severity patterns will dictate what local set up is appropriate.

One illustrative MTP is shown in Fig. 8.9. It is not in use at any specific institution and is different, if similar, to the current protocol used by the UK DMS. It incorporates a targeted approach to TIC using early viscoelastic testing to

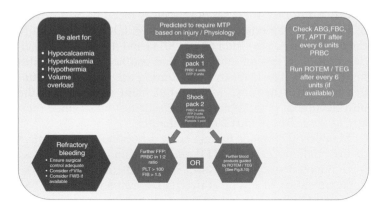

FIGURE 8.9 Illustrative Massive Transfusion Protocol

determine product requirements after an initial empirical administration of blood products. It highlights many of the points made in this chapter, including early use of cryoprecipitate and in variance to current UK DMS practice and based on the latest evidence advocates an initial plasma: PRBC ratio of 1:2, rather than 1:1.

What About the Patient Receiving Anti-coagulant Treatment?

There are now a multitude of anti-coagulant agents available for the treatment and prevention of thromboembolic conditions. Patients receiving these agents who are involved in traumatic injury pose a particular challenge for clinicians. The evidence base for managing reversal of these agents in the context of traumatic haemorrhage is minimal but the current consensus guidelines of the European Task Force for Advanced Bleeding Care in Trauma are shown in Table 8.3. Reversal agents should only be used where there is clinically significant bleeding and wherever possible advice should be sort from a haematology specialist (Fig. 8.10).

TABLE 8.3 Recommendations for reversal of existing pro-coagulants in patients with traumatic haemorrhage

Agent class	Examples	Suggested treatment
Vitamin K dependent anticoagulant	Warfarin	PCC – dose in accordance with INR (20–50 U/kg)
Anti Xa agents	Rivaroxaban, Apixaban	High dose PCC (25–50 U/kg)
Direct Thrombin inhibitors	Dabigatran	No agent has shown efficacy
Antiplatelet agents	Aspirin, Clopidogrel	Desmopressin (DDAVP) 0.3 ug/kg

Taken from Spahn et al. [4]

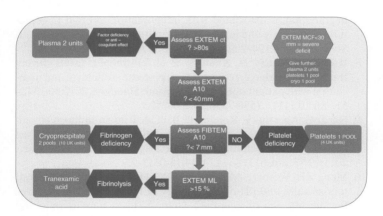

FIGURE 8.10 Flowchart for ROTEM guided therapy as part of a massive transfusion protocol

References

1. MacLeod JBA, Lynn M, McKenney MG, et al. Early coagulopathy predicts mortality in trauma. J Trauma Inj Infect Crit Care. 2003;55:39–44. doi:10.1097/01.TA.0000075338.21177.EF.
2. Brohi K, Singh J, Heron M, Coats T. Acute traumatic coagulopathy. J Trauma Inj Infect Crit Care. 2003;54:1127–30. doi:10.1097/01.TA.0000069184.82147.06.

3. Cohen MJ, Call M, Nelson M, et al. Critical role of activated protein C in early coagulopathy and later organ failure, infection and death in trauma patients. Ann Surg. 2012;255:379–85. doi:10.1097/SLA.0b013e318235d9e6.

4. Spahn DR, Bouillon B, Cerný V, Coats TJ. Management of bleeding and coagulopathy following major trauma: an updated European guideline. Crit Care. 2013;17:R76. doi:10.1186/cc12685.

5. Brohi K, Cohen MJ, Ganter MT, et al. Acute coagulopathy of trauma: hypoperfusion induces systemic anticoagulation and hyperfibrinolysis. J Trauma Inj Infect Crit Care. 2008;64:1211–7. doi:10.1097/TA.0b013e318169cd3c.

6. Rizoli SB, Scarpelini S, Callum J, et al. Clotting factor deficiency in early trauma-associated coagulopathy. J Trauma. 2011;71:S427–34. doi:10.1097/TA.0b013e318232e5ab.

7. Johansson PI, Stensballe J, Rasmussen LS, Ostrowski SR. A high admission syndecan-1 level, a marker of endothelial glycocalyx degradation, is associated with inflammation, protein C depletion, fibrinolysis, and increased mortality in trauma patients. Ann Surg. 2011;254:194–200. doi:10.1097/SLA.0b013e318226113d.

8. Rourke C, Curry N, Khan S, et al. Fibrinogen levels during trauma hemorrhage, response to replacement therapy, and association with patient outcomes. J Thromb Haemost. 2012;10:1342–51. doi:10.1111/j.1538-7836.2012.04752.x.

9. Nardi G, Agostini V, Rondinelli B, et al. Trauma-induced coagulopathy: impact of the early coagulation support protocol on blood product consumption, mortality and costs. Crit Care. 2015;19:83. doi:10.1186/s13054-015-0817-9.

10. Meng ZH, Wolberg AS, Monroe DM, Hoffman M. The effect of temperature and pH on the activity of factor VIIa: implications for the efficacy of high-dose factor VIIa in hypothermic and acidotic patients. J Trauma Inj Infect Crit Care. 2003;55:886–91. doi:10.1097/01.TA.0000066184.20808.A5.

11. Engström M, Schött U, Romner B, Reinstrup P. Acidosis impairs the coagulation: a thromboelastographic study. J Trauma Inj Infect Crit Care. 2006;61:624–8. doi:10.1097/01.ta.0000226739.30655.75.

12. Hußmann B, Lefering R, Taeger G, et al. Influence of prehospital fluid resuscitation on patients with multiple injuries in hemorrhagic shock in patients from the DGU trauma registry. J Emerg Trauma Shock. 2011;4:465–71. doi:10.4103/0974-2700.86630.

13. Schöchl H, Frietsch T, Pavelka M, Jámbor C. Hyperfibrinolysis after major trauma: differential diagnosis of lysis patterns and prognostic value of thrombelastometry. J Trauma. 2009;67:125–31. doi:10.1097/TA.0b013e31818b2483.

14. Saillant NN, Sims CA. Platelet dysfunction in injured patients. Mol Cell Ther. 2014;2:37. doi:10.1186/s40591-014-0037-8.

15. Maegele M, Paffrath T, Bouillon B. Acute traumatic coagulopathy in severe injury: incidence, risk stratification, and treatment options. Dtsch Arztebl Int. 2011;108:827–35. doi:10.3238/arztebl.2011.0827.

16. Tonglet ML, Minon JM, Seidel L, et al. Prehospital identification of trauma patients with early acute coagulopathy and massive bleeding: results of a prospective non-interventional clinical trial evaluating the Trauma Induced Coagulopathy Clinical Score (TICCS). Crit Care. 2014;18:1–8. doi:10.1186/s13054-014-0648-0.

17. ACS TQIP massive transfusion in trauma guidelines. 2013;1–18.

18. Doran CM, Woolley T, Midwinter MJ. Feasibility of using rotational thromboelastometry to assess coagulation status of combat casualties in a deployed setting. J Trauma Inj Infect Crit Care. 2010;69:S40–8. doi:10.1097/TA.0b013e3181e4257b.

19. Borgman MA, Spinella PC, Perkins JG, et al. The ratio of blood products transfused affects mortality in patients receiving massive transfusions at a combat support hospital. J Trauma. 2007;63:805–13. doi:10.1097/TA.0b013e3181271ba3.

20. Gunter OL, Au BK, Isbell JM, et al. Optimizing outcomes in damage control resuscitation: identifying blood product ratios associated with improved survival. J Trauma. 2008;65:527–34. doi:10.1097/TA.0b013e3181826ddf.

21. Holcomb JB, Del Junco DJ, Fox EE, et al. The prospective, observational, multicenter, major trauma transfusion (PROMMTT) study: comparative effectiveness of a time-varying treatment with competing risks. JAMA Surg. 2013;148:127–36. doi:10.1001/2013.jamasurg.387.

22. Holcomb JB, Tilley BC, Baraniuk S, et al. Transfusion of plasma, platelets, and red blood cells in a 1:1:1 vs a 1:1:2 ratio and mortality in patients with severe trauma: the PROPPR randomized clinical trial. JAMA. 2015;313:471–82. doi:10.1001/jama.2015.12.

23. Watson GA, Sperry JL, Rosengart MR, et al. Fresh frozen plasma is independently associated with a higher risk of multiple organ failure and acute respiratory distress syndrome. J Trauma Inj Infect Crit Care. 2009;67:221–30. doi:10.1097/TA.0b013e3181ad5957.

24. Watts S, Nordmann G, Brohi K, et al. Evaluation of prehospital blood products to attenuate acute coagulopathy of trauma in a model of severe injury and shock in anesthetized pigs. Shock. 2015;44 Suppl 1:138–48. doi:10.1097/SHK.0000000000000409.

25. Brown LM, Aro SO, Cohen MJ. A high fresh frozen plasma: packed red blood cell transfusion ratio decreases mortality in all massively transfused trauma patients regardless of admission international normalized ratio. J Trauma Inj Infect Crit Care. 2011;71:S358–63. doi:10.1097/TA.0b013e318227f152.

26. Holcomb JB, Zarzabal LA, Michalek JE, et al. Increased platelet:RBC ratios are associated with improved survival after massive transfusion. J Trauma Inj Infect Crit Care. 2011;71:S318–28. doi:10.1097/TA.0b013e318227edbb.

27. Stinger HK, Spinella PC, Perkins JG, et al. The ratio of fibrinogen to red cells transfused affects survival in casualties receiving massive transfusions at an Army Combat Support Hospital. J Trauma Inj Infect Crit Care. 2008;64:S79–85. doi:10.1097/TA.0b013e318160a57b.

28. Curry N, Rourke C, Davenport R, et al. Early cryoprecipitate for major haemorrhage in trauma: a randomised controlled feasibility trial. Br J Anaesth. 2015;115:aev134–83. doi:10.1093/bja/aev134.

29. CRASH-2 Trial Collaborators, Shakur H, Roberts I, et al. Effects of tranexamic acid on death, vascular occlusive events, and blood transfusion in trauma patients with significant haemorrhage (CRASH-2): a randomised, placebo-controlled trial. Lancet. 2010;376:23–32. doi:10.1016/S0140-6736(10)60835-5.

30. Draxler DF, Medcalf RL. The fibrinolytic system-more than fibrinolysis? Transfus Med Rev. 2015;29:102–9. doi:10.1016/j.tmrv.2014.09.006.

31. Viuff D, Lauritzen B, Pusateri AE, et al. Effect of haemodilution, acidosis, and hypothermia on the activity of recombinant factor VIIa (NovoSeven). Br J Anaesth. 2008;101:324–31. doi:10.1093/bja/aen175.

32. Boffard KD, Riou B, Warren B, et al. Recombinant factor VIIa as adjunctive therapy for bleeding control in severely injured trauma patients: two parallel randomized, placebo-controlled, double-blind clinical trials. J Trauma Inj Infect Crit Care. 2005;59:8–15; discussion 15–8.

33. Hauser CJ, Boffard K, Dutton R, et al. Results of the CONTROL Trial: efficacy and safety of recombinant activated factor VII in the management of refractory traumatic hemorrhage. J Trauma Inj Infect Crit Care. 2010;69:489–500. doi:10.1097/TA.0b013e3181edf36e.

34. Auten JD, Lunceford NL, Horton JL, et al. The safety of early fresh, whole blood transfusion among severely battle injured at US Marine Corps forward surgical care facilities in Afghanistan. J Trauma Acute Care Surg. 2015;79:790–6. doi:10.1097/TA.0000000000000842.

35. Chan CM, Shorr AF, Perkins JG. Factors associated with acute lung injury in combat casualties receiving massive blood transfusions: a retrospective analysis. J Crit Care. 2012;27:419e.7–14. doi:10.1016/j.jcrc.2011.11.010.
36. Rossaint R, Bouillon B, Cerny V, et al. The STOP the bleeding campaign. Crit Care. 2013;17:136. doi:10.1186/cc12579.
37. Surgeon general's operational policy letter. Management of massive haemorrhage on operations, February 2009.
38. Nardi G, Agostini V, Rondinelli BM, et al. Prevention and treatment of trauma induced coagulopathy (TIC). An intended protocol from the Italian trauma update research group. J Anesthesiol Clin Sci. 2013;2:1–10. doi:10.7243/2049-9752-2-22.

Chapter 9
Thoracic Trauma and Management of Ventilation in the Critically Injured Patient

Michael C. Reade

Abstract Blunt chest trauma most commonly affects the chest wall in isolation, but if sufficiently forceful can also damage intrathoracic structures. Conversely, penetrating trauma commonly has minimal substantial effect on the chest wall (other than by creating a pneumothorax), but places intrathoracic structures at risk. Penetrating trauma more commonly requires operative intervention, but this is still only required in 15–20 % of patients presenting alive to hospital. Lung injury, either direct or indirect, is the commonest concern for the intensivist. Many theoretically attractive treatments for the acute respiratory distress

M.C. Reade, MBBS, MPH, DPhil, FANZCA, FCICM
Joint Health Command, Australian Defence Force,
Canberra, ACT 2610, Australia

The Burns, Trauma and Critical Care Research Centre,
University of Queensland and Royal Brisbane
and Women's Hospital, Brisbane, QLD 4029, Australia
e-mail: m.reade@uq.edu.au; Michael.reade@defence.gov.au

S.D. Hutchings (ed.), *Trauma and Combat Critical Care in Clinical Practice*, In Clinical Practice,
DOI 10.1007/978-3-319-28758-4_9,
© Crown Copyright 2016

syndrome have failed in definitive clinical trials, but several approaches reduce mortality and/or morbidity; these include low tidal volume ventilation, permissive hypercapnia, lung recruitment, PEEP strategies and prone positioning. Low dose steroids remain controversial. Rational, guideline-based use of prophylactic and therapeutic antibiotics, along with several non-antibiotic approaches including semi-recumbent positioning, improve patient outcomes and prevent emergence of resistant organisms. Extracorporeal CO_2 removal with or without transmembrane oxygenation await confirmation of benefit in large trials in trauma, but evidence from other settings argues for their use, at least in select patients. Modern ventilators synchronise better to patient effort, allowing lighter sedation, earlier mobilisation and quicker extubation.

Keywords Thoracic trauma • Lung injury • ARDS • Pneumothorax • Haemothorax • Mechanical ventilation • Non-invasive ventilation • Lung protective ventilation • Weaning

Part 1: Management of the Patient with Severe Chest Trauma

What Pathology Should Be Suspected After Blunt Traumatic Injury to the Chest?

Substantial blunt force applied to the chest most commonly results in injury to the chest wall alone, including contusion, fractures of the ribs (which if fractured in two places and over two or more adjacent ribs can produce a flail segment), sternum, clavicles, scapulae, and more rarely, damage to the intercostal vessels. The first and second ribs and the scapula require the greatest anterior-posterior force to fracture, heightening suspicion of injuries to intrathroacic structures. Intrathoracic structures susceptible to injury include:

• The Heart

Manifestations of injury include septal or valvular rupture, coronary artery dissection, myocardial contusion and commotio cordis. The incidence of myocardial contusion is unknown, in part because cardiac troponin is commonly raised in major trauma due to non-cardiac causes, and in part because the heart of asymptomatic patients is not routinely examined by echocardiography. It is likely that mild myocardial contusion is common but rarely clinically significant, especially as there is no specific treatment other than optimisation of haemodynamics. Commotio cordis, the induction of ventricular fibrillation following a direct blow within the 15–30 ms period just prior to the peak of the T wave, is most common when the chest is struck during sport – for example in cricket, baseball, and hockey. Commotio cordis is the only traumatic cause of cardiac arrest that is likely to respond to defibrillation. Despite a structurally normal heart, historical survival rates from commotio cordis (before widespread deployment of Automated External Defibrillators) was only 15 % [1].

• The Great Vessels

Complete disruption almost always leads to death prior to hospital presentation, so the commonest pathology in patients who survive to hospital admission is a traumatic dissection. This is classically identified as a widening of the superior mediastinum (to >8 cm in a supine or >6 cm in an erect chest radiograph), but this sign is neither sensitive nor specific, arguing that patients with substantial chest trauma, along with those with any signs of traumatic dissection, such as unequal radial pulses or brachial arterial pressures, should have this condition excluded by contrast CT of the chest.

- The Chest Wall and Pleural Space

Pathology includes haemothorax, pneumothorax, and tension pneumothorax. In the absence of chest wall penetration, pneumothorax occurs due to disruption of the lung parenchyma. The incidence of pneumothorax in blunt chest trauma patients admitted to hospital is around 30 %, compared to 95 % of penetrating trauma patents.

- The Large Airways

This can result in a bronchopleural fistula, pneumomediastinum (which may be of sufficient pressure to cause a "tension" effect compressing mediastinal structures) or pneumothorax (+/− tension).

- The Lungs [The Principal Topic of Part 2 of This Chapter]

What is the Epidemiology of Chest Injuries?

The incidence of intrathoracic injuries amongst 1490 patients with (predominantly blunt) chest trauma surviving to presentation at an urban trauma centre was: 55 % soft tissue trauma alone; 35 % rib fractures (18 % of whom had associated subcutaneous emphysema), 3 % had a clinically significant flail segment and 18 % a haemothorax or pneumothorax [2]. No injuries to the great vessels, trachea and major airways, or tension pneumothorax were reported. Another study reported on 127 blunt chest trauma patients without bony chest wall injury, finding 16 % with cardiac contusions, 8 % with ruptured diaphragms, 7 % with ruptured aortas, 3 % with cardiac ruptures, 2 % with tracheobronchial injuries, 2 % with pulmonary lacerations and 1 % with injury to the great vessels [3].

Only 20–30 % of admitted patients with blunt chest trauma require insertion of an intercostal catheter, and less than 10 % require operative surgery [4].

What Pathology Should Be Suspected After Penetrating Traumatic Injury to the Chest?

The ratio of penetrating to blunt chest trauma varies markedly according to environment. Penetrating trauma has a greater chance of affecting the intrathoracic structures (heart, lungs, and great vessels) and in one observational series, 34 % of patients with this injury pattern died prior to hospital arrival [5]. Penetrating chest trauma patients who survive to hospital admission have a lower mortality than with blunt trauma as the latter is more often associated with extrathoracic injuries [6]. The pathology amongst 120 patients surviving to presentation at a major trauma hospital with penetrating thoracic trauma (87 % due to gunshot wounds) was: 65 % haemothorax; 21 % haemopneumothorax; 5 % isolated pneumothorax; 4 % pulmonary contusion; 2 % pericardial injury [7]. Injuries to the trachea and major airways, oesophagus, diaphragm, thoracic duct, spinal column and great vessels were not reported in this series, with varying (but low) incidence in other studies. Penetrating wounds below the nipple commonly enter the abdominal cavity.

Pulmonary contusion is common after high-energy wounding but uncommon after stab and low-energy firearm and blast-fragmentation wounds [8]. Low energy wounds may cause haemorrhage from intercostal vessels but rarely affect the chest wall in other ways. Penetrating wounds to the heart typically enter the right ventricle (the most anterior structure). Even small myocardial wounds can cause pericardial tamponade with <100 ml blood. Most penetrating wounds to the great vessels are fatal before intervention is possible.

Amongst military casualties next to exsanguinating haemorrhage (60 %), tension pneumothorax is the second commonest cause (33 %) of preventable death in penetrating trauma [9]. Several case series have shown that needle decompression is frequently an ineffective treatment for tension pneumothorax, leading many to recommend finger thoracostomy followed by intercostal catheter insertion if the required skills and equipment are available. Notably, these figures are often quoted with the suggestion that they should determine priorities for intervention, but this may be misleading. Based on post-mortem studies, these statistics do not account for patients who *would have died* were it not for *successful interventions* such as airway control. Opening the airway (in particular) may be proportionately more important than these figures suggest.

Although more common than with blunt thoracic trauma, only a small minority of patients with penetrating chest injuries (14 % in one series) require surgical management other than the placement of an intercostal catheter [10].

What Imaging Is Recommended After Trauma to the Chest?

A suggested algorithm for determining which imaging is required following traumatic thoracic injury is shown in Fig. 9.1.

- Chest X Ray (CXR)

Patients with substantial chest trauma should have a chest radiograph to screen for intrathoracic pathology. However, plain chest radiographs are not sensitive for many injuries, in one study detecting only 32 % of pneumothoraces subsequently identified on a CT scan [11]. Repeating the chest radiograph after 6 h increases sensitivity.

- Lung Ultrasound

Ultrasound examination of the lung is more sensitive and just as specific for pneumothorax than CXR [12]. Additionally, haemothorax, pericardial fluid, and myocardial filling and function can be assessed. When skills and equipment are available, ultrasound should precede chest radiography.

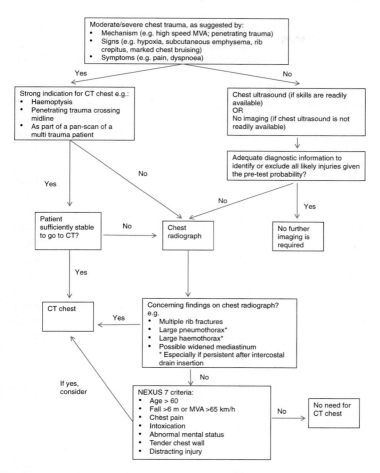

FIGURE 9.1 Algorithm for selecting diagnostic imaging following thoracic trauma

• Chest CT

A CT chest is indicated after substantial blunt trauma if there is chest wall deformity, multiple rib fractures, a large pneumothorax or haemothorax, or an apparently widened mediastinum in chest radiograph. Often CT chest is performed as part of whole body axial imaging, predicated by mechanism of injury. CT findings change management in 20–30 % of patients with chest radiograph abnormalities, but in only 5 % of patients with no plain radiographic abnormalities but a concerning mechanism of injury. One reason to perform a CXR prior to CT is to identify gross intrathoracic pathology that requires treatment prior to the patient leaving a resuscitation or critical care area for the usually less well-resourced CT scanning area. However, if there is a clear indication for a CT chest in a patient who appears physiologically stable, omitting the chest radiograph and proceeding directly to CT is reasonable. *Absence* of several factors (the NEXUS 7 Chest Criteria: age >60 years; rapid deceleration mechanism i.e., fall >6 m; or vehicle crash >65 km/h; chest pain; intoxication; abnormal mental status; tenderness to chest wall palpation; and distracting painful injury) suggests a very low chance of chest injury after blunt trauma, suggesting omission of a CT chest is safe [13]. Penetrating trauma that crosses the midline should be assessed with a CT chest. An abdominal CT is also valuable in assessing abdominal injury from penetration below the level of the nipple.

What Should Be Done for Patients with Marked Shortness of Breath Following Blunt or Penetrating Chest Trauma?

Patients with suspected tension pneumothorax (suggested by dyspnoea, a hyper-resonant chest, absent unilateral breath sounds, elevated JVP and falling arterial blood pressure, deviation of midline structures to the contralateral side, subcutaneous emphysema and confirmed by ultrasound appearance) should have one or both hemithoraces decompressed by finger thoracostomy followed by insertion of an intercostal catheter. This should precede the chest radiograph; however, in trained hands lung ultrasound can provide a rapid and reliable method for excluding pneumothorax in this setting. Only if resources/equipment for finger thoracostomy are unavailable should a needle thoracostomy be considered as an alternative. A 3.2 cm cannula failed to decompress the chest in 65 % of patients in one series, although a 4.5 cm cannula was unsuccessful in only 4 % [14]. Therefore, if a needle thoracostomy is attempted, a long cannula is preferable.

When Is a Thoracotomy Indicated Following Chest Trauma?

Patients with suspected cardiac tamponade, suggested by hypotension, elevated JVP, and muffled heart sounds, and confirmed by echocardiography, should have either a surgical pericardial window or preferably, if cardiac disruption is suspected, an anterolateral or clamshell thoracotomy. Thoracotomy allows pericardial drainage, repair of myocardial rupture, clamping of the aorta, internal cardiac massage and internal defibrillation. Induction of anaesthesia and commencement of positive pressure ventilation classically causes immediate cardiovascular collapse, so the surgical team must be prepared to relieve the tamponade within seconds of this occurring. This is usually preferable to attempted needle aspiration prior to induction; in general, there is no role for needle aspiration of traumatic haemopericardium if a surgical approach is possible with the resources available.

Patients in cardiac arrest following chest trauma, with the exception of patients whose most likely diagnosis is commotio cordis, should have immediate evaluation and treatment for hypovolaemia and tension pneumothorax. The classical signs of these conditions are unreliable, whilst lung ultrasound/echocardiography is both sensitive and specific. If cardiac tamponade or disruption to the major vessels is suspected, an emergency thoracotomy should be considered if equipment and trained personnel are available. There are several guidelines listing indications and contraindications for resuscitative thoracotomy and proposing yet another definitive protocol is unhelpful. As a general guide, cardiac arrest due to penetrating trauma is more likely to respond to emergency thoracotomy than is arrest with blunt trauma. A favourable result is almost never possible even in penetrating trauma if resuscitative thoracotomy is initiated more than 15 min after the onset of cardiac arrest. Whether a clam-shell or anterolateral approach is best will be determined by the pattern of injury or wounding and the available surgical expertise.

A resuscitative thoracotomy may be indicated prior to cardiac arrest – if time allows, ideally by an appropriately trained surgical team in an adequately-equipped operating theatre.

What Is the Management of Myocardial Contusion?

Patients with hypotension or arrhythmia after chest trauma should have an echocardiogram to identify regional wall motion abnormalities (suggesting myocardial contusion) and pericardial blood/fluid. There is no specific treatment for myocardial contusion other than to optimise preload and afterload, and monitor/treat arrhythmias if they occur.

What Is the Management for Traumatic Pneumothoraces, Haemothoraces, Pneumomediastinum and Oesophageal Injury?

Patients with haemothorax or pneumothorax visible on plain radiograph should have a medium to large bore (>32 F) chest tube inserted. There is little, if any, role for percutaneous fine bore chest drainage in trauma. There appears little advantage in placing such drains on suction [15]. The usual insertion point is the fifth intercostal space just anterior to the mid-axillary line, but the second or third intercostal space in mid-clavicular line is an acceptable alternative. Blood accumulating in a haemothorax usually originates in the lung parenchyma or intercostal vessels, so uncommonly requires surgery to correct; disruption of the great vessels rarely results in survival to hospital. If more than 1000–1500 ml drains initially, or more than 200–300 ml subsequently drain per hour, thoracotomy should be considered.

Retained haemothorax despite intercostal catheter drainage is an indication for early video-assisted thoracoscopic surgery to reduce the risk of empyema and fibrosis with consequent reduction in lung function.

Optimal management of patients with an "occult pneumothorax" (visible on CT imaging but not on plain radiograph) is unclear. Only 5–10 % of such pneumothoraces expand to become clinically significant. A reasonable approach is NOT to insert an intercostal catheter for asymptomatic occult pneumothoraces <8 mm long in spontaneously breathing patients unless the patient becomes symptomatic or the pneumothorax expands. There is conflicting trial evidence as to whether mechanical ventilation mandates chest drainage of all occult pneumothoraces. The Eastern Association for the Surgery of Trauma recommends that close observation alone is a reasonable option [16].

Patients with tension mediastinum with signs similar to cardiac tamponade but no pericardial fluid on echocardiography and mediastinal air on chest radiography, must have urgent surgical drainage via a suprasternal incision.

Patients suspected of having penetrating oesophageal injury suggested by the track of the knife/projectile or pneumomediastinum on chest radiograph/CT, should have oesophagoscopy and/or radiographic evaluation with contrast. The risk of further injury with insufflation of air argues against oesophagoscopy if contrast radiography is possible. Oesophageal rupture necessitates urgent insertion of a para-oesophageal drain with or without primary repair of the oesophagus or cervical diversion and tube gastrostomy.

How Should Rib Fractures Be Managed?

Rib fractures are present in 70 % of patients admitted to hospital after vehicle crashes [3]. Most rib fractures heal spontaneously, but some progress to non-union with associated chronic pain on inspiration. Most patients with rib fractures are successfully managed as outpatients using oral +/− parenteral analgesia and instruction +/− physiotherapy assistance in deep breathing. Relative indications for hospital admission include >3 contiguous rib fractures, underlying respiratory disease, smokers and the elderly. Multiple rib fractures or fractures in high-risk patients warrant regional analgesia with a thoracic epidural or paravertebral catheter. These techniques are preferable to repeated intercostal nerve blocks or intrapleural infusion of local anaesthetic. Deterioration in respiratory function often requires mechanical ventilation, typically 24–48 h after injury. Patients with a flail chest (three or more contiguous ribs fractured in two places, producing paradoxical motion and loss of inspiratory strength) commonly (59 % in one study) require mechanical ventilation [17].

What Is the Role for Operative Fixation of Rib Fractures?

A recent meta-analysis of nine studies that compared operative fixation of a flail segment to non-operative management found that operative fixation reduced duration of mechanical ventilation, ICU and hospital length of stay, pneumonia, need for tracheostomy, and mortality [18]. Other indications for rib fixation include pain not responsive to optimal analgesia, chest wall deformity, and, in the subacute setting, non-union.

Part 2: Management of the Critically Ill Patient with Traumatic Lung Injury

The term "acute respiratory distress syndrome" (ARDS) was first coined in 1967 and identified in many casualties of the Vietnam War, most likely due to the practice of aggressive crystalloid resuscitation at that time [19]. ARDS is now defined (according to the "Berlin definition") as an "*acute diffuse, inflammatory lung injury, leading to increased pulmonary vascular permeability, increased lung weight, and loss of aerated lung tissue…[with] hypoxemia and bilateral radiographic opacities, associated with increased venous admixture, increased physiological dead space and decreased lung compliance"* [20]. The onset must be rapid (<1 week), there must be bilateral opacities consistent with pulmonary oedema on CT or plain radiography, the ratio of PaO2 to FiO2 (the P/F ratio) must be <300 (39.9 kPa) at a minimum of 5 cmH2O PEEP, and these features must not be explicable by cardiac failure or fluid overload. Pathological features include loss of alveolar structure, proteinaceous debris and inflammatory cells occluding alveoli and small airways, and inflammatory infiltrate in the extravascular lung parenchyma. 4.5 % of 4397 patients admitted to a level 1 trauma centre developed ARDS after blunt trauma, with independent risk factors found to include Injury Severity Score >25, pulmonary contusion, age >65 years, hypotension on admission, and 24-h transfusion requirement >10 units [21]. Trauma is the cause of 7 % of ARDS cases, with a similar incidence in blunt and penetrating chest trauma [22].

What Mechanisms Lead to Respiratory Impairment Following Severe Traumatic Injury?

Direct Damage

Trauma can cause direct impairment of lung function by:

- Rupture of the visceral pleura or penetration of the chest wall, causing pneumothorax or haemothorax.
- Haemorrhage into the alveolae and extra-alveolar lung parenchyma (lung contusion) (with >20 % of the lung parenchyma on CT marking an inflection point in the incidence of ARDS) [22]. The mechanism of pulmonary contusion is likely to be a combination of alveolar rupture due to overdistension, shear force disruption at gas–liquid interfaces, and dislocation of alveoli from bronchi.
- Atelectasis due to reduced inspiratory effort.
- Inhalation injury.
- Aspiration.

- Predisposition to pneumonia with resulting direct lung function impairment.
- Inability to expand the lung through loss of muscular effort due to a flail segment of the chest wall, or loss of innervation of the intercostal muscles (+/– diaphragm) due to spinal injury.

Indirect Damage

Non-specific systemic inflammation resulting from trauma to the chest and elsewhere, including haemorrhagic shock alone with no tissue damage, can produce effects essentially indistinguishable to those of direct lung injury [23]. The exact pathogenic mechanisms are poorly understood, but probably involve activated neutrophils accumulating in the lung and releasing pro-inflammatory mediators such as TNF, IL-1B, IL-6 and IL-8 along with proteolytic enzymes, reactive oxygen and nitrogen molecules. Pulmonary epithelial cell death appears to be more due to apoptosis than necrosis [23], while pulmonary capillary endothelial cells express adhesion receptors for neutrophils and other inflammatory cells, accompanied with loss of the (presumably protective) glycocalyx. Lymphocytes and dendritic cells are recruited to the lung several days after these initial insults and are thought to contribute to the resolution of inflammation, although this can be accompanied by fibrosis. Fibrotic resolution of lung damage is thought to explain long-term impairments in lung function that persist in many patients after resolution of the acute disease process.

What Pharmacological Treatments are Beneficial in Influencing the Progression of Lung Injury After Trauma?

The only drug therapies convincingly shown to improve the prognosis of ARDS are those that influence the underlying cause – primarily antibiotics for pneumonia. Various other drug treatments have been tried, with at best limited or equivocal evidence of benefit [24].

Inhaled Beta-2 Agonists

Hypothesised to be of benefit by augmenting alveolar fluid clearance, enhancing surfactant secretion and decreasing endothelial permeability. A small trial showed evidence of reduced extravascular water after 7 days treatment. However, two large subsequent trials were prematurely terminated; one for futility as there were fewer ventilator-free days with albuterol than with placebo in the most severe patients [25] and the other due to increased 28-day mortality (34 % vs. 23 %, $p = -0.03$) in the intervention group [26].

Inhaled Heparin

Hypothesised to reduce fibrin deposition. One small study suggested an increase in ventilator-free days in patients at risk for ARDS, but this is yet to be confirmed in a sufficiently powered trial. Inhaled heparin shows promise in preclinical and small clinical trials of inhalational injury [27] and although this awaits confirmation in a definitive trial, is of sufficiently low risk to have been incorporated into the practice of many burns centres.

Neutrophil Elastase Inhibitors

These inhibit the protease thought to damage lung endothelium in ARDS. Despite a positive early study, a subsequent definitive trial and later meta-analysis showed worse 180-day mortality.

HMG CoA – Reductase Inhibitors (Statins)

These agents reduce inflammation and benefit endothelial function in addition to their ability to lower cholesterol.

Small studies have shown improvement in surrogate outcomes, but this was not confirmed in two subsequent multicentre trials [28, 29].

Aspirin

Administration of aspirin prior to hospitalisation for all critically ill patients, not just those after trauma, was associated with a lower incidence of ARDS, thought due to reduced microthrombi deposition in the lung. Early hospital use of aspirin in patients at high risk of ARDS awaits testing in a clinical trial.

Corticosteroids

Despite many large well-designed trials, the use of steroids in ARDS remains controversial [30]. In patients at high risk of ARDS, high dose steroid (e.g. 30 mg/kg methylprednisolone every 6 h) was associated with worse outcomes, although much lower doses (e.g. hydrocortisone 50 mg 6 hourly) have not been fully evaluated as ARDS prophylaxis. Similarly, high-dose steroids are of no benefit in early ARDS, but two large trials [31, 32] found a lower short-term (ICU or 28 day) mortality associated with low dose steroid (e.g. 1 mg/kg methylprednisolone daily or 50 mg hydrocortisone 6 hourly) for 7–14 days. Steroids were thought to hold particular benefit in the fibroproliferative phase of late ARDS, but this theory was not supported by a 180-patient trial of methylprednisolone 2 mg/kg/day for 14 days in patients with late ARDS [33]. There were more ventilator-free and shock-free days during the first 28 days, improved oxygenation, better respiratory-system compliance, and fewer days of vasopressor therapy in patients who received steroids. However, 60 and 180 day mortality in each group was almost identical. In the subset of patients who began steroid treatment at or after 14 days, 60 and 180 day mortality was significantly increased compared to controls. In summary, corticosteroids at low dose (e.g., 50 mg hydrocortisone IV 6 hourly) initiated at <14 days after ARDS onset, appear to improve pulmonary gas exchange but have not been shown to have a consistent effect on medium to long term mortality. There appear to be few complications from such therapy, which is therefore weakly recommended. However, practice surveys show intensivists rarely prescribe steroids for this indication. Corticosteroids at high dose should not be given for ARDS following trauma unless there is another indication for their use, for example immunosuppression indicated for the management of intercurrent disease.

What Is the Role for Non-invasive Ventilation in Patients with Chest Trauma?

Non-invasive ventilation (NIV) reduces the need for intubation and reduces mortality in non-traumatic type II (hypercapnic) respiratory failure, although appears seldom to benefit patients with type I respiratory failure. However, whether this applies to patients with chest trauma is unclear, given differences in pathological mechanisms, premorbid lung function, mechanical chest function and pain. A recent systematic review identified nine studies addressing this question, none of which was of high quality [34]. Tentative conclusions were that either continuous positive pressure or non-invasive ventilation (NIPPV) reduce the requirement for intubation in patients with chest trauma *at risk of* ARDS who are alert, haemodynamically stable and not in established respiratory failure, but that NIV rarely averts the requirement for intubation in trauma patients with established respiratory failure. Therefore, NIV should be considered for alert, haemodynamically stable patients without substantial facial trauma but with significant chest trauma before the onset of respiratory failure. If commenced it should continue for 48–72 h. Patients in established respiratory failure due to chest trauma should be intubated in preference to a trial of NIV.

What Ventilator Strategy Should Be Followed Initially in Patients Receiving Invasive Mechanical Ventilation Following Traumatic Injury?

The approach to invasive ventilation after chest trauma has an important impact on the progression of lung injury and patient outcome including mortality. Although there is very little evidence derived exclusively from a trauma population, several factors identified in general critical care require consideration.

Tidal Volumes

Ventilation with low (6 ml/kg predicted body weight) tidal volumes, compared to what was, at the time of the trial, arguably, the 'conventional' 12 ml/kg is associated with a significantly lower mortality (31.0 % vs. 39.8 %) in patients with established ARDS [35]. This is hypothesised to be due to less 'volutrauma' (over distension of the more compliant alveoli), 'atelectotrauma' (from shear forces that occur when alveoli repeatedly open and collapse), and possibly also the anti-inflammatory effect of the consequent hypercapnia [36]. The higher airway pressure that accompanies higher tidal volumes is no longer thought to have a significant negative effect in ARDS, as much of the pressure is dissipated by flow through narrowed airways – rendering the term 'barotrauma' obsolete. Whether low tidal-volume ventilation protects against the development of ARDS was less clear until the IMPROVE trial which randomised 400 abdominal surgery patients to low tidal volume or conventional ventilation [37]. Ventilation at 6–8 ml/kg vs. 10–12 ml/kg resulted in less requirement for postoperative ventilation and shorter hospital stay. Patients at risk of ARDS should be ventilated at 6–8 ml/kg ideal body weight.

PEEP

Ventilation using an 'open lung' approach with a high positive end expiratory pressure (PEEP), is physiologically attractive if attempting to minimise atelectotrauma and ventilation/perfusion mismatch. ARDS patients have widely varying percentages of lung that is potentially recruitable through PEEP [38], which explains the difficulty in demonstrating benefit of a high-PEEP strategy in clinical trials that do not take this heterogeneity into account. Nonetheless, a meta-analysis of the three high vs. low PEEP trials found higher survival in the subgroup of patients with established ARDS randomised to the higher PEEP strategy [39]. Therefore, patients with or at risk of ARDS should be ventilated using a higher PEEP than other ICU patients. There is no consensus on how best to determine the optimal PEEP for an individual patient with, or at risk of, ARDS. Options include adjustment to optimise the P/F ratio, to a level higher than the lower inflection point of the pressure-volume loop, to a level that maximises static compliance, or to a level determined at the end of a staircase recruitment manoeuvre, such as that shown in Fig. 9.2. The 'optimal' PEEP may be a

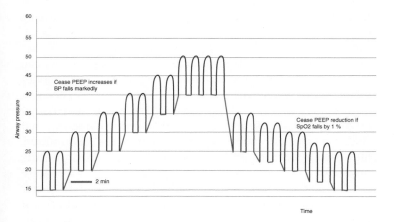

FIGURE 9.2 Graphical representation of a possible lung recruitment strategy

compromise between that which provides the best oxygenation and that which reduces repetitive lung stretch and hyperinflation. No universal recommendation can be made.

Mode of Ventilation

The optimal mode of mandatory mechanical ventilation in the early phase of treatment i.e., prior to weaning, is the subject of much debate. North American ICUs traditionally using assist-control ventilation (ACV) while those in UK, Australia and elsewhere preferring either volume or pressure-targeted synchronised intermittent mandatory ventilation + pressure support ventilation (SIMV + PSV) for any spontaneous breaths above the set mandatory rate. SIMV should not be used without PSV. No trial has demonstrated superiority of one approach over another. Theoretical advantages of SIMV + PSV are greater patient comfort (and less dys-synchrony) and lower mean airway pressures.

There is no overall outcome superiority to targeting breaths to a set pressure or as set volume. In most patients the choice is not important, but some patients breathe more comfortably or have better gas exchange using one or the other. This is often influenced by the characteristics and settings of the ventilator. For example, pressure targeted modes usually (unless able to be set otherwise) deliver their maximum inspiratory flow at the start of inspiration, so as to achieve the set pressure as quickly as possible. However, the same effect can be generated by many ventilators in volume-targeted modes by increasing the maximal flow rate, or changing to a decelerating flow pattern. Without such modifications to volume-targeted modes, there is some older trial evidence that pressure-targeted modes produce better gas distribution, improved synchrony and earlier extubation. Maximal early inspiratory flow maximises gas transfer and may be more comfortable for 'air hungry' patients, but equally may trigger pulmonary inspiratory-off receptors producing a sensation of dyspnoea. The best advice is to choose one mode for most patients in order to maximise staff familiarity, but try the other if synchrony or gas exchange is suboptimal.

Many modern ventilators can sense respiratory effort and compliance breath-to-breath or within a single breath, allowing them to adjust pressure applied such that the targeted tidal volume is achieved with the patient generating as much of the driving pressure as possible. Ventilator manufacturers have a confusing array of names for such "dual control modes" including AutoFlow (Drager), VC+ (Puritan Bennett) and PRVC (Siemens). There is no trial evidence that such modes improve patient outcome, but such trials are difficult to perform and there is seemingly no disadvantage to using these modes if they are available.

Bi-level positive airway pressure (BIPAP, Bi-Vent, BiPhasic, DuoPAP) cycles between a high and low pressure (typically 20 and 5 cmH2O) at a rate that achieves a desired minute volume, but supports extra spontaneous breaths at both the high and low pressures with pressure support. A variant of this is Airway Pressure Release Ventilation (APRV), which differs only in that the time spent at the higher pressure is much greater than that at the lower pressure (around 5:1). Theoretically these modes improve oxygenation by alveolar recruitment while allowing greater patient comfort than a conventional mode with the same mean airway pressure. They have no advantage over pressure-targeted ACV or SIMV + PSV in a patient taking no spontaneous breaths.

Another method of increasing the mean airway pressure using "conventional" ACV or SIMV + PSV, is inverse ratio ventilation. Using this method the inspiratory phase is set longer than expiration; this technique has not convincingly been found to improve oxygenation or outcome.

How Should the Patient with Worsening Lung Compliance Be Managed?

Muscle Relaxants

A randomised controlled trial of 340 patients with early (<48 h from onset) ARDS found muscle relaxation with cis-atracurium for 48 h improved the adjusted 90-day survival and ventilator-free days without increasing muscle weakness

[40]. This is the only large study supporting this strategy, but given the failure of many other treatments for ARDS, muscle relaxation should be strongly considered, especially in patients with early deterioration.

Recruitment Manoeuvres

Recruitment manoeuvres to reduce atelectasis are theoretically appealing but presently lack strong trial evidence. Muscle relaxation, with adequate sedation, is often required for maximal effectiveness and tolerability. One approach, a "staircase" recruitment manoeuvre currently being evaluated in the PHARLAP trial [41], involves a starting pressure control ventilation with plateau <30 cmH2O, tidal volume <6 ml/kg, PEEP 15 cmH2O and FiO2 such that SpO2 is 90–92 %; the PEEP is increased in 5 cmH20 increments every 2 min to a maximum of 40 cmH2O; discontinuing if this precipitates hypotension, then reduced to 25, 22.5, 20, 17.5 and 15 cmH2O, ceasing reduction if there is a drop in the SpO2 of 1 % from the maximum achieved. A graphical representation of this strategy is shown in Fig. 9.2. The manoeuvre ideally increases lung compliance, requiring adjustment of pressure control settings to achieve the same tidal volume as was present at baseline. A pilot study of this technique found it was associated with reduced pro-inflammatory cytokines and better lung compliance and oxygenation. This, or similar, protocols are therefore recommended in patients with worsening respiratory function.

What Strategies Are There for the Patient Who Develops Refractory Hypoxaemia?

Figure 9.3 shows a suggested strategy for escalation of respiratory support in patients with worsening hypoxaemia.

Worsening gas exchange on conventional ventilation

Simple interventions:
- Change from pressure target to volume target, or vice versa
- Increase PEEP from 5 to 10 or 15 cmH2O (titration to oxygenation is the simplest approach; alternatives are listed in the text)
- Chest physiotherapy
- Suction secretions +/- bronchoscopy
- Diuresis to euvolaemia / mild hypovolaemia

Consider hydrocortisone 50mg IV 6 hourly, noting equivocal evidence of mortality benefit, and the current practice of most intensivists not to use corticosteroids in this circumstance.

Muscle relaxation e.g. with cis-atracurium 15 mg IV bolus followed by a continuous infusion of 37.5 mg/h for 48 h.

Recruitment manoeuvre, such as that outlined in Fig 9.2

Prone position ventilation

Options:
- If possible, transfer to a hospital capable of providing ECMO (ideally before ECMO is actually required, although transfer after initiating ECMO at the referring hospital is possible for experienced ECMO retrieval teams.
- Consider ECCOR
- Consider VA or VV ECMO

FIGURE 9.3 Algorithm for managing ventilated patients with lung injury and worsening hypoxaemia

Inhaled Nitric Oxide

This increases oxygenation in some ARDS patients, but convincingly does not improve mortality regardless of the degree of hypoxia [42]. It should not be used.

High-Frequency Oscillatory Ventilation (HFOV)

In early ARDS, <2 weeks from onset of respiratory symptoms, the use of HFOV was associated with a significantly higher (47 % vs. 35 %) mortality than conventional low tidal volume ventilation [43]. Although the trial did not concentrate on patients with life-threatening refractory hypoxia, this increased mortality has led many ICUs to abandon this technique. If used, it should only be employed by those experienced in its use and discontinued should the patient worsen.

Prone Position Ventilation

Prone positioning of patients with severe ARDS significantly decreased 28 and 90 day mortality [44], and so is strongly recommended in general ICU patients. Patients with isolated chest trauma should be able to be positioned prone, and even multi-trauma patients can be successfully treated in this manner [45].

Extra Corporeal CO2 Removal (ECCOR)

Partial lung support using low-impact pump driven venovenous extracorporeal CO_2 removal (ECCOR) devices with relatively small access cannulae to facilitate very low tidal volume (3 ml/kg) ventilation has shown promise in several case series [46], including in military patients injured in the Afghanistan campaign. ECCOR should be strongly considered if the equipment is available.

Extra Corporeal Membrane Oxygenation (ECMO)

The CESAR trial showed transfer of patients with severe respiratory failure to an ECMO centre improved survival without severe disability [47]. The applicability of veno-venous ECMO to trauma patients is often questioned due to the usual requirement for systemic heparinisation, but modern heparin-bonded circuits, allowing minimal or briefly no systemic anticoagulation and careful patient selection at one centre, shows that ECMO should at least be considered as a rescue therapy [48].

What Other Elements of Management Are Important in Ventilated Trauma Patients?

Fluid Strategy

The FACTT trial in 1000 ARDS or lung injury patients compared a "liberal" fluid arm targeting CVP 14 mmHg or PAOP 18 mmHg, which resulted in a +6 L fluid balance over 7 days, with a "conservative" strategy that targeted CVP ≤ 8 mmHg or PAOP 12 mmHg, which resulted in a neutral fluid balance over the same period [49]. Less fluid was associated with better oxygenation and more days free of mechanical ventilation without producing adverse cardiovascular or renal effects. Therefore, patients with (and probably at risk of) ARDS, should not be allowed to become fluid overloaded; consider compensating for an initial 24 h of fluid resuscitation with subsequent active diuresis.

Humidification

Humidification of inspired gases is required to reduce heat loss, prevent occlusion of the endotracheal tube by secretions, and avert respiratory mucosal ulceration. The performance and durability of passive heat-moisture exchangers vary considerably. One study found only 37.5 % produced an absolute humidity above the 30 mgH2O/L required to ensure a low risk

of tube occlusion in most patients. Active humidification produces still higher water content and is indicated for patients
with bloody respiratory secretions, tenacious sputum, or those
whose secretions frequently contaminate a passive HME [50].

Chest Physiotherapy

Chest physiotherapy is essential in thoracic trauma, with an
emphasis on deep or positive-pressure assisted inspirations,
to assist pulmonary toilet. There is some, albeit imperfect,
evidence that closed tracheal suctioning is superior to open
suctioning in reducing the incidence of Ventilator Associated
Pneumonia (VAP) [51].

Prophylactic Antibiotics

Noting substantial controversy, including guidelines to the
contrary from the Eastern Association for the Surgery of
Trauma, a meta-analysis of five high-quality trials found
prophylactic antibiotics in patients with blunt or penetrating
trauma who required an intercostal catheter, in comparison
to placebo, reduced the incidence of empyema and pneumonia [52]. Therefore, antibiotics should be considered for all
patients immediately after insertion of an intercostal catheter. If an antibiotic is to be used, Cefazolin or Co-Amoxiclav
for 24 h is a reasonable choice.

How Can the Risk of Ventilator-Associated Pneumonia (VAP) Be Reduced?

VAP is common, occurring in 9–27 % of ventilated patients,
with a higher incidence in chest trauma [53]. Interventions
that reduce VAP include:

- Sitting the patient 30° head-up.
- Small bowel, as opposed to gastric, feeding.

- Endotracheal tubes with a suction port that allows aspiration of subglottic secretions
- Selective decontamination of the digestive tract with antibiotics and topical oral antiseptics

What Are the Indications for Antibiotics in the Treatment of Suspected VAP?

VAP can be particularly difficult to separate from non-infectious causes of respiratory deterioration and systemic inflammation. Using post-mortem examination as the gold standard, clinical criteria alone have a sensitivity of only 69 % and specificity of 75 %. The Clinical Pulmonary Infection Score (CPIS), shown in Table 9.1, combining clinical, radio-

TABLE 9.1 The Clinical Pulmonary Infection Score (CPIS)

Parameter	Value	Score
Temperature (°C)	36.5–38.4	0
	38.5–38.9	1
	≤35 or 39	2
White cell count (cells/mm^2)	4000–11,000	0
	<4000 or >11,000	1
	≥500 band cells	2
Tracheal secretions	None	0
	Mild/non-purulent	1
	Purulent	2
Chest radiograph (excluding pulmonary oedema and ARDS)	No infiltrate	0
	Diffuse/patchy infiltrate	1
	Localised infiltrate	2
Endotracheal aspirate culture	No or mild growth	0
	Moderate or florid growth	1
	Moderate or florid growth AND pathogen consistent with Gram stain	2
PaO2/FiO2	>240 or ARDS	0
	≤240 and absence of ARDS	2

graphic and laboratory results, is commonly used, but has been criticised for having a low sensitivity and specificity with a diagnostic cut off of 6 [54]. In practice, most clinicians institute antibiotics for VAP when a patient's condition deteriorates and several of the types of features shown in Table 9.1 are present.

Antibiotic selection for VAP depends heavily on local microbiological flora, but in general, onset within the first 4 days of ventilation can often be treated with narrow spectrum agents if an organism is cultured, whereas late VAP is often polymicrobial and due to resistant organisms, requiring broad-spectrum coverage. A safe duration of therapy is 8 days, but there is an increasing trend to even shorter courses if clinical resolution is rapid.

How Should the Patient Be Weaned from Mechanical Ventilation?

The conventional approach to ventilator weaning is to lighten sedation and opioid analgesia as soon as possible and to change from a mandatory rate breathing mode (ACV or SIMV + PSV) to PSV alone. The initial PEEP and pressure support should be the same as that which has been required to deliver mandatory breaths of a satisfactory volume. There is no set recipe for reducing PEEP, pressure support and FiO2; most clinicians change one at a time and observe the effect before altering another.

In the weaning phase while supported on PSV alone, it is common for patients to take variable tidal volumes, some or all of which may be above the 6 ml/kg IBW recommended when delivering a mandatory rate and volume/pressure. There is no evidence that reducing the pressure support in an attempt to reduce tidal volume to 6 ml/kg in this circumstance is beneficial. Indeed, doing so may cause tachypnoea and/or patient distress. PSV should be titrated to patient comfort and respiratory rate rather than an arbitrary tidal volume.

Patients with good gas exchange and strong respiratory effort can be extubated directly from PSV. Typically (in a 70 kg adult) this would not be attempted until an $FiO2 \leq 40\%$, $PEEP \leq 8$ cmH2O, pressure support ≤ 10 cmH2O produces a respiratory rate <20, TV > 6–8 ml/kg, and forced vital capacity >1 L. Various indices and scores (such as the Rapid Shallow Breathing Index [frequency/tidal volume] <65) attempt to predict successful extubation, but many clinicians believe overall clinical impression is more accurate.

An alternative to extubation is to trial a period of no ventilator support, with the patient breathing humidified oxygen through the endotracheal tube. The resistance of the tube imposes a higher work of breathing than is normal once extubated, so if a patient passes this test logic suggests extubation should be safe. However, requiring this extra effort before permitting extubation potentially needlessly prolongs intubation. It is not recommended for most patients.

Adaptive Support Ventilation (ASV) uses an algorithm based on patient sex and height to determine desired minute volume (input as a % of that predicted), adjusting both tidal volume and rate to minimise work of breathing and maximise the proportion of inspiratory effort made by the patient. There is limited trial evidence that this hastens liberation from mechanical ventilation [55].

What Other Aspects of Patient Care Assist Ventilator Weaning?

Approaches known to hasten extubation include:

- Exercise, either in bed or by mobilisation with appropriate support.
- Using an opioid-analgesia-first, delirium treatment, and minimal sedation regimen.
- Daily complete cessation of all sedatives, with re-titration if necessary, is one effective method of minimising sedative use.
- Avoidance of longer-acting sedatives in favour of propofol, dexmedetomidine or remifentanil.

When Should a Tracheostomy Be Inserted?

- The TRACMAN trial found no mortality or length of stay benefit from early (within 4 days) vs. late (after 10 days if still indicated) tracheostomy in patients anticipated to require at least 7 more days of mechanical ventilation [56]. Nearly all patients randomised to early tracheostomy had one inserted, whereas this was true of only 45 % of patients in the late group. In most patients, therefore, insertion of tracheostomy can be safely delayed until after day 10 of mechanical ventilation. The advantages of a tracheostomy at around this time include a reduced sedation requirement, better pulmonary toilet, and a reduced chance of long-term complications of trans-laryngeal intubation such as subglottic stenosis and vocal cord damage.

How Should a Patient Be Weaned from Ventilation Through a Tracheostomy?

A tracheostomy is less of a noxious stimulus than a trans-laryngeal tube, meaning that almost all tracheostomy patients can discontinue all sedatives. This allows more gradual weaning from mechanical ventilation than with an endotracheal tube, allowing the patient to progressively regain respiratory muscle strength. Various tracheostomy weaning options include:

- Progressive gradual reduction in pressure support and PEEP
- Periods off all mechanical support, with humidified oxygen provided either by a T-piece, "trache shield" or "Swedish nose" (heat/moisture exchanger) attached to the tracheostomy. A suggested programme is 10 min off mechanical support every 2–4 h, with increases to 20, 30, and 60 min off support over a period of days. Faster weaning in a co-operative interactive patient can be achieved by allowing unsupported ventilation to persist as long as tolerated, with 2–6 h periods of rest in between. Care must

be taken not to exhaust the patient, as this reduces strength in subsequent spontaneous breathing periods. Initially these approaches occur during waking hours, with a full night of comfortable unsupported breathing being the ultimate goal.

What Special Techniques Might Be Applied to a Patient with a Bronchopleural Fistula?

The primary treatment of a bronchopleural fistula is an intercostal catheter to avert development of a tension pneumothorax. Positive pressure ventilation increases gas leak through a bronchopleural fistula and probably delays the chance of spontaneous resolution. Therefore, the positive pressure applied to the bronchopleural fistula should be minimised. Approaches include simply minimising mean and peak airway pressures by prolonging inspiratory time and reducing minute volume, tolerating hypercapnia, selective lung ventilation using a double-lumen tube and two ventilators or transiently occluding the main bronchus on the affected side with a bronchial blocker. If the fistula is large or has not resolved after several days, an anatomic wedge or non-anatomic partial lung resection may be indicated.

What Can Be Done to Assist Ventilator Weaning in a Patient with Metabolic Alkalosis?

Metabolic alkalosis is not uncommon in patients with chest trauma and acute lung injury, as diuretics, which may cause loss of $H+$ ions, are often prescribed to achieve a neutral or negative fluid balance. The respiratory compensation for metabolic alkalosis is hypoventilation, such that increased CO_2 returns pH towards 7.40. A stimulus to hypoventilation can obviously impede weaning from mechanical ventilation. Acetazolamide (500 mg enteral bd), is a useful treatment that takes 24–48 h to manifest an effect.

References

1. Maron BJ, Estes III NA, Link MS. Task Force 11: commotio cordis. J Am Coll Cardiol. 2005;45(8):1371–3.
2. Liman ST, Kuzucu A, Tastepe AI, Ulasan GN, Topcu S. Chest injury due to blunt trauma. Eur J Cardiothorac Surg. 2003;23(3):374–8.
3. Shorr RM, Crittenden M, Indeck M, Hartunian SL, Rodriguez A. Blunt thoracic trauma. Analysis of 515 patients. Ann Surg. 1987;206(2):200–5.
4. deLesquen H, Avaro JP, Gust L, Ford RM, Beranger F, Natale C, et al. Surgical management for the first 48 h following blunt chest trauma: state of the art (excluding vascular injuries). Interact Cardiovasc Thorac Surg. 2015;20(3):399–408.
5. Lerer LB, Knottenbelt JD. Preventable mortality following sharp penetrating chest trauma. J Trauma. 1994;37(1):9–12.
6. Demirhan R, Onan B, Oz K, Halezeroglu S. Comprehensive analysis of 4205 patients with chest trauma: a 10-year experience. Interact Cardiovasc Thorac Surg. 2009;9(3):450–3.
7. Khan MS, Bilal A. A prospective study of penetrating chest trauma and evaluation of role of thoracotomy. J Postgraduate Med Institute. 2004;18(1):33–9.
8. Cohn SM. Pulmonary contusion: review of the clinical entity. J Trauma. 1997;42(5):973–9.
9. Champion HR. A profile of combat injury. J Trauma. 2003;54: S13–9.
10. Onat S, Ulku R, Avci A, Ates G, Ozcelik C. Urgent thoracotomy for penetrating chest trauma: analysis of 158 patients of a single center. Injury. 2011;42(9):900–4.
11. Nagarsheth K, Kurek S. Ultrasound detection of pneumothorax compared with chest X-ray and computed tomography scan. Am Surg. 2011;77(4):480–4.
12. Blaivas M, Lyon M, Duggal S. A prospective comparison of supine chest radiography and bedside ultrasound for the diagnosis of traumatic pneumothorax. Acad Emerg Med. 2005;12(9): 844–9.
13. Rodriguez RM, Anglin D, Langdorf MI, Baumann BM, Hendey GW, Bradley RN, et al. NEXUS chest: validation of a decision instrument for selective chest imaging in blunt trauma. JAMA Surg. 2013;148(10):940–6.
14. Ball CG, Wyrzykowski AD, Kirkpatrick AW, Dente CJ, Nicholas JM, Salomone JP, et al. Thoracic needle decompression for

tension pneumothorax: clinical correlation with catheter length. Can J Surg. 2010;53(3):184–8.

15. Morales CH, Mejia C, Roldan LA, Saldarriaga MF, Duque AF. Negative pleural suction in thoracic trauma patients: a randomized controlled trial. J Trauma Acute Care Surg. 2014;77(2): 251–5.

16. Mowery NT, Gunter OL, Collier BR, Diaz Jr JJ, Haut E, Hildreth A, et al. Practice management guidelines for management of hemothorax and occult pneumothorax. J Trauma. 2011;70(2):510–8.

17. Dehghan N, de Mestral C, McKee MD, Schemitsch EH, Nathens A. Flail chest injuries: a review of outcomes and treatment practices from the National Trauma Data Bank. J Trauma Acute Care Surg. 2014;76(2):462–8.

18. Leinicke JA, Elmore L, Freeman BD, Colditz GA. Operative management of rib fractures in the setting of flail chest: a systematic review and meta-analysis. Ann Surg. 2013;258(6): 914–21.

19. Ashbaugh DG, Bigelow DB, Petty TL, Levine BE. Acute respiratory distress in adults. Lancet. 1967;2(7511):319–23.

20. Ranieri VM, Rubenfeld GD, Thompson BT, Ferguson ND, Caldwell E, Fan E, et al. Acute respiratory distress syndrome: the Berlin Definition. JAMA. 2012;307(23):2526–33.

21. Miller PR, Croce MA, Kilgo PD, Scott J, Fabian TC. Acute respiratory distress syndrome in blunt trauma: identification of independent risk factors. Am Surg. 2002;68(10):845–50.

22. Bakowitz M, Bruns B, McCunn M. Acute lung injury and the acute respiratory distress syndrome in the injured patient. Scand J Trauma Resusc Emerg Med. 2012;20:54.

23. Perl M, Lomas-Neira J, Venet F, Chung CS, Ayala A. Pathogenesis of indirect (secondary) acute lung injury. Expert Rev Respir Med. 2011;5(1):115–26.

24. Boyle AJ, Mac SR, McAuley DF. Pharmacological treatments in ARDS; a state-of-the-art update. BMC Med. 2013;11:166.

25. Matthay MA, Brower RG, Carson S, Douglas IS, Eisner M, Hite D, et al. Randomized, placebo-controlled clinical trial of an aerosolized beta(2)-agonist for treatment of acute lung injury. Am J Respir Crit Care Med. 2011;184(5):561–8.

26. Gao SF, Perkins GD, Gates S, Young D, McAuley DF, Tunnicliffe W, et al. Effect of intravenous beta-2 agonist treatment on clinical outcomes in acute respiratory distress syndrome (BALTI-2): a multicentre, randomised controlled trial. Lancet. 2012;379(9812): 229–35.

27. Miller AC, Elamin EM, Suffredini AF. Inhaled anticoagulation regimens for the treatment of smoke inhalation-associated acute lung injury: a systematic review. Crit Care Med. 2014;42(2): 413–9.

28. McAuley DF, Laffey JG, O'Kane CM, Perkins GD, Mullan B, Trinder TJ, et al. Simvastatin in the acute respiratory distress syndrome. N Engl J Med. 2014;371(18):1695–703.

29. Truwit JD, Bernard GR, Steingrub J, Matthay MA, Liu KD, Albertson TE, et al. Rosuvastatin for sepsis-associated acute respiratory distress syndrome. N Engl J Med. 2014;370(23): 2191–200.

30. Peter JV, John P, Graham PL, Moran JL, George IA, Bersten A. Corticosteroids in the prevention and treatment of acute respiratory distress syndrome (ARDS) in adults: meta-analysis. BMJ. 2008;336(7651):1006–9.

31. Annane D, Sebille V, Bellissant E. Effect of low doses of corticosteroids in septic shock patients with or without early acute respiratory distress syndrome. Crit Care Med. 2006;34(1): 22–30.

32. Meduri GU, Golden E, Freire AX, Taylor E, Zaman M, Carson SJ, et al. Methylprednisolone infusion in early severe ARDS results of a randomized controlled trial. 2007. Chest. 2009;136(5 Suppl):e30.

33. Steinberg KP, Hudson LD, Goodman RB, Hough CL, Lanken PN, Hyzy R, et al. Efficacy and safety of corticosteroids for persistent acute respiratory distress syndrome. N Engl J Med. 2006;354(16):1671–84.

34. Duggal A, Perez P, Golan E, Tremblay L, Sinuff T. Safety and efficacy of noninvasive ventilation in patients with blunt chest trauma: a systematic review. Crit Care. 2013;17(4):R142.

35. Ventilation with lower tidal volumes as compared with traditional tidal volumes for acute lung injury and the acute respiratory distress syndrome. The Acute Respiratory Distress Syndrome Network. N Engl J Med. 2000;342(18):1301–8.

36. Curley G, Hayes M, Laffey JG. Can 'permissive' hypercapnia modulate the severity of sepsis-induced ALI/ARDS? Crit Care. 2011;15(2):212.

37. Futier E, Constantin JM, Paugam-Burtz C, Pascal J, Eurin M, Neuschwander A, et al. A trial of intraoperative low-tidal-volume ventilation in abdominal surgery. N Engl J Med. 2013;369(5):428–37.

38. Gattinoni L, Caironi P, Cressoni M, Chiumello D, Ranieri VM, Quintel M, et al. Lung recruitment in patients with the acute

respiratory distress syndrome. N Engl J Med. 2006;354(17): 1775–86.

39. Briel M, Meade M, Mercat A, Brower RG, Talmor D, Walter SD, et al. Higher vs lower positive end-expiratory pressure in patients with acute lung injury and acute respiratory distress syndrome: systematic review and meta-analysis. JAMA. 2010;303(9):865–73.

40. Papazian L, Forel JM, Gacouin A, Penot-Ragon C, Perrin G, Loundou A, et al. Neuromuscular blockers in early acute respiratory distress syndrome. N Engl J Med. 2010;363(12):1107–16.

41. Hodgson CL, Tuxen DV, Davies AR, Bailey MJ, Higgins AM, Holland AE, et al. A randomised controlled trial of an open lung strategy with staircase recruitment, titrated PEEP and targeted low airway pressures in patients with acute respiratory distress syndrome. Crit Care. 2011;15(3):R133.

42. Adhikari NK, Dellinger RP, Lundin S, Payen D, Vallet B, Gerlach H, et al. Inhaled nitric oxide does not reduce mortality in patients with acute respiratory distress syndrome regardless of severity: systematic review and meta-analysis. Crit Care Med. 2014;42(2):404–12.

43. Ferguson ND, Cook DJ, Guyatt GH, Mehta S, Hand L, Austin P, et al. High-frequency oscillation in early acute respiratory distress syndrome. N Engl J Med. 2013;368(9):795–805.

44. Guerin C, Reignier J, Richard JC, Beuret P, Gacouin A, Boulain T, et al. Prone positioning in severe acute respiratory distress syndrome. N Engl J Med. 2013;368(23):2159–68.

45. Voggenreiter G, Neudeck F, Aufmkolk M, Fassbinder J, Hirche H, Obertacke U, et al. Intermittent prone positioning in the treatment of severe and moderate posttraumatic lung injury. Crit Care Med. 1999;27(11):2375–82.

46. Morimont P, Batchinsky A, Lambermont B. Update on the role of extracorporeal CO_2 removal as an adjunct to mechanical ventilation in ARDS. Crit Care. 2015;19(1):117.

47. Peek GJ, Mugford M, Tiruvoipati R, Wilson A, Allen E, Thalanany MM, et al. Efficacy and economic assessment of conventional ventilatory support versus extracorporeal membrane oxygenation for severe adult respiratory failure (CESAR): a multicentre randomised controlled trial. Lancet. 2009;374(9698): 1351–63.

48. Ried M, Bein T, Philipp A, Muller T, Graf B, Schmid C, et al. Extracorporeal lung support in trauma patients with severe chest injury and acute lung failure: a 10-year institutional experience. Crit Care. 2013;17(3):R110.

49. Wiedemann HP, Wheeler AP, Bernard GR, Thompson BT, Hayden D, de Boisblanc B, et al. Comparison of two fluid-management strategies in acute lung injury. N Engl J Med. 2006;354(24):2564–75.
50. Gross JL, Park GR. Humidification of inspired gases during mechanical ventilation. Minerva Anestesiol. 2012;78(4): 496–502.
51. Kuriyama A, Umakoshi N, Fujinaga J, Takada T. Impact of closed versus open tracheal suctioning systems for mechanically ventilated adults: a systematic review and meta-analysis. Intensive Care Med. 2015;41(3):402–11.
52. Sanabria A, Valdivieso E, Gomez G, Echeverry G. Prophylactic antibiotics in chest trauma: a meta-analysis of high-quality studies. World J Surg. 2006;30(10):1843–7.
53. Kalanuria AA, Zai W, Mirski M. Ventilator-associated pneumonia in the ICU. Crit Care. 2014;18(2):208.
54. Schurink CA, Van Nieuwenhoven CA, Jacobs JA, Rozenberg-Arska M, Joore HC, Buskens E, et al. Clinical pulmonary infection score for ventilator-associated pneumonia: accuracy and inter-observer variability. Intensive Care Med. 2004;30(2): 217–24.
55. Kirakli C, Naz I, Ediboglu O, Tatar D, Budak A, Tellioglu E. A randomized controlled trial comparing the ventilation duration between Adaptive Support Ventilation and Pressure Assist/Control Ventilation in medical ICU patients. Chest. 2015; 147:1503–9.
56. Young D, Harrison DA, Cuthbertson BH, Rowan K. Effect of early vs late tracheostomy placement on survival in patients receiving mechanical ventilation: the TracMan randomized trial. JAMA. 2013;309(20):2121–9.

Chapter 10
Management of Blast Related Injuries

Emrys Kirkman and Michael C. Reade

Abstract Blast related injuries are common in military conflict and can also result from action by terrorist groups against civilian targets. The pattern of injury depends on the type of explosive, with high explosives capable of causing unique effects through the action of the blast wave. The environment is critically important in determining the effects of blast injury, with blast in enclosed spaces or underwater magnifying the

E. Kirkman, OBE, PhD (✉)
Defence Science and Technology Laboratory, Porton Down,
Salisbury SP4 0JQ, UK
e-mail: EKIRKMAN@mail.dstl.gov.uk

M.C. Reade, MBBS, MPH, DPhil, FANZCA, FCICM
Joint Health Command, Australian Defence Force,
Canberra, ACT 2610, Australia

The Burns, Trauma and Critical Care Research Centre,
University of Queensland and Royal Brisbane and
Women's Hospital, Brisbane, QLD 4029, Australia

S.D. Hutchings (ed.), *Trauma and Combat Critical Care
in Clinical Practice*, In Clinical Practice,
DOI 10.1007/978-3-319-28758-4_10,
© Crown Copyright 2016

effect of blast wave force transmission. Blasts can also cause ballistic injury by energising projectiles, blunt trauma from structural collapse, and thermal and toxic injuries. "Blast Lung" is imprecisely defined but results from damage at the alveolar capillary interface with the predominant feature being pulmonary haemorrhage. Death is most commonly caused by severe cardiovascular impairment resulting from arterial gas embolism. The incidence of severe respiratory failure in survivors of blast injury is probably quite low. Management is essential supportive and similar to that applied to other forms of lung injury in critically injured patients. Attention should be paid to lung protective ventilation and a conservative fluid management strategy. Specific novel therapies such as pro or anti- coagulants and steroids remain unproven.

Keywords   Blast injury • Blast lung • ARDS • Pulmonary haemorrhage • High explosives • Military conflict • Trauma • Critical illness

Introduction

Recent military conflicts have highlighted the importance of injuries caused by blast, although the frequent use of high explosive by terrorist organisations means that these injuries are not limited to the military population. Although many blast related injuries from the recent conflict in Afghanistan involved severe damage to the lower extremities, the additional effects of thoracic blast can produce clinical features which are unusual and sometimes unique. In this chapter we discuss blast related injury with a particular focus on the thoracic and pulmonary effects.

What Is an Explosive?

An explosive is a substance that, once initiated, is capable of rapid, self-propagating, decomposition into gaseous products with violent release of energy in the form of pressure and heat. Explosives are commonly divided into "high" and "low" explosives. There is no clear dividing line between these categories but as a generalisation it is said that a high explosive "detonates" while a low explosive "deflagrates" (i.e. burns). This distinction relates to the rate at which the chemical reaction (which forms the front at which the material decomposes) travels through the explosive material. In a high explosive this front, known as a detonation wave, travels through the material at, or higher than, the speed of sound, while in a low explosive the decomposition front travels subsonically. An example of a high explosive is TNT (trinitrotoluene), while a low explosive is exemplified by black powder (or gunpowder).

The vast majority of clinical reports of blast trauma are based on injuries resulting from the detonation of high explosives. Far fewer experimental studies are based on high explosives, in part because of the difficulties associated with conducting experimental studies using high explosives. Many experimental studies of the medical/biological consequences of explosive injuries utilise components of an explosion such as those generated using equipment like "shock tubes". This latter approach can be very informative when attempting to study specific elements of explosive injury. However, care must be taken to avoid over-interpretation of the results as they often lack the interaction between injury modalities that are important in the overall clinical picture.

How Do Explosives Cause Injury?

Injuries from explosions are complex and usually consist of several parts that are defined according to the component of the explosion that caused them [1]. To understand these injuries we must therefore consider the component parts of an explosion and how they interact with the body.

When an explosive detonates it generates an extremely rapid increase in pressure in the immediate vicinity of the explosion; this rise in pressure is almost instantaneous with a rise time of a few microseconds. With conventional explosives, the pressure rise at a static point lasts only a few milliseconds.

"Enhanced" blast munitions prolong this elevated pressure to amplify force transmission. The wave of pressure (called the 'peak overpressure') travels outwards at supersonic velocities. This is called the 'shock wave'. However, the magnitude of the peak overpressure declines rapidly as it travels away from the site of the explosion. Because of this rapid decay of the peak overpressure, the incidence of injuries amongst survivors from this particular element of an explosion in a free field is low because the victim needs to be relatively close to the explosion to receive a sufficient "dose" of shock wave to cause damage. However, a shock wave can be amplified when it encounters a reflecting surface (such as a wall that does not collapse when exposed to the wave), and can reverberate within a confined space. Fluid transmits the shock wave more efficiently than air. Consequently, the incidence of injuries due to shock waves are much higher if the casualties are near reflecting surfaces, within enclosed spaces, or underwater.

As the shock wave produced by conventional explosives is a very brief event it does not cause the casualty to move any great distance; this is not the part of the explosion that 'throws things around'. The shock wave can, however, cause serious injury defined as 'primary blast injuries'. These are almost, but not completely, unique to injuries caused by explosions. Gas containing organs are particularly susceptible, and traditionally the lungs, bowel and ears have been areas of medical concern.

Fragments of the munition casing, pre-formed fragments contained within the device and surrounding debris energized by the explosion, are propelled outwards and can collide with the casualty. Injuries from these fragments and debris are defined as 'secondary blast injury' which essentially are conventional blunt and penetrating injuries resulting in tissue damage and haemorrhage.

In addition, the explosion gives rise to a very large volume of hot gas. This literally pushes air and debris outwards, causing more projectile hazards, and acts over a sufficiently long time course to physically throw casualties against other objects, causing blunt injuries classified as 'tertiary blast injuries'. This movement of air is called the 'blast wind'. The shock wave and the blast wind are sometimes collectively (but confusingly) called the 'blast wave'.

Other injuries which include burns, responses to toxic chemicals associated with the blast and exaggerated inflammatory responses fall into quaternary and quinary categories [1, 2]. Table 10.1 summarises these categories of blast injury.

A victim of explosive injury is therefore likely to suffer a mixture of these blast-related injuries. Secondary blast injuries account for the majority of injuries in survivors, particularly when the explosion has occurred in an open space. A clinically significant minority of the seriously injured survivors also exhibit blast lung, which is described in detail later in this chapter. When the explosion occurs in a confined space the proportion of seriously injured survivors exhibiting blast lung increases dramatically [4, 5] because the shock wave can be amplified and reflected near solid structures, increasing exposure. We are therefore faced with a casualty who is likely to have extensive tissue damage and severe blood loss, and in

TABLE 10.1 Classification and nature of the components of blast injuries

Category	Cause
Primary	Shock wave causing injuries particularly in gas containing organs such as lung and bowel, but possibly in other organs such as brain
Secondary	Ballistic wounds from primary fragments (from the device) and secondary fragments (from the environment). Penetrating and blunt injuries.
Tertiary	Blast wave propels individuals onto other structures. Mainly blunt injuries.
Quaternary	Other explosion-related injuries, illnesses or disease
Quinary	Injuries resulting from specific additives such as bacteria and radiation ("dirty bombs")

Adapted from Champion et al. [3]

a proportion of these casualties, blast lung resulting in varying degrees of respiratory failure.

The mechanisms of injury outlined in this section are based on those expected from exposure to high-explosives and these must be distinguished from the low explosive events that are much more common in civilian practice: for example explosion of fireworks, a fuel/air mixture from an domestic gas bottle opened in an enclosed space, or when the vapour inside a liquid fuel tank ignites. Despite the high level of suspicion amongst clinicians treating such patients, there are almost no published reports of blast wave damage to the lung in these circumstances. Although pulmonary complications commonly ensue, these are usually explained by inhalation of heated or toxic gases or the ARDS that can develop after extensive burns.

What Is Blast Lung?

Blast lung is a primary blast injury that is characterised by pulmonary contusion and the rapid development of pulmonary oedema, with a consequent reduction in pulmonary gas transfer [6, 7]. The shock wave causes an immediate lung injury involving rupture of alveolar capillaries, the influx of blood, and extravasation of oedema fluid into lung tissue [8, 9] giving rise to haemorrhagic foci which can be substantial. The intrapulmonary haemorrhage and oedema contribute to the initial respiratory compromise in blast lung [10]. The problem is exacerbated because free haemoglobin (Hb) from extravasated blood induces free radical reactions which can cause oxidative damage [10] and initiate/augment a pro-inflammatory response [11]. Free Hb also causes an accumulation of inflammatory mediators and chemotactic attractants [12] thereby amplifying the problem. The combined influence of pulmonary haemorrhage and oedema reduces pulmonary gas transfer and leads initially to hypoxaemia and, with worsening blast lung, hypercarbia.

Clinical Features of Blast Lung

Although blast lung can be defined as a pathophysiological entity, clinical classification is difficult as lung injury in critically ill trauma patients is almost always multi-factorial. There is no formal definition of blast lung in contrast, for example, to ARDS. The term generally refers to a spectrum of pulmonary effects that follow exposure to a blast wave. Clinical features can include:

- haemoptysis
- expectorated frothy sputum
- dyspnoea, hypoxia and hypercapnia
- subcutaneous emphysema
- retrosternal chest pain
- radiographic abnormalities. The classic chest radiograph appearance is a bilateral 'bats wing' perihilar infiltrate, although unilateral signs may be present if the patient has been oriented side-on to the blast wave. These features typically appear within a few hours, take 24–48 h to reach maximum intensity, and persist for 7–10 days. Pulmonary barotrauma can result in pneumothorax, haemothorax, pneumomediastinum, and surgical emphysema.

The tympanic membrane is the air/tissue interface most likely to be damaged by primary blast injury. This fact misleadingly suggested to some authors that examination of the tympanic membrane might be an effective screening tool to identify patients at risk of blast lung. Regrettably, several case series have shown convincingly that this is not the case. For example, of 647 survivors of explosions, 193 had primary blast injury of whom 18 (9.3 %) had no tympanic membrane perforation. One-forty-two had isolated tympanic membrane perforation with no lung injury [13]. The tympanic membranes of all blast survivors should be examined but the only initial management likely to be required is topical antibiotics. Seventy-five percent of blast-associated tympanic membrane perforations heal spontaneously. Those that have not healed by 8 weeks post injury should be referred for ENT opinion and management.

What Pathophysiological Changes Occur Following Thoracic Blast Exposure?

A number of experimental studies and clinical reports have indicated that primary blast injury to the thorax produces a characteristic triad comprising bradycardia, prolonged hypotension and apnoea followed by rapid shallow breathing [7].

The bradycardia and apnoea seen immediately after blast are both thought to be mediated by a vagal reflex [14, 15]. However, the aetiology of the hypotension seen after primary blast injury is more complex and appears to be due to a fall in peripheral resistance and cardiac output, the latter because of a myocardial impairment which can last many hours after blast injury [16]. Although the autonomic nervous system plays some part in the hypotension it is not solely responsible. Recent findings have suggested that primary blast injury causes a rapid release of the potent vasodilator nitric oxide (NO) from the pulmonary circulation [17–19], which could in theory lead to a systemic response that includes vasodilatation.

The combined effects of hypoxia and altered cardiovascular reflexes that follow thoracic blast exposure can have profound effects on the ability of the casualty to respond to concomitant or further events such as haemorrhage and resuscitation [20].

The immediate cause of death following primary blast injury, in the absence of obvious external injuries, has been the subject of much debate in the literature and a number of theories have been advocated [21–24]. Leaving aside deaths due to the total disruption of the body very close to the point of detonation [22] and secondary changes such as the development of ARDS and perforation peritonitis, the chief causes of death can be classified as respiratory and cardiovascular. Evidence for these phenomena comes almost exclusively from animal experimental work.

Cardiovascular Mortality

Generally it has been thought that death is secondary to obstruction of the pulmonary capillary bed [21–24] and a greatly dilated right ventricle is often found at post-mortem. Primary cardiac injury has also been implicated but evidence for commotio cordis or sufficient myocardial contusion as the immediate cause of death is scarce [21, 25].

Air embolism in blast injury is the result of air entering the circulation through the damaged alveoli. In animals dying within some minutes of blast injury, air is frequently found intravascularly [23]. The air bubbles are found, often in large quantities, and always in the arterial side of the circulation. Furthermore, air emboli are only found in animals that die rapidly after exposure and never in those animals that survive to be sacrificed [23]. Air is most commonly found in the coronary arteries, the left side of the heart and in brain vessels, especially the basilar vessels and in the choroid plexuses. Therefore, in some cases of immediately fatal primary blast injury, air emboli, especially of the coronary arteries, is likely to be the cause of death. Fat embolism as a cause of death has been suggested [26, 27] and refuted [21, 28] and the time course of haemorrhagic shock from disrupted solid organs is considered too slow to account for immediate death following blast injury.

Respiratory Mortality

In severe pulmonary blast injury there is massive pulmonary contusion and haemorrhage into the bronchial tree. A post mortem example from an animal exposed to blast injury is shown in Fig. 10.1. Bleeding is frequently observed through

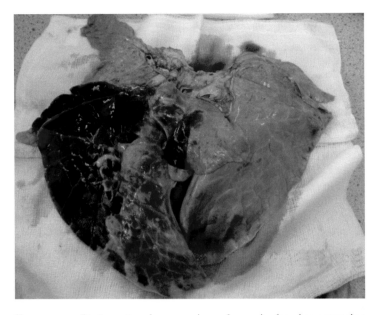

FIGURE 10.1 Post mortem lung specimen from pig showing extensive contusional changes soley resulting from blast exposure

the mouth and nose [29] and the experimental animals are seen to make a few, terminal, maximally forced respiratory movements for air as they suffocate in extravasated blood or fluid resulting from fulminant pulmonary oedema [21, 22, 30]. These observations suggest that there is no respiratory centre damage [21] as had originally been suggested by earlier workers [31].

The original view was that in animals that do not obstruct the airways with blood and froth, early pulmonary pathology is not usually sufficient to account for death [32, 33]. The development of pulmonary oedema supervening on a physiological shunt through non-aerated contused lung may disturb the pulmonary gas exchange sufficiently to be incompatible with life [33] Clemedson supported the view of

Benzinger [33] that respiratory symptoms are not the cause of death but are the consequence of the circulatory failure [34]. More recent studies conducted on rabbits (*Cernak I*, personal communication) have shown that the reflex apnoea can in some circumstances be sufficiently prolonged to cause death in studies conducted on anaesthetised rabbits. It is unknown whether this could be a cause of death in human casualties.

What Is the Incidence of Blast Lung in Survivors of a Blast Event?

As we have seen high-explosive blast commonly causes widespread damage to the lung and wider cardiovascular system. However, the most severely affected patients die almost immediately either from the cardio-respiratory effects of the blast itself, or from secondary or tertiary blast injury. The incidence of blast lung amongst patients who survive to hospital care is quite low and determined by the category of blast event (e.g. open space, closed space, underwater, associated with structural collapse) and type of explosive device (conventional vs. enhanced blast munition). Several studies support these statements:

- A study of published data of 3,357 victims of terrorist bombings found that of immediate fatalities, 47 % had post-mortem evidence of blast lung, while the incidence of blast lung in immediate survivors was only 0.6 % [35].
- A study of published data of 29 terrorist bombings involving 8,364 casualties analysed the incidence of pulmonary blast injury classified by blast event type and by severity [36]. As expected, a relatively high proportion (21 %) of survivors of blast in an enclosed space had some form of lung injury (including pneumothorax and pulmonary contusion), but only 16 % had "blast lung syndrome" (i.e. lung injury sufficiently severe to meet the criteria of ARDS or

require mechanical ventilation). In contrast, blast in open air only affected the lung in 7 % of survivors, with 5 % developing blast lung syndrome. Survivors of blast that caused structural collapse were even less likely to have lung involvement, with only 1 % developing blast lung syndrome.

- Of 107 patients admitted to a tertiary ICU after blast injury in Afghanistan 2008–2010, 13.1 % had "blast lung"; however, this cohort was a subset of 412 blast wound survivors, the remainder of whom survived without significant pulmonary complications. The incidence of blast lung in survivors was therefore 3.6 % [37].

Blast waves are more efficiently propagated through water than through air, while fragmentation and displacement are diminished. Consequently, underwater blast causes a much greater incidence of blast lung injury in initial survivors. For example, of 32 survivors of an Israeli destroyer sunk in 1967 who were subsequently exposed to the blast of a missile detonating in the water nearby, 27 (84 %) had blast lung injury [38].

Ballistic armour plates are effective in protecting the thorax against blast-fragmentation wounds to the chest. There is some evidence that by creating reflections of blast wave energy in close proximity to the chest, there is a small increase in the chance of primary blast wave injury when wearing body armour. However, the overall low incidence of blast lung quoted above in British troops from Afghanistan [37], nearly all of whom would have been wearing body armour, suggests the substantial benefit outweighs this theoretical risk.

The expected mortality of patients who survive to hospital admission meeting various definitions of "blast lung" is probably around 10 % [39]. Patients who survive hospital admission usually have no long term pulmonary consequences. A study of 11 blast survivors 1 year after injury found none had symptoms or appreciable signs, and most had normal tests of lung function [40].

How Should Blast Lung Injury Be Managed?

The pathogenesis of blast lung is quite different to that of most other causes of ARDS. However, conducting clinical trials in this patient population is difficult, as blast events are mostly unpredictable and often managed in hospitals ill-equipped to recruit into research studies. In the absence of better evidence, blast lung is essentially managed according to the principles outlined for ARDS in Chap. 9. In addition, however, the following considerations should guide initial management of blast lung:

- The high incidence of pneumothorax and the low sensitivity of chest radiographs in detecting this condition suggest particular care should be taken prior to any aeromedical transfer. Prophylactic chest drain insertion is preferable to tension pneumothorax at altitude.
- Fluid overload exacerbates ARDS and may be particularly detrimental in blast lung. Guiding fluid management using more sophisticated endpoints than pulse, blood pressure and lactate is therefore potentially more important in blast lung than in other forms of ARDS. The techniques for assessing and optimising volume status, outlined in Chap. 6, should be rigorously applied.
- There is a theoretical risk of air embolism with positive pressure ventilation. However, a patient who requires intubation and mechanical ventilation should not have this delayed by paying this concern undue attention. Peak and mean airway pressures should be minimised, with tolerance of permissive hypercapnia. Ventilation at 6 ml/kg Ideal Body Weight (as for other patients at risk of ARDS) should be sufficient. PEEP should be high enough to achieve required oxygenation, but not higher. Because of this consideration, logic suggests blast lung should lead to a lower threshold to initiate extracorporeal CO_2 removal or ECMO, as was used successfully in ten military casualties [41]; however trial evidence to support this is unlikely to be available.
- Blast applied preferentially to one side of the body may result in severe effects in one lung (including pulmonary

haemorrhage and reduced compliance) with relatively normal compliance and gas exchange in the other. This may be managed best with differential lung ventilation using a double lumen endotracheal tube, with each lumen connected to an individually-set ventilator. Alternatively, bronchial blockers introduced under direct vision with a bronchoscope can isolate pulmonary haemorrhage. Positioning on one side such that the better lung is dependent (and so receives the greater proportion of cardiac output) is often helpful.

• The rule regarding non-invasive ventilation described for chest injury in general applies equally to blast lung. A patient in hypercarbic respiratory failure may benefit, but most patients with blast lung will not be hypercarbic; hypoxia in such patients is better managed with intubation and mechanical ventilation.

How Should the Patient with Suspected Gas Embolism Be Managed?

A deteriorating patient with blast lung should be treated in essentially the same manner as any other with chest trauma, as is described in Chap. 9. An additional early consideration nearly-unique to lung blast injury is arterial gas embolus. Arterial gas emboli most typically affect the cerebral circulation (causing stroke) and coronary vessels (casing myocardial ischaemia or infarction). While these conditions most commonly lead to rapid death, as outlined earlier in this chapter, the alveolar-vascular communications opened by blast can remain open for up to half an hour, resulting in delayed presentations and the opportunity for therapy.

• The patient should be positioned supine (in contrast to venous gas emboli, for which patients are traditionally positioned head-down and left lateral decubitus).
• The patient should inspire the highest possible FiO2: if spontaneously breathing either through a reservoir mask or a high-flow mask with a flow that exceeds peak inspira-

tory flow rate, and if mechanically ventilated using 100 % oxygen. De-nitrogenating the circulating blood in this manner will, theoretically, draw nitrogen from the bubbles of air back into the circulating blood volume, leaving the oxygen in the bubbles to be absorbed as cells metabolise.

- Hyperbaric oxygen accelerates the removal of nitrogen from air emboli, but is rarely available in the few hours after blast when it would be most useful.
- Cardiovascular collapse due to myocardial ischaemia from coronary air emboli should be treated using inotropes (e.g. adrenaline) titrated to conventional indices, such as Cardiac Index.

What Specific Strategies Have Been Advanced for the Treatment of Blast Lung Injury?

Several therapies are suggested by the pathological mechanisms outlined above, but all lack supporting high quality evidence.

Pro-coagulants (e.g. Clotting Factors or Recombinant Factor VIIa)

Pulmonary haemorrhage is a component of blast lung, and is likely to be exacerbated by the endogenous Trauma Induced Coagulopathy detected in around 30 % of major trauma patients. Haemostatic resuscitation applied in this setting may be of benefit in the management of lung injury but trial data is lacking. The use of novel pro-coagulants (e.g. recomcivbinant factor VIIa) in this setting is controversial. Very small clinical case series have shown a benefit of both systemic and intra-bronchial rVIIa on oxygenation [42]. However, animal trials have shown no convincing benefit and larger clinical trials are very unlikely to be performed.

Heparin and Other Anticoagulants

Although coagulopathy is likely to worsen pulmonary contusion and haemorrhage in the initial hours after blast injury, anticoagulation in later stages may have a role. The anti-inflammatory properties of heparin (either inhaled or systemic) are best supported by case series in inhalation injury [43] – and inhalation injury is difficult to distinguish from primary blast lung in many patients. Judging optimal timing of heparin administration is a substantial impediment to testing this therapy in a clinical trial.

Corticosteroids

The role of corticosteroids in ARDS is controversial, based on assessments of several large clinical trials and meta-analyses. Whether the inflammation that accompanies blast lung might be particularly responsive to either low-dose or high-dose steroids is not likely to be answered by a clinical trial. Therefore, advice on the role of steroids is likely to parallel advice in other forms of ARDS.

Antibiotics

Patients injured by primary blast also typically have penetrating wounds that warrant prophylactic antibiotics in the perioperative period following debridement. However, primary blast injury *per se* is not an indication for antibiotics.

Analgesia

Possibly the most effective adjuvant treatment for blast lung is to optimise respiratory mechanics by effective regional or parenteral analgesia. Approaches to analgesia, following thoracic trauma are discussed in Chap. 16.

References

1. Belanger HG, Scott SG, Scholten J, Curtiss G, Vanderploeg RD. Utility of mechanism-of-injury-based assessment and treatment: blast injury program case illustration. J Rehabil Res Dev. 2005;42(4):403–12.

2. Finlay SE, Earby M, Baker DJ, Murray VSG. Explosions and human health: the long-term effects of blast injury. Prehosp Disaster Med. 2012;27(4):385–91.

3. Champion HR, Holcomb JB, Young LA. Injuries from explosions: physics, biophysics, pathology, and required research focus. J Trauma. 2009;66(5):1468–77; discussion 1477.

4. de Ceballos JPG, Turégano-Fuentes F, Pérez-Díaz D, Sanz-Sánchez M, Martin-Llorente C, Guerrero-Sanz JE. 11 March 2004: the terrorist bomb explosions in Madrid, Spain--an analysis of the logistics, injuries sustained and clinical management of casualties treated at the closest hospital. Crit Care. 2005;9(1):104–11.

5. Martí M, Parrón M, Baudraxler F, Royo A, Gómez León N, Alvarez-Sala R. Blast injuries from Madrid terrorist bombing attacks on March 11, 2004. Emerg Radiol. 2006;13(3):113–22.

6. Elsayed NM, Gorbunov NV, Kagan VE. A proposed biochemical mechanism involving hemoglobin for blast overpressure-induced injury. Toxicology. 1997;121(1):81–90.

7. Kirkman E, Watts S. Characterization of the response to primary blast injury. Philos Trans R Soc Lond B Biol Sci. 2011;366(1562):286–90.

8. Elsayed NM. Toxicology of blast overpressure. Toxicology. 1997;121(1):1–15.

9. Almogy G, Luria T, Richter E, Pizov R, Bdolah-Abram T, Mintz Y, et al. Can external signs of trauma guide management?: Lessons learned from suicide bombing attacks in Israel. Arch Surg. 2005;140(4):390–3.

10. Gorbunov NV, Asher LV, Ayyagari V, Atkins JL. Inflammatory leukocytes and iron turnover in experimental hemorrhagic lung trauma. Exp Mol Pathol. 2006;80(1):11–25.

11. Gorbunov NV, Elsayed NM, Kisin ER, Kozlov AV, Kagan VE. Air blast-induced pulmonary oxidative stress: interplay among hemoglobin, antioxidants, and lipid peroxidation. Am J Physiol. 1997;272(2 Pt 1):L320–34.

12. Gorbunov NV, McFaul SJ, Januszkiewicz A, Atkins JL. Pro-inflammatory alterations and status of blood plasma iron in a model of blast-induced lung trauma. Int J Immunopathol Pharmacol. 2005;18(3):547–56.

13. Leibovici D, Gofrit ON, Shapira SC. Eardrum perforation in explosion survivors: is it a marker of pulmonary blast injury? Ann Emerg Med. 1999;34(2):168–72.
14. Ohnishi M, Kirkman E, Guy RJ, Watkins PE. Reflex nature of the cardiorespiratory response to primary thoracic blast injury in the anaesthetised rat. Exp Physiol. 2001;86(3):357–64.
15. Irwin RJ, Lerner MR, Bealer JF, Mantor PC, Brackett DJ, Tuggle DW. Shock after blast wave injury is caused by a vagally mediated reflex. J Trauma. 1999;47(1):105–10.
16. Harban F, Kirkman E, Kenward CE, Watkins PE. Primary thoracic blast injury causes acute reduction in cardiac function in the anaesthetised pig. J Physiol (Lond). 2001;533:81.
17. Žunić G, Romić P, Vueljić M, Jovanikić O. Very early increase in nitric oxide formation and oxidative cell damage associated with the reduction of tissue oxygenation is a trait of blast casualties. Vojnosanit Pregl. 2005;62(4):273–80.
18. Žunić G, Pavlović R, Maličević Ž, Savić V, Cernak I. Pulmonary blast injury increases nitric oxide production, disturbs arginine metabolism, and alters the plasma free amino acid pool in rabbits during the early posttraumatic period. Nitric Oxide. 2000;4(2):123–8.
19. Gorbunov NV, Das DK, Goswami SK, Gurusami N, Atkins JL. Nitric oxide (NO), redox signalling, and pulmonary inflammation in a model of polytrauma. Proceedings of the XIII Congress of the Society for Free Radical Research International. Davos, Switzerland. 2006, pp. 2–4.
20. Kirkman E, Watts S, Cooper G. Blast injury research models. Philos Trans R Soc Lond B Biol Sci. 2011;366(1562):144–59.
21. Clemedson CJ. An experimental study of air blast injuries. Acta Physiol Scand. 1949;18:1–200.
22. Krohn PL, Whitteridge D, Zuckerman S. Physiological effects of blast. Lancet. 1942;i:252–8.
23. Clemedson CJ, Hultman HI. Air embolism and the cause of death in blast injury. Mil Surg. 1954;114(6):424–37.
24. Clemedson CJ, Pettersson H. Genesis of respiratory and circulatory changes in blast injury. Am J Physiol. 1953;174(2):316–20.
25. Clemedson CJ, HULTMAN H. Cardiac output in early phase of blast injury in rabbits. Am J Physiol. 1958;194(3):601–6.
26. Hooker DR. Physiological effects of air concussion. Am J Physiol. 1924;67:219–73.
27. Robb-Smith AHT. Pulmonary fat embolism. Lancet. 1941;i:135.
28. Cohen H, Biskind GR. Pathologic aspects of atmospheric blast injuries in man. Arch Pathol (Chic). 1946;42:12–34.

29. Zuckerman S. Experimental study of blast injuries to the lung. Lancet. 1940;ii:219–24.
30. Zuckerman S. Discussion on the problem of blast injuries. Proc R Soc Med. 1941;34:171–88.
31. Mott FW. The effects of high explosives upon the central nervous system. Lancet. 1916;187(4826):441–49.
32. Clemedson CJ. Shock wave transmission to the central nervous system. Acta Physiol Scand. 1956;37(2–3):204–14.
33. Benzinger T. Physiological effects of blast in air and water. German aviation medicine in World War II, Vol 2. Washington, DC: US Government Printing Office; 1950, pp. 1225–59.
34. Clemedson CJ, Hultman H, Gronberg B. Respiration and pulmonary gas exchange in blast injury. J Appl Physiol. 1953;6(4): 213–20.
35. Frykberg ER, Tepas III JJ. Terrorist bombings. Lessons learned from Belfast to Beirut. Ann Surg. 1988;208(5):569–76.
36. Arnold JL, Halpern P, Tsai MC, Smithline H. Mass casualty terrorist bombings: a comparison of outcomes by bombing type. Ann Emerg Med. 2004;43(2):263–73.
37. Mackenzie IM, Tunnicliffe B. Blast injuries to the lung: epidemiology and management. Philos Trans R Soc Lond B Biol Sci. 2011;366(1562):295–9.
38. Huller T, Bazini Y. Blast injuries of the chest and abdomen. Arch Surg. 1970;100(1):24–30.
39. Conventional Warfare: Ballistic, Blast, and Burn Injuries (Textbook of Military Medicine Series on Combat Casualty Care, Part 1 Volume 5). Washington, DC: Office of the Surgeon General of the U.S. Army; 1991.
40. Hirshberg B, Oppenheim-Eden A, Pizov R, Sklair-Levi M, Rivkin A, Bardach E, et al. Recovery from blast lung injury: one-year follow-up. Chest. 1999;116(6):1683–8.
41. Bein T, Zonies D, Philipp A, Zimmermann M, Osborn EC, Allan PF, et al. Transportable extracorporeal lung support for rescue of severe respiratory failure in combat casualties. J Trauma Acute Care Surg. 2012;73(6):1450–6.
42. Heslet L, Nielsen JD, Nepper-Christensen S. Local pulmonary administration of factor VIIa (rFVIIa) in diffuse alveolar hemorrhage (DAH) – a review of a new treatment paradigm. Biologics. 2012;6:37–46. doi:10.2147/BTT.S25507.
43. Miller AC, Elamin EM, Suffredini AF. Inhaled anticoagulation regimens for the treatment of smoke inhalation-associated acute lung injury: a systematic review. Crit Care Med. 2014; 42(2):413–9.

Chapter 11
Managing Severe Traumatic Brain Injury Outside of the Neurosciences Critical Care Unit

George Evetts and Sam D. Hutchings

Abstract Traumatic brain injury (TBI) can commonly present to medical facilities without specialist neuroscience services and clinicians at these centers will be required to perform early stabilization and treatment. Early optimisation of cerebral perfusion pressure and oxygen delivery prevents secondary brain injury and has an important impact on mortality and long term outcomes. Important basic support measures have been shown to have positive mortality benefits, including optimal ventilation, prevention of pyrexia, and normoglycaemia, but management of intra-cranial hypertension is paramount given the association with

G. Evetts, MBBS, BSc, MRCP, FRCA (✉)
Defence Medical Services, Imperial School of Anaesthesia,
London, UK
e-mail: George.evetts@gmail.com

S.D. Hutchings, MRCS, FRCA, FFICM, DICM, DipIMC
Department of Critical Care, Kings College Hospital,
Denmark Hill, London SE5 9RS, UK

S.D. Hutchings (ed.), *Trauma and Combat Critical Care in Clinical Practice*, In Clinical Practice,
DOI 10.1007/978-3-319-28758-4_11,
© Crown Copyright 2016

245

poor outcomes. In specialist centers this is usually guided by the use of invasive intracranial pressure (ICP) monitoring; such techniques may not be available in a non-specialist centre. A method of TBI management based upon regular imaging and clinical examination (ICE) has been shown to be a comparable management strategy and is the standard of care used by the United Kingdom Defence Medical Services (UK DMS) when more advanced monitoring is not available. A developing method of measuring deterioration in ICP is the use of optic nerve sheath ultrasound, but the requirement for training, operator dependency, and current paucity of evidence prevents widespread adoption. This chapter will discuss the provision of basic support and homeostasis measures for the management of severe TBI outside of specialist centers, along with a suggested protocol for the management of intracranial hypertension in the absence of specialist expertise and monitoring.

Keywords Traumatic brain injury • Intracranial hypertension • Cerebral perfusion pressure • Osmotherapy • Intracranial pressure monitoring • Primary brain injury • Secondary brain injury • Optic nerve sheath ultrasound

Introduction

Severe traumatic brain injury (TBI), which may be defined as a GCS of <8 on presentation or subsequent assessment, will often be managed within a dedicated neurosciences intensive care unit in the developed world. There is good evidence that such a strategy has a beneficial effect on outcome [1]. However, many patients worldwide do not have access to such specialist facilities, and even within sophisticated trauma networks patients may initially present to trauma units that lack dedicated neurological critical care support.

Predicting outcome in young patients with severe TBI is difficult and a significant proportion of those with seemingly catastrophic injuries at presentation go on to defy the odds and achieve a good neurological outcome. According to some studies nearly half of all patients in this group have no, or minimal functional deficit at 12 months post injury [2].

Given the importance of early effective intervention in this cohort it is important that clinicians who are responsible for their care in these non-specialist centers have an effective framework to guide early management. The Defence Medical Services of the United Kingdom (UK DMS) has managed many patients with severe TBI during recent combat operations in Iraq and Afghanistan and have developed a protocolised approach for management, in the absence of dedicated cerebral monitoring, prior to transfer to neurosurgical facilities. The approach outlined in this chapter is based upon those guidelines.

Whole books have been dedicated to the subject of neuro-critical care and this chapter does not attempt to provide a comprehensive guide to the management of such patients. Instead it outlines an approach that may be of use to clinicians who work outside of neurocritical care, but who nonetheless may find themselves in the position of managing patients with severe TBI for a period of time.

What Is Primary and Secondary Brain Injury?

The cranium is a rigid box of constant volume, which provides protection for it's contents: blood, cerebrospinal fluid, and brain tissue. The Munro-Kellie hypothesis states that the total volume of the cranium's contents remains constant and that an increase in any of the constituents must be offset by a decrease in another. This can only be achieved to a limit of 150–200 ml, any further expansion causing a rapid increase in intracranial pressure. Since Cerebral Perfusion Pressure (CPP) is equal to Mean Arterial Pressure (MAP) - Intra

Cranial Pressure (ICP), any increase in ICP can be detrimental to cerebral blood flow and oxygen delivery.

Primary brain injury is the damage to neurological tissue that occurs at the time of the initial injury and can be focal or diffuse. Focal injuries are more obvious on axial imaging and may take the form of contusions with surrounding areas of oedema or discrete areas of haemorrhage, either within the brain parenchyma or extra cerebral. These extra cerebral haematomas often exert a mass effect which if not surgically treated can lead to a progressive rise in intra cranial pressure. Recognition and management of such treatable lesions is vital at an early stage in the management of patients with severe TBI. Diffuse brain injury, sometimes termed Diffuse Axonal Injury (DAI), is more difficult to diagnose with CT imaging. It is associated with shear forces causing widespread distortion to the white matter and multiple small petechial haemorrhages resulting from damage to the intraparenchymal small blood vessels. Finally, the mechanism of primary brain injury is important. Penetrating injuries, such as those resulting from gun shot wounds, are associated with significantly worse outcome than damage caused by blunt trauma [3].

With the exception of surgical intervention to treat mass lesions, little can be done to ameliorate the immediate effects of primary brain injury. The focus of the intensive care specialist is mainly directed towards the prevention and mitigation of secondary brain injury. Secondary brain injury refers to the damage that can occur to the potentially viable brain tissue surrounding the area of primary damage. Such tissue is frequently swollen and vulnerable to any reduction in perfusion. Any increase in tissue death will lead to further swelling with consequent reduction in cerebral perfusion and this can rapidly turn into a downward spiral, leading to irreversible loss of brain tissue and generalized cerebral oedema. The management strategy outlined in the rest of this chapter is focused on recognising and treating cerebral hypo-perfusion in order to arrest this chain of events.

Why Is the Detection and Management of Intracranial Hypertension of Such critical Importance?

Raised intracranial pressure is a sign of brain tissue injury and swelling. Left untreated, it contributes to a self perpetuating cycle of secondary brain injury. Augmentation of MAP to increase CPP is a common treatment in patients with severe TBI, but raised ICP has a strong independent correlation with poor outcome in its own right, independent of any effects on CPP. In other words, just increasing MAP in an attempt to overcome a rising ICP is not as efficacious as preventing the ICP rise in the first instance. One retrospective analysis found that an ICP > 20 mmHg was a powerful predictor of poor outcome and that this remained true even when CPP was maintained at >60 mmHg [4]. Another study showed a mortality rate of 47 % in those with an ICP ≥ 20 mmHg, at any time, compared to 17 % in those without intra-cranial hypertension [5].

Standard practice, as recommended by the US Brain Trauma Foundation, is the use of invasive intra cerebral pressure monitoring for patients with a GCS of <8 and radiological evidence of a primary brain injury [6]. Controversy still exists as to the usefulness of ICP monitoring with some retrospective cohort data failing to show any difference in outcome compared to matched controls with similar injury severity [7, 8]. However, other studies have supported its use [9–11]. The first randomised trial comparing ICP monitoring with a group of patients monitored using CT Imaging and Clinical Examination (ICE), demonstrated non-inferiority of the ICE approach [12]. Although this trial may not apply to all patient populations, it does lend support to the use of an ICE strategy as best practice in the absence of specialist monitoring. It is the ICE arm of this study that provides the basis for the ICP management guidelines adopted by the UK DMS which are discussed later in this chapter.

Part One: General Therapeutic Measures for the Management of Severe TBI

Careful attention to the maintenance of physiology with the aim of minimising rises in ICP and maintaining haemodynamic stability are vital in achieving oxygen delivery to the injured brain and preventing secondary brain injury. Specific factors include optimisation of gas exchange, ensuring adequate cerebral perfusion pressure through control of systemic haemodynamics, patient positioning and homeostasis during the stress response. Prevention of secondary problems such as seizures and venous thromboembolism are also crucial. Patients who still have brain swelling after the application of these therapies will require additional management, outlined later in this chapter.

All patients with severe TBI should have the core treatment measures shown in Table 11.1 applied as soon as possible following injury.

What Is an Appropriate PaO_2 for Patients with Severe TBI?

Patients with severe TBI will almost universally require invasive ventilation for both airway protection and control of gas exchange. Oxygenation should be continually monitored with pulse oximetry and regular arterial blood gas analysis, with rigorous avoidance of hypoxaemia ($SaO_2 > 95\%$ and $PaO_2 > 10$ kPa). Whilst there is no high quality evidence relating to hypoxemia and TBI, there are several data sets that have shown associations with mortality from secondary brain injury. Information from the United States Traumatic Coma Data Bank, showed an association between hypoxaemia, which occurred in 22.4% of severe TBI patients, and mortality [13]. The study included 717 pre-hospital patients and classified hypoxaemia as a $PaO_2 < 60$ mmHg (7.9 KPa). In-hospital data also supports the finding that a period of

TABLE 11.1 General treatment measures applied to all patients with severe TBI

$PaO_2 > 10$ kPa, $PaCO_2$ 4.5–5 kPa
Na+ >140 mmol/l
Glucose 6–10 mmol/l
Avoid Pyrexia (Temperature <37.5 °C)
VTE prophylaxis with intermittent calf compression stockings. Avoid pharmacological thromboprophylaxis for 48 h post injury.
Levetiracetam 500 mg bd for seizure prophylaxis.
In the absence of ICP monitoring, maintenance of MAP >80, in order to maintain a cerebral perfusion pressure of >60 mmHg (assuming an ICP of 20 mmHg).
Systolic blood pressure >90 mmHg at all times.

hypoxaemia leads to increased mortality; a study examining 71 patients finding that duration of $SaO_2 < 90$ % was an independent predictor of mortality [14]. Given the critical dual effects of hypoxaemia, namely increased cerebral blood flow and reduced oxygen delivery, we recommend that a target be adopted in excess of the level that is known to cause these effects.

What Is an Appropriate $PaCO_2$ for Patients with Severe TBI?

$PaCO_2$ is one of the critical determinants of cerebral blood flow and hence brain volume. A reduction in $PaCO_2$ decreases ICP and common practice is to aim for a $PaCO_2$ of 4.5–5.0 kPa. Further decreases in $PaCO_2$ continue to decrease brain volume, but at the expense of cerebral blood flow with below normal $PaCO_2$ being associated with worse outcomes [15]. However, targeted short term hyperventilation may have a role on the management of refractory intra-cranial hypertension, this is covered in more detail in Part 2 of this chapter.

Is the Application of Positive End Expiratory Pressure (PEEP) Safe in Patients with Severe TBI?

Patients with TBI are at increased risk of acute lung injury, in which the use of PEEP is widely accepted and has been shown to be beneficial along with low tidal volume ventilation [16]. Several small non randomized studies have indicated that the application of PEEP in patients with severe TBI is safe and not associated with increases in ICP [17–19]. Therefore, the level of PEEP should be determined by the patient's respiratory status without reference to the presence of brain injury.

What Should Be the Strategy for Haemodynamic Management in the Patient with Severe TBI?

Patients with severe TBI should be maintained in a euvolaemic state using blood products or suitable isotonic or hypertonic fluids. Hypotonic fluids should be avoided as these can contribute to worsening brain swelling and secondary brain injury. There is some limited evidence that patients with severe TBI resuscitated with albumin rather than normal saline have worse outcomes [20], but evidence relating to the use of other colloids in this setting is scarce. We suggest that following initial resuscitation in which the use of blood products may be appropriate, 0.9 % saline should be the fluid of choice for patients with severe TBI.

Hypotension has been shown to have a significant impact on outcome in patients with TBI. In one pre-hospital study using the United States Traumatic Coma Data Bank, a single systolic BP of <90 mmHg was a powerful predictor of poor outcome, being associated with a two fold increase in mortality compared with matched controls without hypotension [13]. Further work looking at in-hospital hypotension supports this association with one study showing that the odds ratio for death increases from 2.1 to 8.1 with repeated episodes of hypotension [21]. For this reason, early continuous invasive blood pressure monitoring is strongly advised with a low threshold for pharmacological augmentation of blood pressure to maintain a systolic BP of >90 mmHg and MAP > 80 mmHg.

Which Sedative and Anaesthetic Agents Are Appropriate for Use in Patients with Severe TBI?

Adequate sedation is important to minimise increases in ICP from painful and noxious stimuli, and to maintain compliance with ventilation. A decrease in cerebral metabolic rate and oxygen demand of brain tissue may also serve to prevent secondary brain injury since cerebral blood flow tends to follow demand. There is very little evidence to suggest superiority of particular pharmacological agents and so the choice of sedative agent will depend on evidence of brain swelling and the predicted time course of ventilation.

Shorter acting agents such as Propofol and the synthetic opioids (Fentanyl or Remifentanil) are preferred as first line agents. Propofol is a commonly used agent and has the advantage of maintaining any remaining cerebral auto-regulation as well as decreasing the cerebral metabolic rate. It has also been shown to significantly decrease day three ICP when compared to morphine, although this was not associated with a difference in neurological outcome or mortality [22]. Longer term use at higher doses has been associated with Propofol infusion syndrome (see Chap. 16), and introduction of other agents should be considered at an early stage.

The longer acting agents such as Morphine, Midazolam or Thiopentone should be introduced in a tiered fashion based on evidence of brain swelling, as discussed later in this chapter. Midazolam has a stable haemodynamic profile in moderate dose, and has been shown to have similar outcomes to Propofol with less sedation failure [23]. It may therefore be a useful additive, especially in patients who require higher dose sedation because of proven or suspected brain swelling.

The synthetic opioids are also commonly used agents. It has been reported that Fentanyl can increase ICP [24], but this has been shown not to cause cerebral ischaemia [25]. Remifentanil has an advantageous pharmacokinetic profile, potentially enabling earlier assessment and extubation in those patients with minimal injures on axial imaging [17].

Barbituates should be reserved as a second line treatment for patients with proven brain swelling. Their use is covered later in this chapter.

There is no evidence that muscle relaxants affect ICP or alter outcome in patients with TBI, however coughing and ventilator dys-synchrony can produce very abrupt rises in ICP which may be detrimental. Two studies showed no increase in ICP with atracurium and cis-atracurium [18, 19] and an animal study showed no increase in ICP with atracurium or suxamethonium [26].

Which Severe TBI Patients Should Receive Seizure Prophylaxis and Which Agent Should Be Used?

It is desirable to prevent post-traumatic seizures, which can contribute to secondary brain injury by increasing both ICP and cerebral metabolic demand. However, there are side affects to anti-epileptic medications and a balance of risk and benefit must be sought. A randomised, double blind study of over 400 patients compared post-traumatic phenytoin prophylaxis with placebo, and found a significant reduction in seizures during the first week in the phenytoin group (3.6 vs 14.2 %), but no significant difference after day 8 [27]. The trial also reported no increase in adverse effects between those treated with phenytoin and a placebo. Other agents have also been investigated, with sodium valproate having a similar efficacy to phenytoin, but associated with a higher mortality [28]. Levetiracetam has also been shown to be equally efficacious [29, 30], and cheaper than phenytoin [31], with the added advantage of not requiring therapeutic monitoring.

Do Patients with Severe TBI Require Special Positioning?

Head up tilt is a common maneuver for aiding venous drainage of the cranium and has been shown to decrease cerebral blood volume [32]. Any compression or manipulation of the neck can cause interruption of venous drainage and increased ICP. Although no trials have studied effects on outcome, there have been reported increases in ICP associated with cervical collar usage [33, 34]. Clearing the C-spine should be a priority in these patients, and if not possible then other means of stabilization such as blocks and tape are advocated [34].

What Temperature Should Routinely Be Targeted in Patients with Severe TBI?

Hyperthermia has been shown to worsen secondary brain injury in animal models [35] and there is an association with worse outcomes in humans [36]. Although a different patient cohort, evidence from patients in a comatose state following cardiac arrest, suggests that a policy of targeted temperature control to 36° is as efficacious as therapeutic hypothermia to 32° with regard to improving neurological recovery [37]. We advocate routine control of temperature to normothermia following severe TBI. The use of therapeutic hypothermia to control ICP is covered in Part 2 of this chapter.

Is Stress Ulcer Prophylaxis Required in Patients with Severe TBI?

Early enteral feeding and prompt resuscitation decrease the risk of stress ulceration, but all critically ill patients remain at risk, particularly those who are mechanically ventilated and coagulopathic [38]. Pharmacological prophylaxis with Histamine-2 receptor antagonists is commonly used in critically ill patients and has been shown to be superior to Sucralfate [39]. Proton pump inhibitors are another possibility with some meta-analyses showing them to be superior [40, 41], whilst others show no difference in efficacy [42, 43]. Based upon this, either agent can be used.

What Is an Appropriate Haemoglobin Concentration in Patients with Severe TBI?

With oxygen delivery based upon saturation, haemoglobin concentration and cardiac output, maintenance of an adequate haemoglobin concentration is important for the prevention of secondary brain injury. There are no trials specific for haemoglobin targets in TBI. The TRICC study [44] which led to the widespread adoption of a more restrictive transfusion policy in critically ill patients, only included a small number of trauma patients and does not specify how many of these had severe TBI. In acute TBI patients, where anaemia may be due to blood loss rather than critical illness, it may be prudent to maintain a higher haemoglobin level. We advocate a level of 10 g/dl, whilst acknowledging that this is based on no real evidence of benefit.

What Is the Importance of Glycaemic Control in Patients with Severe TBI?

Hyperglycaemia is common in patients with TBI and appears to be associated with increased mortality [45]. However 'tight' glycaemic control has been shown to increase periods of critical reduction of brain glucose and has also not been shown to be beneficial to outcome in patients with TBI [46]. There is also evidence that episodes of hypoglycaemia are associated with worse outcomes in critically ill patients [47]. Patients with traumatic brain injury, in common with other critically ill patients, should therefore be managed with a broad glycaemic control target of 6–10 mmol/l.

Part Two: Detecting and Treating Brain Swelling Without Dedicated ICP Monitoring

As discussed in the introduction to this chapter, the use of ICP monitoring is widespread within neuroscience critical care units. However, there will be circumstances where, even in mature trauma systems, patients may not immediately present to such a facility. Furthermore, in remote parts of the world, or in developing countries, clinicians may not have access to such resources. In the remainder of this chapter we describe an approach to the management of such patients which has been developed by the UK DMS.

What Strategy Should Be Used for Detecting Intracranial Hypertension in the Absence of Dedicated ICP Monitoring?

Current evidence would suggest a method based upon Imaging and Clinical Examination (ICE) is best practice in the absence of invasive ICP monitoring. This strategy was described in a study by Chesnut et al. in the first prospective randomised controlled trial of the effectiveness of invasive ICP monitoring [12]. Three-hundred and twenty-four patients were randomised to either standard care with invasive ICP monitoring, or a didactic protocol based upon ICE. Baseline characteristics were similar in both groups. Survival time and functional status at 3 and 6 months were not significantly different between the groups. However, the patients in the ICE arm did receive significantly more interventions, principally hyperventilation and hyperosmolar therapy.

The ICE strategy relies upon regular CT imaging at specified pre-determined time points and as required based upon evidence of neurological deterioration, termed 'neuroworsening' by the authors. Signs of neuroworsening were defined as:

- Decrease in the motor component of the GCS score of >2
- New loss of pupil reactivity
- Interval development of pupil asymmetry of >2 mm
- New focal motor deficit
- Herniation syndrome

Clearly such a strategy requires regular and prompt access to axial imaging and consequently has clear implications for unit workload. If brain swelling is detected on CT examination then treatment should be escalated, for example by increasing sedation, increasing the amount of prescribed hyperosmolar therapy or by performing short term targeted hyperventilation.

The adapted ICE strategy, used by the UK DMS is shown in Fig. 11.1.

What Are the Signs of Brain Swelling on CT Scan?

Signs of brain swelling can be obvious but may also be subtle. It is therefore important that, if at all feasible, such CT images be reviewed by a specialist neuro-radiologist. In a remote environment this may require the use of data uplinks.

Three image patterns that are associated with brain swelling are shown in Figs. 11.2, 11.3 and 11.4.

Can Optic Nerve Sheath Ultrasound Be Used for Monitoring Changes in ICP?

The optic nerve is part of the central nervous system and the optic nerve sheath continuous with the subarachnoid space. Intra cerebral pressure changes are therefore transmitted through the CSF to the optic nerve sheath, which enlarges as ICP increases. The optic nerve sheath diameter (ONSD) is easy to measure using ultrasound at the bedside and is a potentially useful tool for detecting rises in ICP, particularly in settings where ICP monitoring is

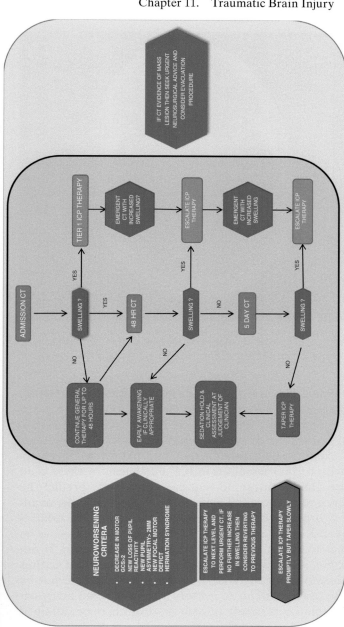

Figure 11.1 Protocol based approach to the management of severe TBI in the absence of invasive ICP monitoring (Based on UK DMS Clinical Guidelines for Deployed Critical Care)

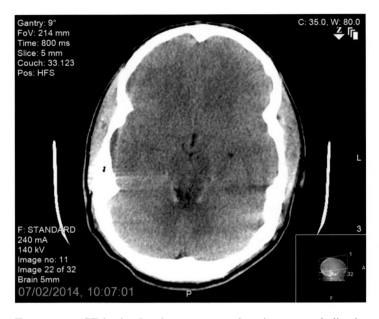

FIGURE 11.2 CT brain showing compressed peri-mesencephalic cisterns (Courtesy of Dr Tom Hurst, King's College Hospital, London)

unavailable. Several studies have confirmed that ONSD can detect the difference between significantly elevated ICP (>20 mmHg) and lower ICP (<20 mmHg) [48–50]. What is less clear is whether changes in ONSD in patients with existing significant intracranial hypertension correlate with further increases in ICP. Furthermore, there is no precise ONSD threshold that can confidently predict the presence of intracranial hypertension. Studies in the available literature have suggested a range of thresholds between 5 and 7 mm [48–50]. ONSD could be used as an adjunct to the ICE strategy when ICP monitoring is not available; it could also be used in the pre-hospital setting. It is however, strongly advised that the technique not be used to triage patients to centers with or without neurosciences facilities; a falsely reassuring result may be obtained

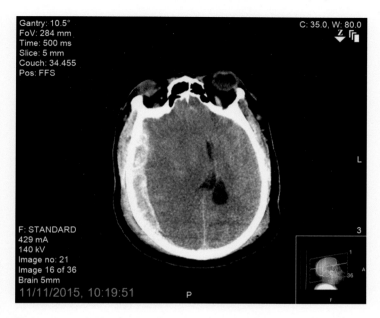

FIGURE 11.3 CT brain showing an acute sub dural haemoatoma and associated midline shift (Courtesy of Dr Tom Hurst, King's College Hospital, London)

early in the course of severe TBI or in the presence of an evolving mass lesion. The decision to transfer to a neuroscience critical care facility should still be made on clinical findings, such as GCS, alongside a consideration of the mechanism of injury.

How Is Optic Nerve Sheath Ultrasound Performed?

It is important that the technique should only be used by those with adequate training and previous experience and that all measurements should ideally be performed by the same individual to minimise inter-observer variation.

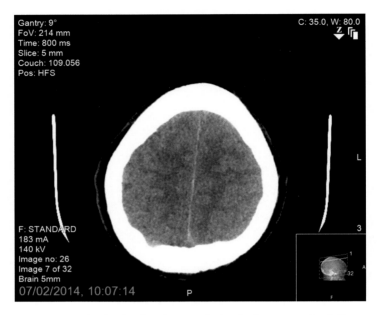

FIGURE 11.4 CT brain showing cortical sulcal compression/efface-ment (Courtesy of Dr Tom Hurst, King's College Hospital, London)

- Measurements should be performed using a linear ultra-sound probe and care should be taken to avoid any pressure on the globe. Large amounts of gel are required in order to optimize acoustic windows and minimise probe contact with the globe itself.
- Measurements should be performed around the time of the initial CT scan and any subsequent CT scan in order to attempt a correlation between CT evidence of intra cranial hypertension and the caliber of the ONS.
- Three measurements should be taken from each globe and the mean value recorded. Measurements should be made at 3 mm behind the globe in line with the perpendicular axis of the optic nerve as shown in Fig. 11.5.
- ONSD diameters of above 5.5 mm usually indicate significant intracranial hypertension but in the absence of a

reliable threshold clinicians are advised to use the ONSD measurement, in conjunction with other signs of neuro-worsening, to guide management.

What Therapeutic Measures Should Be Used to Control Brain Swelling and Intra Cranial Hypertension?

There are a variety of strategies used to control brain swelling above and beyond those basic measures outlined in Part 1 of this chapter.

Osmotherapy

Hyperosmolar therapy in the form of mannitol and hypertonic saline is often first line treatment in the management of raised intracranial pressure. Creation of an osmotic gradient between the blood and brain tissue causes a decrease in brain tissue oedema. Both agents also cause an immediate increase in cardiac output through plasma expansion, and a decrease in plasma viscosity which could assist with microvascular blood flow. There is no strong evidence to suggest benefit of one agent over the other, but hypertonic saline has the advantage of prolonged volume expansion aiding systemic haemodynamic stability, in contrast to mannitol which causes a profound diuresis and significant hypovolaemia if unchecked. There is evidence that hypertonic saline is safe and decreases ICP [51–53], but there is no recorded outcome difference between mannitol and hypertonic saline [54, 55]. There is also a reported risk of renal failure when osmolarity exceeds 320 mOsm/L using mannitol, but sodium levels have also been reported as high as 180 mmol/L with no adverse affects [56]. In general, 320 mOsm/L is the recommended maximum osmolarity when using either agent.

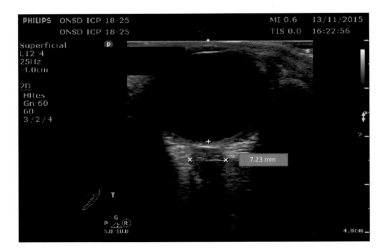

FIGURE 11.5 Ultrasound image of the optic nerve sheath. The diameter has been measured 3 mm behind the globe and is 7.2 mm. This patient had intracranial hypertension with an average ICP of around 20 mmHg but occasional spikes to around 30 mmHg

Sedation

As previously discussed, adequate sedation to avoid an ICP surge from noxious stimuli, allow ventilation, and decrease brain tissue oxygen demand is an important tenet of TBI management. Each sedative agent has advantages and disadvantages and their different mechanisms of action can be exploited to summate their ICP lowering affects, or used in a tiered approach to manage intracranial hypertension refractory to basic measures. Propofol and a short acting opioid are useful first line agents allowing prompt wake up, but with evidence of raised ICP, tiered introduction of further agents such as benzodiazepines and barbituates can be used. Barbituates have a highly suppressive affect on cerebral metabolic rate and ICP, causing an isoelectric EEG at therapeutic doses. They do not however have a very favourable pharmacokinetic profile for sedation due to their long context sensitivity half life and propensity to cause haemodynamic instability. There is minimal evidence for routine use of barbituates. A trial by Schwartz et al. [57] comparing initial treatment of raised ICP (>25 mmHg for more than 15 min) with barbituates or mannitol showed a worse outcome with barbituates (mortality 77 % vs 41 %). A systematic review of the small number of published studies failed to show a convincing benefit although many of the studies were several decades old and none examined the use of barbituates as a third line sedative agent [58]. Use of barbituates for refractory ICP management may have some benefit, with a trial by Eisenberg et al. [59] showing a survival rate of 92 % for barbituate responders compared to 17 % for non-responders when used after other methods of ICP control had failed. It seems rational to reserve barbituate use for the management of refractory intra cranial hypertension, paying careful attention to cardiovascular stability upon introduction.

Therapeutic Hypothermia

The role of therapeutic hypothermia, usually cooling to 32–35 °C, has yielded conflicting results. Some small trials have shown long term outcome benefits, including improved mortality [60]. However larger multi-center randomised controlled trials and meta-analyses have failed to show either mortality or long-term neurological benefits [61–64]. The EUROTHERM 3235 trial [65] ceased recruitment early due to safety concerns in the study group. In this study, therapeutic hypothermia was implemented as a first line ICP controlling mechanism at 32–35 °C until ICP was <20, with further measures if required. Both groups were well matched at baseline but favourable outcomes (Glasgow outcome score 5–8) were 25.7 % in the hypothermia group compared to 36.5 % in the control group, with mortality also being higher in the hypothermia group. There was less use of stage 3 ICP treatments, such as barbituate therapy, in the hypothermia group but use of decompressive craniectomy was similar.

ICPs and cerebral perfusion pressures were not significantly different, and there were no differences in rates of pneumonia. This study would therefore suggest that hypothermia could cause harm, both in mortality and functional outcome. Therefore we do not recommend that therapeutic hypothermia be used in patients with severe TBI.

Hyperventilation

Since cerebral blood flow follows $PaCO_2$ in a linear fashion control of $PaCO_2$ is not only paramount to avoid an unnecessary surge in ICP, but also to avoid potentially damaging cerebral ischaemia if $PaCO_2$ is allowed to reach sub-normal levels. A prospective interventional study by Coles et al. [66], showed a significantly higher volume of hypo-perfused brain on positron emission tomography after decreasing $PaCO_2$ from 4.8 to 3.9 kPa. Coupled with several small observational studies that have shown cerebral blood flow to be particularly sub-optimal in the first 24 h following injury and that hyperventilation worsened perfusion [67], it would be reasonable to assume that hypocapnia is detrimental. However, cerebral metabolic rate is reduced in TBI, and so perfusion below the norm, may not necessarily cause harm. In a study by Diringer et al. [68], cerebral blood flow, oxygen extraction fraction and cerebral metabolic rate for oxygen ($CMRO_2$) were measured by positron emission tomography in patients subjected to different levels of hypocapnia for intermittent periods. Even at cerebral blood flows of 10 ml/100 g/min $CMRO_2$ remained unchanged suggesting that oxygen delivery matched demand and implying that any reduced blood flow should not in theory cause further secondary brain injury.

Based on the above evidence, brief periods of hyperventilation (less than 60 min) in the presence of refractory intracranial hypertension could be advocated as a temporary measure, and may not be harmful. It should be withdrawn if it has no therapeutic affect and other therapeutic measures instituted to prevent prolonged use.

Decompressive Craniectomy

Removal of a bone flap, allowing brain tissue, to swell is not infrequently used in the treatment of intracranial hypertension. Decompressive craniectomy (DC) has clearly been shown to decrease ICP [69, 70], but most published evidence up until recently have been case reports, animal studies and retrospective cohort studies, with some concern that although DC may improve survival, it is at the expense of lifelong severe disability [71]. One trial of DC in 27 children showed a non-significant trend towards improved functional outcome, but the larger Decompressive Craniectomy (DECRA) trial failed to show mortality or other outcome benefits [72]. Patients in the DECRA trial were randomised to treatment after reaching an ICP of 20 mmHg for only 10 min, causing some to argue that this did not reflect true severe persistent intra cranial hypertension. Results are awaited from the RESCUE ICP trial (Randomised Evaluation of Surgery with Craniectomy for Uncontrollable Elevation of Intra-Cranial Pressure) which is examining outcomes in 400 patients with ICP>25 mmHg for more than 1 h who have failed to respond to second tier medical therapy. This situation more closely mirrors current clinical practice and the results will be of interest.

Performing a decompressive craniectomy in the absence of neurosurgical expertise is fraught with hazard and cannot be advocated. However, emergency 'burr holes' by trained non-specialist surgeons has been suggested as beneficial in the patient with proven extra-axial haematoma with a significant mass effect who faces a prolonged transfer time to specialist neurosurgical care [73]. Evidence consists only of case reports [74] and retrospective data series [75–77], one of which showed a worse outcome with intervention.

Suggested Management Protocol for Severe TBI Outside of the Neuroscience Critical Care Unit

All patients with severe TBI should have the basic measures outlined in Part 1 of this chapter instituted. Following detection of brain swelling therapeutic measures to control this should be

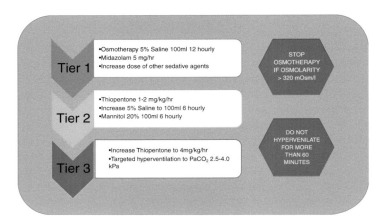

FIGURE 11.6 Hierarchical therapeutic approach to the management of brain swelling (Based on UK DMS Clinical Guidelines for Deployed Critical Care)

instituted or escalated to the next level. The UK DMS uses three escalating therapeutic tiers to manage brain swelling associated with severe TBI and these are shown in Fig. 11.6.

Wherever possible close liaison with neurosciences critical care and neurosurgical specialists is strongly advised, especially when patients have intracranial mass lesions detected on axial imaging.

Where experience exists with ONSD US this can augment the treatment pathway shown in Fig. 11.1. An increasing trend in ONSD should trigger an emergent CT scan. However, it remains unclear whether ONSD US can accurately track intra cranial hypertension in patients with more chronic brain swelling and it should be used with caution if adopted.

Conclusion

Patients with severe TBI who, for whatever reason, cannot be immediately managed in dedicated neuroscience critical care units are at increased risk of worse outcomes. However, attention to detail and the adoption of a management strategy based on Imaging and Clinical Examination can go someway towards mitigating the clinical risk. Future strategies being investigated by military healthcare providers include expanding the scope of ONSD US and the use of small transportable CT scanners which can be deployed in "forward" medical treatment facilities.

References

1. Patel HC, Menon DK, Tebbs S, Hawker R, Hutchinson PJ, Kirkpatrick PJ. Specialist neurocritical care and outcome from head injury. Intensive Care Med. 2002;28(5):547–53.
2. Myburgh JA, Cooper DJ, Finfer SR, Venkatesh B, Jones D, Higgins A, et al. Epidemiology and 12-month outcomes from traumatic brain injury in Australia and New Zealand. J Trauma. 2008;64(4):854–62.
3. Part 2: prognosis in penetrating brain injury. J Trauma. 2001;51(2 Suppl):S44–86.
4. Juul N, Morris GF, Marshall SB, Marshall LF. Intracranial hypertension and cerebral perfusion pressure: influence on neurological deterioration and outcome in severe head injury. The Executive Committee of the International Selfotel Trial. J Neurosurg. 2000;92(1):1–6.
5. Balestreri M, Czosnyka M, Hutchinson P, Steiner LA, Hiler M, Smielewski P, et al. Impact of intracranial pressure and cerebral perfusion pressure on severe disability and mortality after head injury. Neurocrit Care. 2006;4(1):8–13.
6. Bratton SL, Chestnut RM, Ghajar J, McConnell Hammond FF, Harris OA, Hartl R, et al. Guidelines for the management of severe traumatic brain injury. VI. Indications for intracranial pressure monitoring. J Neurotrauma. 2007;24 Suppl 1:S37–44.
7. Cremer OL, van Dijk GW, van Wensen E, Brekelmans GJ, Moons KG, Leenen LP, et al. Effect of intracranial pressure monitoring and targeted intensive care on functional outcome after severe head injury. Crit Care Med. 2005;33(10):2207–13.
8. Shafi S, Diaz-Arrastia R, Madden C, Gentilello L. Intracranial pressure monitoring in brain-injured patients is associated with worsening of survival. J Trauma. 2008;64(2):335–40.

9. Dawes AJ, Sacks GD, Cryer HG, Gruen JP, Preston C, Gorospe D, et al. Intracranial pressure monitoring and inpatient mortality in severe traumatic brain injury: a propensity score-matched analysis. J Trauma Acute Care Surg. 2015;78(3):492–501; discussion 501 – 2.

10. Farahvar A, Gerber LM, Chiu YL, Carney N, Hartl R, Ghajar J. Increased mortality in patients with severe traumatic brain injury treated without intracranial pressure monitoring. J Neurosurg. 2012;117(4):729–34.

11. Alali AS, Fowler RA, Mainprize TG, Scales DC, Kiss A, de Mestral C, et al. Intracranial pressure monitoring in severe traumatic brain injury: results from the American College of Surgeons Trauma Quality Improvement Program. J Neurotrauma. 2013;30(20):1737–46.

12. Chesnut RM, Temkin N, Carney N, Dikmen S, Rondina C, Videtta W, et al. A trial of intracranial-pressure monitoring in traumatic brain injury. N Engl J Med. 2012;367(26):2471–81.

13. Chesnut RMML, Klauber MR, et al. The role of secondary brain injury in determining outcome from severe head injury. J Trauma. 1993;34:216–22.

14. Jones PAAP, Midgely S, et al. Measuring the burden of secondary insults in head injured patients during intensive care. J Neurosurg Anesthesiol. 1994;6:4–14.

15. Muizelaar JP, Marmarou A, Ward JD, Kontos HA, Choi SC, Becker DP, et al. Adverse effects of prolonged hyperventilation in patients with severe head injury: a randomized clinical trial. J Neurosurg. 1991;75(5):731–9.

16. Network TARDS. Ventilation with lower tidal volumes as compared with traditional tidal volumes for acute lung injury and the acute respiratory distress syndrome. N Engl J Med. 2000;342(18):1301–8.

17. Karabinis A, Mandragos K, Stergiopoulos S, Komnos A, Soukup J, Speelberg B, et al. Safety and efficacy of analgesia-based sedation with remifentanil versus standard hypnotic-based regimens in intensive care unit patients with brain injuries: a randomised, controlled trial [ISRCTN50308308]. Crit Care (London, England). 2004;8(4):R268–80.

18. Minton MD, Stirt JA, Bedford RF, Haworth C. Intracranial pressure after atracurium in neurosurgical patients. Anesth Analg. 1985;64(11):1113–6.

19. Schramm WM, Jesenko R, Bartunek A, Gilly H. Effects of cisatracurium on cerebral and cardiovascular hemodynamics in

patients with severe brain injury. Acta Anaesthesiol Scand. 1997;41(10):1319–23.

20. Myburgh J, Cooper DJ, Finfer S, Bellomo R, Norton R, Bishop N, et al. Saline or albumin for fluid resuscitation in patients with traumatic brain injury. N Engl J Med. 2007;357(9):874–84.

21. Manley G, Knudson MM, Morabito D, Damron S, Erickson V, Pitts L. Hypotension, hypoxia, and head injury: frequency, duration, and consequences. Arch Surg (Chicago, Ill: 1960). 2001;136(10):1118.

22. Kelly DF, Goodale DB, Williams J, Herr DL, Chappell ET, Rosner MJ, et al. Propofol in the treatment of moderate and severe head injury: a randomized, prospective double-blinded pilot trial. J Neurosurg. 1999;90(6):1042–52.

23. Sandiumenge Camps A, Sanchez-Izquierdo Riera JA, Toral Vazquez D, Sa Borges M, Peinado Rodriguez J, Alted LE. Midazolam and 2% propofol in long-term sedation of traumatized critically ill patients: efficacy and safety comparison. Crit Care Med. 2000;28(11):3612–9.

24. Albanese J, Viviand X, Potie F, Rey M, Alliez B, Martin C. Sufentanil, fentanyl, and alfentanil in head trauma patients: a study on cerebral hemodynamics. Crit Care Med. 1999;27(2):407–11.

25. Sperry RJ, Bailey PL, Reichman MV, Peterson JC, Petersen PB, Pace NL. Fentanyl and sufentanil increase intracranial pressure in head trauma patients. Anesthesiology. 1992;77(3):416–20.

26. Haigh JD, Nemoto EM, DeWolf AM, Bleyaert AL. Comparison of the effects of succinylcholine and atracurium on intracranial pressure in monkeys with intracranial hypertension. Can Anaesth Soc J. 1986;33(4):421–6.

27. Temkin NR, Dikmen SS, Wilensky AJ, Keihm J, Chabal S, Winn HR. A randomized, double-blind study of phenytoin for the prevention of post-traumatic seizures. N Engl J Med. 1990;323(8):497–502.

28. Temkin NR, Dikmen SS, Anderson GD, Wilensky AJ, Holmes MD, Cohen W, et al. Valproate therapy for prevention of post-traumatic seizures: a randomized trial. J Neurosurg. 1999;91(4):593–600.

29. Jones KE, Puccio AM, Harshman KJ, Falcione B, Benedict N, Jankowitz BT, et al. Levetiracetam versus phenytoin for seizure prophylaxis in severe traumatic brain injury. Neurosurg Focus. 2008;25(4):E3.

30. Szaflarski JP, Sangha KS, Lindsell CJ, Shutter LA. Prospective, randomized, single-blinded comparative trial of intravenous levetiracetam versus phenytoin for seizure prophylaxis. Neurocrit Care. 2010;12(2):165–72.
31. Caballero GC, Hughes DW, Maxwell PR, Green K, Gamboa CD, Barthol CA. Retrospective analysis of levetiracetam compared to phenytoin for seizure prophylaxis in adults with traumatic brain injury. Hosp Pharm. 2013;48(9):757–61.
32. Lovell AT, Marshall AC, Elwell CE, Smith M, Goldstone JC. Changes in cerebral blood volume with changes in position in awake and anesthetized subjects. Anesth Analg. 2000;90(2): 372–6.
33. Mobbs RJ, Stoodley MA, Fuller J. Effect of cervical hard collar on intracranial pressure after head injury. ANZ J Surg. 2002;72(6):389–91.
34. Ho AM, Fung KY, Joynt GM, Karmakar MK, Peng Z. Rigid cervical collar and intracranial pressure of patients with severe head injury. J Trauma. 2002;53(6):1185–8.
35. Sakurai A, Atkins CM, Alonso OF, Bramlett HM, Dietrich WD. Mild hyperthermia worsens the neuropathological damage associated with mild traumatic brain injury in rats. J Neurotrauma. 2012;29(2):313–21.
36. Rincon F, Patel U, Schorr C, Lee E, Ross S, Dellinger RP, et al. Brain injury as a risk factor for fever upon admission to the intensive care unit and association with in-hospital case fatality: a matched cohort study. J Intensive Care Med. 2015;30:107–14.
37. Nielsen N, Wetterslev J, Cronberg T, Erlinge D, Gasche Y, Hassager C, et al. Targeted temperature management at 33°C versus 36°C after cardiac arrest. N Engl J Med. 2013;369(23): 2197–206.
38. Cook DJ, Fuller HD, Guyatt GH, Marshall JC, Leasa D, Hall R, et al. Risk factors for gastrointestinal bleeding in critically ill patients. Canadian Critical Care Trials Group. N Engl J Med. 1994;330(6):377–81.
39. Cook D, Guyatt G, Marshall J, Leasa D, Fuller H, Hall R, et al. A comparison of sucralfate and ranitidine for the prevention of upper gastrointestinal bleeding in patients requiring mechanical ventilation. Canadian Critical Care Trials Group. N Engl J Med. 1998;338(12):791–7.
40. Barkun AN, Bardou M, Pham CQ, Martel M. Proton pump inhibitors vs. histamine 2 receptor antagonists for stress-related mucosal bleeding prophylaxis in critically ill patients: a meta-analysis. Am J Gastroenterol. 2012;107(4):507–20; quiz 521.

41. Alhazzani W, Alenezi F, Jaeschke RZ, Moayyedi P, Cook DJ. Proton pump inhibitors versus histamine 2 receptor antagonists for stress ulcer prophylaxis in critically ill patients: a systematic review and meta-analysis. Crit Care Med. 2013;41(3):693–705.
42. Lin PC, Chang CH, Hsu PI, Tseng PL, Huang YB. The efficacy and safety of proton pump inhibitors vs histamine-2 receptor antagonists for stress ulcer bleeding prophylaxis among critical care patients: a meta-analysis. Crit Care Med. 2010;38(4):1197–205.
43. Pilkington KB, Wagstaff MJ, Greenwood JE. Prevention of gastrointestinal bleeding due to stress ulceration: a review of current literature. Anaesth Intensive Care. 2012;40(2):253–9.
44. Hébert PC, Wells G, Blajchman MA, Marshall J, Martin C, Pagliarello G, et al. A multicenter, randomized, controlled clinical trial of transfusion requirements in critical care. N Engl J Med. 1999;340(6):409–17.
45. Griesdale DE, Tremblay MH, McEwen J, Chittock DR. Glucose control and mortality in patients with severe traumatic brain injury. Neurocrit Care. 2009;11(3):311–6.
46. Green DM, O'Phelan KH, Bassin SL, Chang CW, Stern TS, Asai SM. Intensive versus conventional insulin therapy in critically ill neurologic patients. Neurocrit Care. 2010;13(3):299–306.
47. Krinsley JS, Grover A. Severe hypoglycemia in critically ill patients: risk factors and outcomes. Crit Care Med. 2007;35(10):2262–7.
48. Cammarata G, Ristagno G, Cammarata A, Mannanici G, Denaro C, Gullo A. Ocular ultrasound to detect intracranial hypertension in trauma patients. J Trauma. 2011;71(3):779–81.
49. Dubourg J, Javouhey E, Geeraerts T, Messerer M, Kassai B. Ultrasonography of optic nerve sheath diameter for detection of raised intracranial pressure: a systematic review and meta-analysis. Intensive Care Med. 2011;37(7):1059–68.
50. Geeraerts T, Launey Y, Martin L, Pottecher J, Vigue B, Duranteau J, et al. Ultrasonography of the optic nerve sheath may be useful for detecting raised intracranial pressure after severe brain injury. Intensive Care Med. 2007;33(10):1704–11.
51. Huang SJ, Chang L, Han YY, Lee YC, Tu YK. Efficacy and safety of hypertonic saline solutions in the treatment of severe head injury. Surg Neurol. 2006;65(6):539–46; discussion 546.
52. Horn P, Munch E, Vajkoczy P, Herrmann P, Quintel M, Schilling L, et al. Hypertonic saline solution for control of elevated intracranial pressure in patients with exhausted response to mannitol and barbiturates. Neurol Res. 1999;21(8):758–64.

53. Berger S, Schurer L, Hartl R, Messmer K, Baethmann A. Reduction of post-traumatic intracranial hypertension by hypertonic/hyperoncotic saline/dextran and hypertonic mannitol. Neurosurgery. 1995;37(1):98–107; discussion 107–8.

54. Cottenceau V, Masson F, Mahamid E, Petit L, Shik V, Sztark F, et al. Comparison of effects of equiosmolar doses of mannitol and hypertonic saline on cerebral blood flow and metabolism in traumatic brain injury. J Neurotrauma. 2011;28(10):2003–12.

55. Ichai C, Armando G, Orban JC, Berthier F, Rami L, Samat-Long C, et al. Sodium lactate versus mannitol in the treatment of intracranial hypertensive episodes in severe traumatic brain-injured patients. Intensive Care Med. 2009;35(3):471–9.

56. Bratton SL, Chestnut RM, Ghajar J, McConnell Hammond FF, Harris OA, Hartl R, et al. Guidelines for the management of severe traumatic brain injury. II. Hyperosmolar therapy. J Neurotrauma. 2007;24 Suppl 1:S14–20.

57. Schwartz ML, Tator CH, Rowed DW, Reid SR, Meguro K, Andrews DF. The University of Toronto head injury treatment study: a prospective, randomized comparison of pentobarbital and mannitol. Can J Neurol Sci. 1984;11(4):434–40.

58. Roberts I, Sydenham E. Barbiturates for acute traumatic brain injury. Cochrane Database Syst Rev. 2012;(12):CD000033.

59. Eisenberg HM, Frankowski RF, Contant CF, Marshall LF, Walker MD. High-dose barbiturate control of elevated intracranial pressure in patients with severe head injury. J Neurosurg. 1988;69(1):15–23.

60. Jiang J, Yu M, Zhu C. Effect of long-term mild hypothermia therapy in patients with severe traumatic brain injury: 1-year follow-up review of 87 cases. J Neurosurg. 2000;93(4):546–9.

61. Clifton GL, Valadka A, Zygun D, Coffey CS, Drever P, Fourwinds S, et al. Very early hypothermia induction in patients with severe brain injury (the National Acute Brain Injury Study: Hypothermia II): a randomised trial. Lancet Neurol. 2011;10(2):131–9.

62. Clifton GL, Miller ER, Choi SC, Levin HS, McCauley S, Smith Jr KR, et al. Lack of effect of induction of hypothermia after acute brain injury. N Engl J Med. 2001;344(8):556–63.

63. Adelson PD, Wisniewski SR, Beca J, Brown SD, Bell M, Muizelaar JP, et al. Comparison of hypothermia and normothermia after severe traumatic brain injury in children (Cool Kids): a phase 3, randomised controlled trial. Lancet Neurol. 2013;12(6):546–53.

64. Georgiou AP, Manara AR. Role of therapeutic hypothermia in improving outcome after traumatic brain injury: a systematic review. Br J Anaesth. 2013;110(3):357–67.
65. Andrews PJD, Sinclair HL, Rodriguez A, Harris BA, Battison CG, Rhodes JKJ, et al. Hypothermia for intracranial hypertension after traumatic brain injury. N Engl J Med. 0(0):null.
66. Coles JP, Minhas PS, Fryer TD, Smielewski P, Aigbirihio F, Donovan T, et al. Effect of hyperventilation on cerebral blood flow in traumatic head injury: clinical relevance and monitoring correlates. Crit Care Med. 2002;30(9):1950–9.
67. Sioutos PJ, Orozco JA, Carter LP, Weinand ME, Hamilton AJ, Williams FC. Continuous regional cerebral cortical blood flow monitoring in head-injured patients. Neurosurgery. 1995;36(5):943–9; discussion 949–50.
68. Diringer MN, Videen TO, Yundt K, Zazulia AR, Aiyagari V, Dacey Jr RG, et al. Regional cerebrovascular and metabolic effects of hyperventilation after severe traumatic brain injury. J Neurosurg. 2002;96(1):103–8.
69. Aarabi B, Hesdorffer DC, Ahn ES, Aresco C, Scalea TM, Eisenberg HM. Outcome following decompressive craniectomy for malignant swelling due to severe head injury. J Neurosurg. 2006;104(4):469–79.
70. Timofeev I, Czosnyka M, Nortje J, Smielewski P, Kirkpatrick P, Gupta A, et al. Effect of decompressive craniectomy on intracranial pressure and cerebrospinal compensation following traumatic brain injury. J Neurosurg. 2008;108(1):66–73.
71. Timofeev I, Hutchinson PJ. Outcome after surgical decompression of severe traumatic brain injury. Injury. 2006;37(12):1125–32.
72. Cooper DJ, Rosenfeld JV, Murray L, Arabi YM, Davies AR, D'Urso P, et al. Decompressive craniectomy in diffuse traumatic brain injury. N Engl J Med. 2011;364(16):1493–502.
73. Wilson MH, Wise D, Davies G, Lockey D. Emergency burr holes: "How to do it". Scand J Trauma Resusc Emerg Med. 2012;20:24.
74. Motohashi O, Kameyama M, Shimosegawa Y, Fujimori K, Sugai K, Onuma T. Single burr hole evacuation for traumatic acute subdural hematoma of the posterior fossa in the emergency room. J Neurotrauma. 2002;19(8):993–8.
75. Rinker CF, McMurry FG, Groeneweg VR, Bahnson FF, Banks KL, Gannon DM. Emergency craniotomy in a rural Level III trauma center. J Trauma. 1998;44(6):984–9; discussion 989–90.

76. Treacy PJ, Reilly P, Brophy B. Emergency neurosurgery by general surgeons at a remote major hospital. ANZ J Surg. 2005;75(10):852–7.
77. Wester K. Decompressive surgery for "pure" epidural hematomas: does neurosurgical expertise improve the outcome? Neurosurgery. 1999;44(3):495–500; discussion 500–2.

Chapter 12
Management of the Critically Ill Burns Patient

Anthony D. Holley

Abstract   Burn injuries in military personnel during combat are well recognized, historically accounting for approximately 5–20 % of conventional warfare military casualties. It is therefore vitally important that military health professionals have an effective strategy for caring for these patients. The initial approach is the same as for all major trauma, with special attention to airway patency given the risk of airway burns. The respiratory assessment and management must address the potential for significant inhalational injury. The pathophysiology of major burns is complex leading to shock, which is predominantly hypovolaemic in origin, but often

A.D. Holley, MBBCh, DipDHM, FACEM, FCICM
Department of Intensive Care Medicine, Royal Brisbane and
Women's Hospital, Brisbane, Australia

Burns, Trauma and Critical Care Research Centre, The University
of Queensland, Brisbane, Australia

Professional Liaison Officer for Emergency Medicine, Anaesthesia
and Intensive Care Medicine for the Royal Australian Navy,
Canberra, Australia
e-mail: anthony.holley@health.qld.gov.au

S.D. Hutchings (ed.), *Trauma and Combat Critical Care*
in Clinical Practice, In Clinical Practice,
DOI 10.1007/978-3-319-28758-4_12,

multifactorial. Fluid resuscitation should proceed in a timely and predetermined manner with carefully selected goals/endpoints. The consequences of both under and over resuscitation must be appreciated by the clinician and the need for escharotomy or fasciotomy identified. The mechanism of injury must be considered such that special attention can be provided in the setting of chemical and electrical burns. The surgical principles of deep burn management require early debridement and subsequent surface cover. The debrided areas are ultimately skin grafted, but in the interim maybe covered by a range of biological or synthetic products. The burn patient is at risk of a wide range of complications and therefore requires meticulous intensive care management. This chapter provides a comprehensive strategy for the care of a burns victim.

Keywords Burns • Pathophysiology • Resuscitation • Inhalation • Airway • Assessment • Military • Fluids • Ventilation

Introduction

Burn injuries in military personnel during combat are well recognized. In modern conventional conflicts injuries commonly include burns from explosions or penetrating injuries from small arms fire. Historically burn injuries account for approximately 5–20 % of conventional warfare military casualties [1]. During World War II, 1.5 % casualties resulted from burns injury [2, 3]. In the Korean War, burns accounted for 1 % of all battle casualties increasing to 4.6 % in the Vietnam War. The nature of the conflict has substantial impact on injury patterns [4]. In the Yom Kippur Israeli War, characterised by tank battles, 8.1 % of the casualties' sustained burns. Similarly, in the Falklands War, there was a comparatively high incidence of burn injuries seen (14 %) most of which occurred in the setting of burning ships. Burn injuries constituted 2.5 % of casualties from the recent

Afghanistan War [5]. Despite a significant reduction in the lethality of burn injuries over the last three decades resulting from rapid, focused resuscitation and advances in surgical strategies, burns can be devastating injuries which require substantial resources and protracted treatment [6]. It is reasonable for military health care providers to anticipate an increasing incidence of burns casualties with the changing nature of war. Optimal care of the critically burned patient requires prompt assessment of the patient and evaluation of the burn.

Table 12.1 summarises the potential mechanisms of burn injury.

What Is the Pathophysiology of Burn Injury?

The "Jackson Burn Wound Model" assists in understanding the pathophysiology of a burn wound at a local level. In 1947 Jackson described three zones of a burn wound. The primary injury is the **zone of coagulation** nearest the heat source [7]. This zone has irreversible tissue necrosis at the centre of the burn due to exposure to heat, chemicals or electricity. The extent of this injury depends on duration of exposure and the maximal temperature (or concentration). Immediately adjacent to the central zone of necrosis, is the **zone of stasis** in which there is a reduced dermal perfusion, this tissue although damaged is potentially viable.

The principle goal of burn resuscitation is to increase tissue perfusion to this area and prevent the damage from becoming irreversible [8]. This ischaemic zone may progress to full necrosis unless perfusion is re-established [9, 10]. At the periphery of the burn is a third zone, the **zone of hyperaemia** characterised by a reversible increase in blood flow and inflammation. It is important to conceptualise these three zones of a burn in three dimensions (Fig. 12.1) and so if there is further loss of viable tissue it results in both wound deepening and surface extension [11].

The pathophysiology of large surface area burns (>20 %) is extremely complex and requires a detailed understanding

TABLE 12.1 Mechanisms of burn injury

Mechanism	Situation
Flame burns	Secondary to burning fuel, vehicles, buildings, or shelters that were ignited by explosives. Often associated with inhalational injury and other concomitant trauma. Tend to be deep dermal or full thickness
Flash injury	High temperatures generated by explosives
Incinerating materials	Napalm or phosphorus munitions
Contact burns	Hot environmental objects
Steam or hot liquid burns	Steam or hot fluids released by damaged machinery
Chemical burns	Agents of warfare or leakage of chemicals used/stored in the immediate environment. Chemical burns tend to be deep, as the corrosive agent continues to cause coagulative necrosis until completely removed. Alkalis tend to penetrate deeper and continue damaging tissue for a longer duration than acids.
Electrical/laser burns	Equipment accidents.
Radiation burns	Exposure to nuclear weapons.

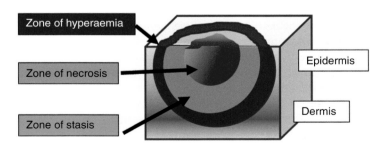

FIGURE 12.1 Schematic representation of local burn zones

TABLE 12.2 Factors influencing the degree of "Burn Shock" which may develop following injury

Patient age
Depth of burn
Surface extent of burn
Presence of inhalation injury
Need for escharotomies/fasciotomies
Time delay to resuscitation
Associated injuries

in order to facilitate appropriate resuscitation. Patients are at risk of developing "burn shock" is if they have greater than 20 % of their total body surface area (TBSA) involved with deep or partial thickness burns [12, 13]. The severity of the shock not only depends on the depth and extent of the burn [14], but also on other factors as shown in Table 12.2.

Burn pathophysiology is characterised by a series of predictable phases [14]. The principle insult is the loss of the integument and hence body fluid and temperature homeostasis. The initial phase of injury is characterized by increased capillary permeability and transmembrane cellular changes. The increased capillary permeability results from a massive and sustained cytokine release into the systemic circulation following injury and includes vasoactive substances, interleukins, histamine and prostaglandins [14]. This results in a distributive shock pattern, which is further exacerbated by fluid loss into the interstitium [15]. Increased capillary permeability, mediated by these cytokines, also results in a loss of intravascular proteins and oncotic pressure [16]. Concomitantly the interstitial oncotic pressure may rise, further encouraging volume loss from the intravascular compartment. It is highly likely that this initial "cytokine storm" may have directly negative effects on both myocardial and renal function [14, 17–19]. The cytokine mediated decrease in myocardial contractility leads to a depressed cardiac output which is further exacerbated by impaired intracellular calcium homeostasis. These factors are summarized in Fig. 12.2

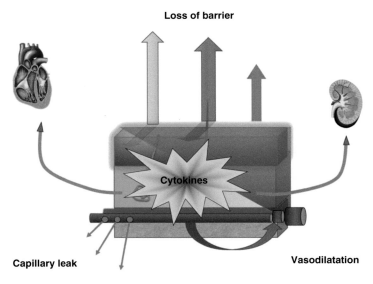

FIGURE 12.2 Burn shock: local and systemic effects of severe burns leading to multifactorial shock

How Should the Patient with Severe Burns Be Assessed?

The assessment of a burns patient is challenging and requires a disciplined and methodical approach. The approach is no different to any other patient with severe multi trauma, but is then followed up by a detailed evaluation of the depth and extent of the burn. See Table 12.3. In order to make an accurate assessment of the burn severity the clinician requires experience, but more importantly diligence. The evolving nature of a burn makes it essential to reassess the wounds frequently within the first 48 h as the exudate and oedema start to resolve.

TABLE 12.3 General approach to burns resuscitation

Primary survey	Assessment of the airway, breathing, circulation, neurological status with full exposure.
Adjuncts to primary survey	Securing reliable intravenous access. Insertion of urinary catheter
Secondary survey	Detailed clinical examination detecting all injuries
Detailed evaluation of the burn	Depth- very rarely homogeneous so all anatomical areas require evaluation. Extent- TBSA (%)

Assessing Burn Depth

Establishing the depth of a burn is critical to developing a formal resuscitation plan [20, 21] and is important in determining the potential for subsequent wound healing and prognosis. The history and injury pattern often afford the clinician a good indication as to the likely severity of injury. On examination of the burn the extent and speed of capillary refill is useful in helping establish burn depth. The clinician needs to be cognisant that burn wound evolution frequently results in increased depth of burn injury when subsequently reviewed. Depending on the depth of tissue damage, burns are classified as either epidermal, superficial dermal partial thickness, deep dermal partial thickness or full thickness as shown in Table 12.4.

Superficial burns and severe deep burns are readily diagnosed; it is those of intermediate or mixed thickness that are more problematic. It is also important to recognise that most burn wounds, especially those involving larger surface areas, are not homogenous in depth. They are often a composite of areas of different depths and only diligent, frequent clinical examination will establish the true extent of injury [13].

Assessing Burn Area

The establishment of burn surface area is an important component of the initial assessment and is critical in determining resuscitation requirements and the need for transfer to a specialist burns centre [22]. The extent of injury is documented using the percentage of the total body surface area that is affected by the burn. It is important that erythematous areas (superficial burn) are not be included when calculating burn area [7].

Several studies have compared a range of methods of estimating burn surface area. The surface area of a patient's palm (including fingers) is about 1 % total body surface area (Fig. 12.3). The accuracy of this method, however tends to decline when used to estimate larger surface areas. It remains a useful strategy in difficult or austere environments.

The Lund & Browder charts (Fig. 12.4) appear more accurate than either the Wallace Rule of Nines (Fig. 12.5) or palm size in determining the percentage of body surface area involved in a burn [7]. The Rule of Nines is however convenient and easily applied in burn patients with the caveat that it is potentially less accurate in children or obese people.

How Should the Patient with Severe Burns Be Resuscitated?

Initial Management

The presentation of severe burn injuries can be startling even for experienced clinicians and they therefore have the potential to be the ultimate distracting injury. Frequently other injuries may coexist, especially when there is a history of:

- Blast or explosion
- Motor vehicle accident
- High voltage electrical injury

It is therefore vital that the attending clinician conduct an effective primary and secondary survey. The patient must be removed from any sources of heat or ongoing thermal injury. Any clothing that is burned, covered with chemicals, or that is constricting must be removed with due attention to the medical providers own safety. It is also important to recognise that inhalation of the toxic products of combustion and hypoxia may cause a decreased level of consciousness.

Burns that are less than three hours old should be cooled using standard tap water, if available (15–18 °C is adequate) for at least 20 min [23] and then the patient should be carefully dried. The patient should then be covered with a clean

TABLE 12.4 Classifying burn depth and its impact on management and prognosis

Burn depth	Clinical features	Prognosis
Superficial epidermal burns: Involves the epidermis	Hyperaemic, erythematous and painful. Blister formation and skin desquamation are delayed for few days.	The stratified layers of the epidermis are lost and healing occurs by regeneration of the epidermis from the basal layer. Heals within 7 days without scarring.
Superficial dermal partial thickness burns: Involves the epidermis And Papillary dermis. Skin overlying the blister is dead and separated from the base by inflammatory oedema fluid	Very painful secondary to sensory nerve exposure. Capillary return brisk with preserved vasculature. Blisters characteristic- on the pink papillary dermis is exposed. Desiccation of exposed dermis can increase the depth of tissue loss.	Spontaneous healing by epithelialisation within 14 days.

(continued)

TABLE 12.4 (continued)

Burn depth	Clinical features	Prognosis
Deep dermal partial thickness burns: Extensive destruction of the dermal vascular plexus. Exposed reticular dermis. The dermal nerve endings are also damaged.	These burns tend to be dry, with diminished fluid exudates. Characterised by the early (within hours) development of extensive blisters, which rupture early to expose deep damaged dermis. Exposed reticular dermis is pale in colour due to damage to dermal blood vessels or red secondary to extravasation of red blood cells from damaged vessels. Markedly decreased capillary return, with no or sluggish blanching. Sensation is reduced	Requires grafting in order to heal
Full thickness burns: Epidermis and dermis destroyed. May penetrate more deeply into underlying structures- fat, muscle and bone.	Dense white, waxy or even charred appearance. The sensory nerves in the dermis are destroyed in a full thickness burn, and so sensation is lost. The coagulated dead skin, which has a leathery appearance is referred to as an eschar.	Requires grafting in order to heal

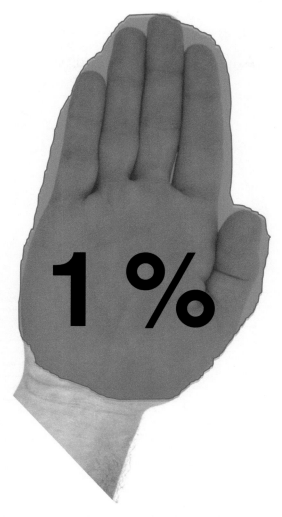

FIGURE 12.3 Palmer surface for estimating burn size

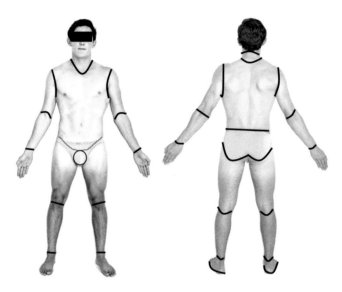

	Birth 1 year	1–4 years	5–9 years	10–14 years	15 years	Adult	Burn size estimate
Head	19	17	13	11	9	7	
Neck	2	2	2	2	2	2	
Anterior trunk	13	13	13	13	13	13	
Posterior trunk	13	13	13	13	13	13	
Right buttock	2.5	2.5	2.5	2.5	2.5	2.5	
Left buttock	2.5	2.5	2.5	2.5	2.5	2.5	
Genitalia	1	1	1	1	1	1	
Right upper arm	4	4	4	4	4	4	
Left upper arm	4	4	4	4	4	4	
Right lower arm	3	3	3	3	3	3	
Left lower arm	3	3	3	3	3	3	
Right hand	2.5	2.5	2.5	2.5	2.5	2.5	
Left hand	2.5	2.5	2.5	2.5	2.5	2.5	
Right thigh	5.5	6.5	8	8.5	9	9.5	
Left thigh	5.5	6.5	8	8.5	9	9.5	
Right leg	5	5	5.5	6	6.5	7	
Left leg	5	5	5.5	6	6.5	7	
Right foot	3.5	3.5	3.5	3.5	3.5	3.5	
Left foot	3.5	3.5	3.5	3.5	3.5	3.5	

Total BSAB _____

FIGURE 12.4 The Lund & Browder Chart

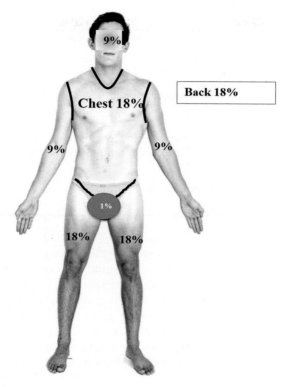

FIGURE 12.5 Wallace Rule of Nines

dry sheet or blanket to prevent hypothermia and all rings and constricting jewellery or garments must be removed.

Airway

The patient's airway remains the priority, and this should include protection of the cervical spine if the mechanism of injury is conducive to vertebral injury. The principle airway concern in the burns patient is the risk of obstruction due to subsequent swelling of the oropharynx and soft tissues of the neck. It is now recognised that more patients than actually

TABLE 12.5 Indications for intubation in burns patients

Stridor is an immediate indication for intubation

Difficulty with phonation is an immediate indication for intubation

Uncooperative/combative/disoriented patient

Significant oral/facial burns

Prophylactic' intubation prior to transfer if history or signs indicate likelihood of inhalation and thus possible airway obstruction

Increasing swelling of head and neck

Unprotected airway

require intubation are intubated, but this situation is preferable to a more conservative approach that may result in delayed unsalvageable airway obstruction [24]. It is important to recognise that airway injury/swelling may not be recognised acutely, but becomes progressively more obvious with time and fluid resuscitation. There are several clinical signs or situations that mandate early intubation as shown in Table 12.5.

A wide range of agents and combinations are available for induction of anaesthesia, including Ketamine, Propofol, Fentanyl and Midazolam, the anaesthetic combination utilised however, needs to account for the significant potential to induce profound hypotension secondary to the loss of sympathetic response in the setting of volume depletion and vasodilatation [25]. The choice of muscle relaxant is similarly extensive, importantly it is safe to use suxamethonium in the first 24 h. The intubating physician must be fully prepared to encounter a difficult airway and be capable and confident of proceeding to a surgical airway [26].

Following successful intubation the endotracheal tube needs to be reliably secured, initially with anaesthetic ties. It is our practice to insert alveolar ridge screws (Fig. 12.6) during the patient's first visit to the operating theatre. This provides a reliable strategy for securing the airway, with the added advantage of avoiding ongoing trauma to facial burns.

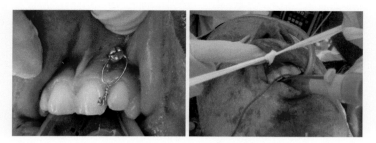

FIGURE 12.6 Alveolar screw providing a secure attachment of the endotracheal tube

TABLE 12.6 Features suggestive of inhalational injury

Facial burns or singed facial/nasal hair is present
Stridor, hoarse voice
Intra- oral oedema
Carbonaceous sputum
Soot or mucosal inflammatory changes in the mouth or nose
The patient was in a confined space at the time of accident

Ventilation

All patients should be evaluated for possible inhalation injury, this includes a detailed review of the history and a reliable clinical examination. Features suggestive of inhalational injury are shown in Table 12.6.

Bronchoscopy

Early bronchoscopy can be valuable in evaluating the extent/presence of inhalation injury [27]. *Masanes* used biopsy histologic findings as the "gold standard," to evaluate the utility of bronchoscopy [28, 29]. Bronchoscopy proved to be sensitive (sensitivity, 0.79) and highly specific (specificity, 0.94) for the

TABLE 12.7 Bronchoscopic grading of inhalation injury [30]

Grade	Severity	Features on bronchoscopy
Grade 0	No injury	Absence of carbonaceous deposits, erythema, oedema, bronchorrhea, or obstruction.
Grade 1	Mild injury	Minor or patchy areas of erythema, carbonaceous deposits in proximal or distal bronchi.
Grade 2	Moderate injury	Moderate degree of erythema, Carbonaceous deposits, bronchorrhea, with or without compromise of the bronchi.
Grade 3	Severe injury	Severe inflammation with friability, copious carbonaceous deposits, bronchorrhea, bronchial obstruction.
Grade 4 [30]	Massive injury	Evidence of mucosal sloughing, necrosis, endoluminal obliteration.

diagnosis of inhalation injury and was more reliable than the circumstances of the injury or the clinical findings. In this study bronchoscopy-proven inhalation injury was one of the most strongly predictive variables for the onset of ARDS and death. *Endorf* and *Gamelli* [30] developed a grading system for inhalational injury (Table 12.7) that provides an objective and clinically useful approach to evaluating the patient with suspected inhalation.

Ventilatory Strategy

There is no ideal respiratory support strategy for the patient with inhalation injury or indeed with severe burns. A practical approach is to provide a protective lung strategy that delivers tidal volumes of 4–6 ml/kg, avoids plateau pressures greater than 30 cmH$_2$O and avoids hyperoxia. Limitation of pressure, acceptance of permissive hypercapnia and strategies to manage secretions are all important. Patients with smoke inhalation are at significant risk of developing ventilator associated pneumonia or acute respiratory distress syndrome [31].

Standard strategies to mitigate this risk should be employed and include: elevation of the head of the bed to 30–45°, frequent position changes and fastidious oral care. Antibiotic prophylaxis has no role and may increase infection rates. There may be a role for extracorporeal membrane oxygenation as an extreme rescue therapy, however there is currently insufficient evidence to make firm recommendations. Prone ventilation can be logistically challenging, but is effective and practical in the hypoxic patient [32].

The efficacy of aerosolised heparin in the adult burn and inhalation injury population remains unclear, however a number of centres continue to use regular nebulised heparin in order to decrease the tenacity of secretions and provide an anti-inflammatory effect [33].

The burn patient may have mechanical factors that impede respiration or precipitate respiratory failure. Deep circumferential burns of the chest or abdomen can restrict chest expansion sufficiently to compromise ventilation and require escharotomy as demonstrated in Fig. 12.7.

What Is an Appropriate Fluid Resuscitation Strategy Following Severe Burn Injury?

While conducting the primary survey reliable intravenous access must be established. Intravenous cannulas may be placed through the burned area if there is no other viable option, it is then necessary to suture the cannula in place to prevent dislodgement. Intraosseous access is an excellent short term alternative while more reliable access is achieved.

The extent of the burn is assessed with respect to percentage body surface area involved and depth. This allows for utilisation of one of the many formulae available (Table 12.8) to guide the initial resuscitation [34, 35].

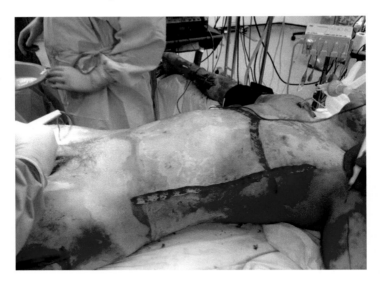

FIGURE 12.7 Escharotomy for circumferential chest burn compromising ventilation

TABLE 12.8 Examples of burn resuscitation formulae

Formula	Strategy
Brooke	First 24 h Lactated Ringers at 1.5 ml/kg/% TBSA burn and colloid at 0.5 ml/kg/% TBSA burn.
Modified Brooke	First 24 h: Lactated Ringers at 2 ml/kg/% TBSA burn. Half in the first 8 h and half in the remaining 16 h.
Parkland	First 24 h Lactated Ringers at 4 ml/kg/%TBSA. Half in first 8 h and half in the remaining 16 h.
Rule of tens	%TBSA × 10 = Initial Fluid Rate mL/h For every 10 kg > 80 kg increase rate by 100 mL/h

The Parkland formula remains the most commonly used formula in the United Kingdom, Ireland, United States and Canada where clinicians report using this formula in 78 % of all burns cases [36].

It is important that maintenance fluids should be added over and above the Parklands formula for children weighing less than 30 kg.

The initial fluid rate selected is not as important as the resuscitation itself, which must be closely monitored and adjusted by a diligent clinician [21]. For burns > 20 % TBSA we would recommend the following:

1. Insert a central venous catheter
2. Insert a urinary (Foley) catheter
3. Use advanced haemodynamic monitoring (e.g. echocardiography to guide resuscitation)
4. Monitor intra-abdominal (bladder) pressure every four hours during the initial resuscitation

The principle aim of fluid resuscitation following a severe burn is to ensure appropriate end-organ tissue perfusion and minimise extension of the injury in the zone of stasis. This task can be extremely difficult to efficiently achieve because of the complex pathophysiology involved in a burn injury. Resuscitation should focus on optimizing global flow and perfusion as outlined in Chap. 6.

Most resuscitation formulae call for the use of isotonic crystalloids. However, there have been proponents of hypertonic solutions and colloids [3, 37]. Studies have demonstrated that colloids provide little clinical benefit when given in the first 24 h post burn and may have detrimental effects on pulmonary function and potentially worsen tissue oedema. The term "fluid creep" has been coined [38], suggesting that some patients are over-resuscitated with resultant complications. Over-resuscitation can result in "resuscitation morbidity", a term used to describe complications secondary to excess fluid delivery including pulmonary oedema and orbital/extremity/abdominal compartment syndromes [39–41]. All of these are associated with increased morbidity and mortality.

Signs of extremity compartment syndrome need to be actively reviewed on an ongoing basis throughout the resuscitation. They may include:

(a) Severe pain at rest
(b) 'Tight' muscle compartments in limbs
(c) Increased pain on passive extension of digits
(d) Decreased distal sensation
(e) Decreased distal perfusion

Early multi-compartment fasciotomy, such as shown in Fig. 12.8 may be limb saving in this setting. The eschar of a burn wound consists of leathery dead skin producing a non-elastic exoskeleton which impedes perfusion. In general, escharotomies are required for circumferential full-thickness extremity burns in which distal perfusion has been compromised or as mentioned for chest burns in which the eschar impedes respiration.

Escharotomies are easily be performed at the bedside with either a scalpel or the use of electrocautery following recognised landmarks as shown in Fig. 12.9. It is important that the incision extends only through the eschar and not through the muscle fascia. Adequate release is apparent by separation of the eschar and improved distal perfusion.

In those situations, where it appears that excess crystalloid has been given, for example patients who exceed the Parkland formula calculation by more than 1.5 times or 6 ml/kg/%TBSA, some suggest "colloid rescue" be employed [42]. The colloid rescue formula advocates 1/3 of the Parkland volume be given as given as albumin and two thirds be given as Lactated Ringer's solution. This formula has been shown by some studies to decrease fluid requirements without any associated increase in mortality or renal failure. The use of hypertonic saline in burn patients has been limited by the

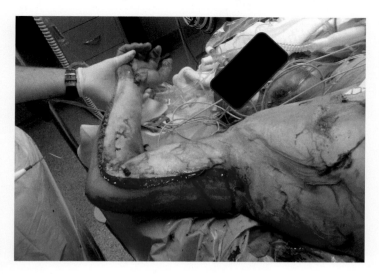

FIGURE 12.8 Upper limb Fasciotomy

concern of hypernatraemia, renal failure and increased mortality [43]. Therefore at the current time it cannot be recommended.

How Should Patients with Electrical Burns Be Managed?

Electrical injuries are classified as low (<1000 V) or high (>1000 V) voltage injuries. Low voltage injuries are usually the result of domestic (240 V single phase AC) or industrial (415 V 3 phase AC) accidents. High voltage electrical injuries usually result from contact with overhead powerlines and other sources of high voltage electrical currents [44].

Electrical burn severity is determined by:

• Voltage
• Current
• Type of current

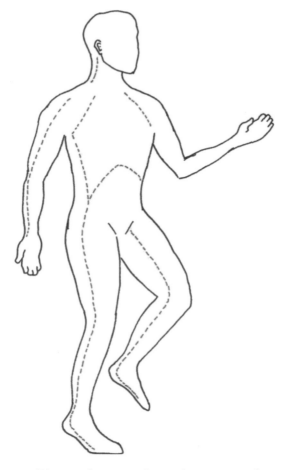

FIGURE 12.9 Diagram demonstrating surface anatomy for escharotomy incisions

- Presence of water
- Duration of contact
- Resistance at contact points

Low voltage injuries are associated with localized areas of tissue destruction, while high voltage injuries tend to be characterized by deep and extensive tissue damage and are frequently associated with other injuries.

Three general patterns of injury are described:

1. 'True' electrical injury caused by current flow
2. Electrical arc injury caused by arc of current from the source to an object
3. Flame injury secondary to the ignition of clothes/garments

The management of these injuries is similar to that of standard burns injury, except for the need to isolate power at the scene and the need to recognise potential associated injuries. Importantly these patients are at high risk of myocardial injury and dysrhythmias. Daily determination of creatinine kinase levels and myoglobin is useful in assessing for occult rhabdomyolysis. Electrical burns may be deceptive with fluid resuscitation requirements that are often greater than that predicted by the area of the cutaneous burn. The extent of the burn and associated muscle damage may not be fully appreciated resulting in fluid loss which is not accounted for by the standard burns formula. It is extremely important to be vigilant for the development of rhabdomyolysis, myoglobinuria, and potential acute kidney injury. Continual clinical review to identify early limb compartment syndrome is also critical.

What Are the Principles of Burn Wound Management?

Thermal injury removes the protective barrier function of the skin and therefore dressings are required to protect the body against evaporative heat loss and environmental microbes. Initially a clean sheet or plastic wrap is useful. Superficial and superficial partial-thickness burns classically will heal without surgical excision and grafting. Regular dressing changes and wound baths remove necrotic debris and enhance heal-

TABLE 12.9 Examples of burn wound care products

Product	Indication
Adherent dressings e.g., Opsite or Duoderm	Superficial burns
Bacitracin, Neomycin, Polymyxin B	Superficial burns Facial burns Burns close to mucosal surfaces
Multiday dressings e.g. Mepilex and Acticoat	Superficial burns and partial thickness burns. Also used post debridement
Silver sulpurdiazine (SSD)	Deep dermal and full thickness burns (away from face and mucosal surfaces).

ing that should be established by two weeks. Superficial wounds require a dressing that provides a moist environment to optimise epithelialization and this is easily achieved with the application of ointments or lotions. With partial-thickness and full-thickness wounds, however, it is necessary to include agents that protect against microbial colonization. It is important to acknowledge that systemic antibiotic prophylaxis has absolutely no role in the management of acute burn wounds and use of prophylactic antibiotics in burn patients is associated with increased infection risk [45]. A comparison of burn wound dressings is shown in Table 12.9.

When managing deep and full thickness burns it is necessary for the patient to be under the care of a surgeon. Early wound excision and closure reduce the incidence of infection and improve survival. It has been increasingly recognised that early removal of dead and severely damaged tissue controls the dramatic systemic inflammatory response that is characteristic of deep burns. Early excision of deep burn wounds also appears to decrease hypertrophic scarring.

The standard modern approach is early staged excision commencing as early as post burn day two. Subsequent operations are conducted at intervals of 2–3 days until the entire eschar is removed and full wound coverage is achieved. The debrided wounds are temporarily covered with biologic dressings or cadaveric allograft until further autogenous donor sites are regenerated [46, 47]. Donor sites usually epithelialise within about 2 weeks allowing new skin to be reharvested.

What Are the Other General Principles of Burn Injury Management in the Intensive Care Unit?

It is important to recognise that this is a highly labour and resource intensive process with large burns often remaining in intensive care for weeks to months. These patients are at substantial risk of hypothermia, anaemia, deep vein thrombosis [48–50] stress ulceration, nutritional deprivation, decubitus and corneal ulceration and so require diligent critical care [34].

Burn victims have multiple factors which may contribute to deep venous thrombosis and pulmonary embolism risk. Patients with greater than 40 % TBSA burn appear to be at highest venous thromboembolic (VTE) risk (2.4 %). The combination of increased TBSA burn and ICU admission predicts those patients at highest risk. Patients with these risk factors probably benefit from early, aggressive VTE prophylaxis [51].

Effective nutritional support is required in patients with severe burn injury, which is characterised by a dramatic elevation in plasma catecholamines, cortisol, and inflammatory mediators resulting in a prolonged and pronounced hypermetabolic response. The risk of inadequate provision of nutrition is rapid whole-body catabolism, muscle wasting, and severe cachexia. Furthermore, nutritional support is an essential component of burn care to prevent ileus and stress ulceration. The American Burn Association practice [15] guidelines recommend the commencement of enteral feeding as soon as practical. Adults are able to maintain their body weight after a significant burn injury only with adequate and continuous

TABLE 12.10 Summary of key points

Burn injury requires a standard trauma approach to avoid missing associated injuries

The burn needs to be carefully evaluated with respect to depth and percentage surface area.

Burn formulae are simply a guide

Endpoints/Goals need to be frequently reviewed to avoid over/under resuscitation

Compartment syndromes need to be excluded

Prophylactic antibiotics are contraindicated.

Early and sequential debridement is indicated for deep and full thickness burns

nutrition of 25 kcal per kilogram body weight per day and an additional 40 kcal per percent total body surface area burn per day. Aggressive protein delivery, providing approximately 20 % of calories from protein, has been associated with improved mortality and morbidity. However, it is important to recognise that the provision of excess calories and/or protein is not only ineffective and but likely to increase complications such as hyperglycaemia and overfeeding syndrome [52–55].

Summary

The thermally injured patient presents significant challenges for the clinical team that requires a coordinated response to resuscitation and vigilance for a wide range of complications. The patient is initially evaluated as for all major trauma. The surface area and depth of burn involved then dictate the initial resuscitation, which is continually modified based on the clinical response. Early surgical involvement is critical and allows for expedient debridement and subsequent coverage. The critical care physician requires a diligent and methodical approach to these complex patients. Key points in the management of severe burns are shown in Table 12.10

References

1. Gomez R, Murray CK, Hospenthal DR, et al. Causes of mortality by autopsy findings of combat casualties and civilian patients admitted to a burn unit. J Am Coll Surg. 2009;208:348–54.
2. Polskin LJ. Burns of World War II. Chic Med Sch Q. 1945;7:15–9.
3. Thomas SJ, Kramer GC, Herndon DN. Burns: military options and tactical solutions. J Trauma. 2003;54:S207–18.
4. Foster MA, Moledina J, Jeffery SL. Epidemiology of U.K. military burns. J Burn Care Res Off Publ Am Burn Assoc. 2011;32:415–20.
5. Roeder RA, Schulman CI. An overview of war-related thermal injuries. J Craniofac Surg. 2010;21:971–5.
6. Saeman MR, Hodgman EI, Burris A, et al. Epidemiology and outcomes of pediatric burns over 35 years at Parkland Hospital. Burns J Int Soc Burn Inj. 2016;42:202–8.
7. Hettiaratchy S, Dziewulski P. ABC of burns: pathophysiology and types of burns. BMJ. 2004;328:1427–9.
8. Middelkoop E, Vloemans AF. Response to burns in the elderly: what is pathophysiology and what is physiology? EBioMedicine. 2015;2:1314–5.
9. Salibian AA, Rosario AT, Severo LA, et al. Current concepts on burn wound conversion – a review of recent advances in understanding the secondary progressions of burns. Burns. 2016. pii: S0305-4179(15)00385-X. doi:10.1016/j.burns.2015.11.007. [Epub ahead of print]
10. Schmauss D, Rezaeian F, Finck T, Machens HG, Wettstein R, Harder Y. Treatment of secondary burn wound progression in contact burns-a systematic review of experimental approaches. J Burn Care Res Off Publ Am Burn Assoc. 2015;36:e176–89.
11. Ganapathy M. Body's response to heat – pathophysiology of burns. Nurs J India. 2012;103:279–81.
12. Peeters Y, Vandervelden S, Wise R, Malbrain ML. An overview on fluid resuscitation and resuscitation endpoints in burns: Past, present and future. Part 1 – historical background, resuscitation fluid and adjunctive treatment. Anaesthesiol Intensive Ther. 2015;47 Spec No:6–14.
13. Murphy P, Colwell C, Pineda G, Bryan T. Burning issues. By understanding the pathophysiology of burns, providers can give patients their best chance at good outcomes. EMS Mag. 2009;38:83–90.

14. Keck M, Herndon DH, Kamolz LP, Frey M, Jeschke MG. Pathophysiology of burns. Wiener Medizinische Wochenschrift. 2009;159:327–36.
15. Pham TN, Cancio LC, Gibran NS, American BA. American Burn Association practice guidelines burn shock resuscitation. J Burn Care Res Off Publ Am Burn Assoc. 2008;29:257–66.
16. Ruiz-Castilla M, Roca O, Masclans JR, Barret JP. Recent advances in biomarkers in severe burns. Shock. 2016;45:117–25.
17. Abu-Sittah GS, Sarhane KA, Dibo SA, Ibrahim A. Cardiovascular dysfunction in burns: review of the literature. Ann Burns Fire Disasters. 2012;25:26–37.
18. Ibrahim AE, Sarhane KA, Fagan SP, Goverman J. Renal dysfunction in burns: a review. Ann Burns Fire Disasters. 2013;26:16–25.
19. Jeschke MG, Patsouris D, Stanojcic M, et al. Pathophysiologic response to burns in the elderly. EBioMedicine. 2015;2:1536–48.
20. Williams D. Nomograms to aid fluid resuscitation in acute burns. Burns J Int Soc Burn Inj. 2011;37:543–5.
21. Tricklebank S. Modern trends in fluid therapy for burns. Burns J Int Soc Burn Inj. 2009;35:757–67.
22. Collis N, Smith G, Fenton OM. Accuracy of burn size estimation and subsequent fluid resuscitation prior to arrival at the Yorkshire Regional Burns Unit. A three year retrospective study. Burns J Int Soc Burn Inj. 1999;25:345–51.
23. Wood FM, Phillips M, Jovic T, et al. Water first aid is beneficial in humans post-burn: evidence from a Bi-national cohort study. PLoS One. 2016;11:e0147259.
24. Romanowski KS, Palmieri TL, Sen S, Greenhalgh DG. More than one third of intubations in patients transferred to burn centers are unnecessary: proposed guidelines for appropriate intubation of the burn patient. J Burn Care Res. 2015. [Epub ahead of print]
25. Patterson DR, Hoffman HG, Weichman SA, Jensen MP, Sharar SR. Optimizing control of pain from severe burns: a literature review. Am J Clin Hypn. 2004;47:43–54.
26. Caruso TJ, Janik LS, Fuzaylov G. Airway management of recovered pediatric patients with severe head and neck burns: a review. Paediatr Anaesth. 2012;22:462–8.
27. Marek K, Piotr W, Stanislaw S, et al. Fibreoptic bronchoscopy in routine clinical practice in confirming the diagnosis and treatment of inhalation burns. Burns J Int Soc Burn Inj. 2007;33:554–60.

28. Masanes MJ, Legendre C, Lioret N, Maillard D, Saizy R, Lebeau B. Fiberoptic bronchoscopy for the early diagnosis of subglottal inhalation injury: comparative value in the assessment of prognosis. J Trauma. 1994;36:59–67.

29. Masanes MJ, Legendre C, Lioret N, Saizy R, Lebeau B. Using bronchoscopy and biopsy to diagnose early inhalation injury. Macroscopic and histologic findings. Chest. 1995;107:1365–9.

30. Endorf FW, Gamelli RL. Inhalation injury, pulmonary perturbations, and fluid resuscitation. J Burn Care Res Off Publ Am Burn Assoc. 2007;28:80–3.

31. Belenkiy SM, Buel AR, Cannon JW, et al. Albumin in burn shock resuscitation: a meta-analysis of controlled clinical studies. J Burn Care Res. 2016;37(3):e268–78.

32. Lee JM, Bae W, Lee YJ, Cho YJ. The efficacy and safety of prone positional ventilation in acute respiratory distress syndrome: updated study-level meta-analysis of 11 randomized controlled trials. Crit Care Med. 2014;42:1252–62.

33. Yip LY, Lim YF, Chan HN. Safety and potential anticoagulant effects of nebulised heparin in burns patients with inhalational injury at Singapore General Hospital Burns Centre. Burns J Int Soc Burn Inj. 2011;37:1154–60.

34. Endorf FW, Ahrenholz D. Burn management. Curr Opin Crit Care. 2011;17:601–5.

35. Burd A. Fluid resuscitation in burns. Burns J Int Soc Burn Inj. 2010;36:1316–7; author reply.

36. Bodger O, Theron A, Williams D. Comparison of three techniques for calculation of the Parkland formula to aid fluid resuscitation in paediatric burns. Eur J Anaesthesiol. 2013;30:483–91.

37. Cocks AJ, O'Connell A, Martin H. Crystalloids, colloids and kids: a review of paediatric burns in intensive care. Burns J Int Soc Burn Inj. 1998;24:717–24.

38. Rogers AD, Karpelowsky J, Millar AJ, Argent A, Rode H. Fluid creep in major pediatric burns. Eur J Pediatr Surg Off J Austrian Assoc Pediatr Surg [et al]=Zeitschrift fur Kinderchirurgie 2010;20:133–8.

39. Azzopardi EA, McWilliams B, Iyer S, Whitaker IS. Fluid resuscitation in adults with severe burns at risk of secondary abdominal compartment syndrome – an evidence based systematic review. Burns J Int Soc Burn Inj. 2009;35:911–20.

40. Oda J, Yamashita K, Inoue T, et al. Resuscitation fluid volume and abdominal compartment syndrome in patients with major burns. Burns J Int Soc Burn Inj. 2006;32:151–4.

41. Endorf FW, Dries DJ. Burn resuscitation. Scand J Trauma Resusc Emerg Med. 2011;19:69.
42. Navickis RJ, Greenhalgh DG, Wilkes MM. Albumin in Burn Shock Resuscitation: A Meta-Analysis of Controlled Clinical Studies. J Burn Care Res. 2016;37(3):e268–78.
43. Greenhalgh DG. Burn resuscitation: the results of the ISBI/ABA survey. Burns J Int Soc Burn Inj. 2010;36:176–82.
44. Aghakhani K, Heidari M, Tabatabaee SM, Abdolkarimi L. Effect of current pathway on mortality and morbidity in electrical burn patients. Burns J Int Soc Burn Inj. 2015;41:172–6.
45. Church D, Elsayed S, Reid O, Winston B, Lindsay R. Burn wound infections. Clin Microbiol Rev. 2006;19:403–34.
46. Nguyen DQ, Dickson WA. A review of the use of a dermal skin substitute in burns care. J Wound Care. 2006;15:373–6.
47. Chua A, Song C, Chai A, Kong S, Tan KC. Use of skin allograft and its donation rate in Singapore: an 11-year retrospective review for burns treatment. Transplant Proc. 2007;39:1314–6.
48. Sebastian R, Ghanem O, DiRoma F, Milner SM, Price LA. Pulmonary embolism in burns, is there an evidence based prophylactic recommendation? Case report and review of literature. Burns J Int Soc Burn Inj. 2015;41:e4–7.
49. Iskander GA, Nelson RS, Morehouse DL, Tenquist JE, Szlabick RE. Incidence and propagation of infrageniculate deep venous thrombosis in trauma patients. J Trauma. 2006;61:695–700.
50. Satahoo SS, Parikh PP, Naranjo D, et al. Are burn patients really at risk for thrombotic events? J Burn Care Res Off Publ Am Burn Assoc. 2015;36(1):100–4.
51. Fecher AM, O'Mara MS, Goldfarb IW, et al. Analysis of deep vein thrombosis in burn patients. Burns J Int Soc Burn Inj. 2004;30:591–3.
52. Guo YN, Li H, Zhang PH. Early enteral nutrition versus late enteral nutrition for burns patients: a systematic review and meta-analysis. Burns. 2015. pii: S0305-4179(15)00317-4. doi:10.1016/j.burns.2015.10.008. [Epub ahead of print]
53. Khorasani EN, Mansouri F. Effect of early enteral nutrition on morbidity and mortality in children with burns. Burns J Int Soc Burn Inj. 2010;36:1067–71.
54. Masters B, Wood F. Nutrition support in burns – is there consistency in practice? J Burn Care Res Off Publ Am Burn Assoc. 2008;29:561–71.
55. Wolf SE. Nutrition and metabolism in burns: state of the science, 2007. J Burn Care Res Off Publ Am Burn Assoc. 2007;28:572–6.

Chapter 13
General Surgical Problems in the Critically Injured Patient

David N. Naumann and Mark Midwinter

Abstract Critically injured patients requiring surgical management often require complex multi-organ support in the intensive care unit. In order to achieve best possible patient outcomes a multidisciplinary approach is required between surgical and critical care specialists in order to optimise the care of the patients from arrival to discharge. Familiarity with the patient pathway, their injury severity, surgical management, and possible complications are paramount in the overall care of these patients. Trauma to the abdomen may result in solid organ, hollow viscus or major vascular injury,

D.N. Naumann, MA, MB, BChir, DMCC, MRCS (✉)
• M. Midwinter, BMedSci, Dip App Stats MD, FRCS
NIHR Surgical Reconstruction and Microbiology Research Centre,
Queen Elizabeth Hospital, Birmingham B15 2TH, UK

Academic Department of Military Surgery and Trauma, Royal
Centre for Defence Medicine, Queen Elizabeth Hospital,
Birmingham B15 2TH, UK
e-mail: david.naumann@nhs.net

S.D. Hutchings (ed.), *Trauma and Combat Critical Care*
in Clinical Practice, In Clinical Practice,
DOI 10.1007/978-3-319-28758-4_13,
© Crown Copyright 2016

most commonly the liver, spleen, kidneys, pancreas, as well as the large and small bowel and vascular structures including major retroperitoneal vessels. These injures are graded in severity according to the American Association of Surgery for Trauma (AAST) which relates to both management strategies and outcomes. Damage control surgery (DCS) is now routine for battlefield abdominal trauma, and this philosophy has heavily influence current civilian practice. The five-stage sequence of DCS includes (i) patient selection, (ii) intra-operative, (iii) critical care, (iv) return to theatre; and (v) formal closure. This has been incorporated in to a broader philosophy of Damage Control Resuscitation. An understanding of the decision making and sequence of surgical management, as well as that of the abdominal compartment syndrome and open abdomen are important features of the management of the surgical patient in critical care, and are discussed in this chapter.

Keywords Organ injury • Damage control surgery • Abdominal compartment syndrome • Abdominal closure • Selective non-operative management

How Should Intra Abdominal Injuries Be Classified?

Intra-abdominal injuries may be sustained either in isolation or as part of a polytraumatic pattern of injury. Since the abdomen contains both solid and hollow viscus organs, each must be considered individually and in concert with the rest during the diagnosis of and subsequent management of injuries. Major vascular structures within the abdomen may also be injured in blunt and penetrating trauma. Since appropriate management may include surgery, interventional radiology and/or selective non-operative management, accurate diagnosis is paramount, and may utilise scoring systems for risk stratification and guidance of treatment. Modern ultrasound and cross-sectional imaging techniques allow the anatomical delineation of injuries in order to aid this diagnostic and decision making process. Indeed, availability of radiological adjuncts such as Focussed Assessment with Sonography in Trauma (FAST) and Computed Tomography (CT) can improve outcomes [1], and prevent unnecessary surgery even following battlefield injury [2]. The former is useful in the overall assessment of patients and decision making, whereas the latter may enable delineation of anatomical injuries.

Solid Organ Injury

The most commonly injured solid organs include the liver, spleen, and kidneys [3]. Specific Organ Injury Scales (OIS) relating to each of these organs have been assigned by the American Association for the Surgery of Trauma (AAST) [4, 5]. These facilitate the reporting and comparison of management strategies and outcomes but do not directly relate to specific management of individual patients, which is more dictated by haemodynamic parameters and stability over time. These OIS are illustrated in Table 13.1 (Liver), Table 13.2 (Spleen), Table 13.3 (Kidney), and Table 13.4 (Pancreas). Blunt splenic trauma (even higher grades of injury) may be treated selectively by non-operative strategies [6]. Although this may be suitable for some penetrating splenic injuries, the vast majority are still managed surgically [7]. Both blunt [8, 9] and penetrating [10] hepatic injuries may also be managed non-operatively with the caveat that certain associated risk factors, such as other injuries, peritoneal signs, and high injury severity scores increase the risk of the requirement for surgery [8]. Kidney trauma is most commonly managed non-operatively, with the exception that Grade V injuries are likely to require surgery [11]. Pancreatic injury management may also be managed selectively non-operatively but this needs to tempered by the high incidence of associated duodenal and vascular injury and complications from major pancreatic duct disruption.

TABLE 13.1 AAST liver injury scale

Grade[*]	Type	Description of injury
I	Hematoma	Subcapsular <10 % surface area
	Laceration	Capsular tear <1 cm parenchymal depth
II	Hematoma	Subcapsular, 10–50 % surface area intraparenchymal <10 cm in diameter
	Laceration	Capsular tear 1–3 parenchymal depth <10 cm in length
III	Hematoma	Subcapsular, >50 % surface area of ruptured subcapsular or parenchymal hematoma; intraparenchymal hematoma >10 cm or expanding
	Laceration	>3 cm parenchymal depth
IV	Laceration	Parenchymal disruption involving 25–75 % hepatic lobe or 1–3 segments
V	Laceration	Parenchymal disruption involving >75 % of hepatic lobe or >3 segments within a single lobe
	Vascular	Juxtahepatic venous injuries; i.e., retro-hepatic vena cava/central major hepatic veins
VI	Vascular	Hepatic avulsion

[*]Advance one grade for multiple injuries up to grade III

Hollow Viscus Injury

A high index of suspicion is warranted for hollow viscus injury following abdominal trauma, including following blunt trauma [12]. The presence of a solid organ injury is predictive of hollow viscus injury [13], and therefore it is important to consider all contents of the abdomen rather than the most obviously injured organ. Classification of small bowel and colonic injuries according to AAST [14] are illustrated in Table 13.5. Hollow viscus injury with

TABLE 13.2 AAST spleen injury scale

Grade*	Type	Description of injury
I	Hematoma	Subcapsular <10 % surface area
	Laceration	Capsular tear <1 cm parenchymal depth
II	Hematoma	Subcapsular, 10–50 % surface area intraparenchymal <5 cm in diameter
	Laceration	Capsular tear, 1–3 cm parenchymal depth that does not involve a trabecular vessel
III	Hematoma	Subcapsular, >50 % surface area or expanding; ruptured subcapsular or parecymal hematoma; intraparenchymal hematoma ≥5 cm or expanding
	Laceration	>3 cm parenchymal depth or involving trabecular vessels
IV	Laceration	Laceration involving segmental or hilar vessels producing major devascularization (>25 % of spleen)
V	Laceration	Completely shattered spleen
	Vascular	Hilar vascular injury with devascularizes spleen

*Advance one grade for multiple injuries up to grade III

peritoneal leakage of bowel contents following trauma must be treated surgically in order to prevent sepsis and multi-organ failure. Very early CT scan may show the solid organ injury but miss associated hollow viscus injury as radiological signs for this take time to develop (bowel thickening, changes in perfusion, associated fluid collection etc.). Therefore a high index of suspicion for associated hollow viscus injury in patients with solid organ injury managed non-operatively must be maintained and rescanning considered if there is any doubt.

TABLE 13.3 AAST kidney injury scale

Grade*	Type	Description of injury
I	Contusion	Microscopic or gross hematuria, urologic studies normal
	Hematoma	Subcapsular, nonexpanding without parenchymal laceration
II	Hematoma	Nonexpanding perirenal hematoma confirmed to renal retroperitoneum
	Laceration	<1.0 cm parenchymal depth of renal cortex without urinary extravagation
III	Laceration	<1.0 cm parenchymal depth of renal cortex without collecting system rupture or urinary extravagation
IV	Laceration	Parenchymal laceration extending through renal cortex, medulla, and collecting system
	Vascular	Main renal artery or vein injury with contained hemorrhage
V	Laceration	Completely shattered kidney
	Vascular	Avulsion of renal hilum which devascularizes kidney

*Advance one grade for bilateral injuries up to grade III

Retroperitoneal Vascular Injury

Retroperitoneal trauma may cause vascular injury, bleeding, and formation of haematoma that may further injure the retroperitoneal anatomical structures. Such haematomas can be divided into three zones in terms of the anatomical relationships. The decision to manage retroperitoneal injuries with surgery or conservative treatment depends on the likely structures that may have been injured, and the mechanism of injury:

(a) **Zone 1** (central and medial; may lead to pancreaticoduodenal injury and/or major abdominal vascular injury). If

TABLE 13.4 AAST pancreas injury scale

Grade*	Type	Description of injury
I	Hematoma	Minor contusion without duct injury
	Laceration	Superficial laceration without duct injury
II	Hematoma	Major contusion without duct injury or tissue loss
	Laceration	Major laceration without duct injury or tissue loss
III	Laceration	Distal transection or parenchymal injury with duct injury
IV	Laceration	Proximal? transection or parenchymal injury involving ampulla
V	Laceration	Massive disruption of pancreatic head
I	Hematoma	Minor contusion without duct injury
	Laceration	Superficial laceration without duct injury

*Advance one grade for multiple injuries up to grade III

TABLE 13.5 AAST small bowel and colon injury score

Grade*	Type	Description of injury
I	Hematoma	Contusion or hematoma without devascularization
	Laceration	Partial thickness, no perforation
II	Laceration	Laceration <50 % of circumference
III	Laceration	Laceration ≥50 % of circumference without transection
IV	Laceration	Transection of the bowel
V	Laceration	Transection of the bowel with segmental tissue loss
	Vascular	Devascularized segment

*Advance one grade for multiple injuries up to grade III

the mechanism of injury is penetrating, then Zone 1 injuries must be explored surgically due to risk of injury to the aorta, vena cava, coeliac trunk, and superior mesenteric artery. Blunt trauma may be managed conservatively, but with a high index of suspicion.

(b) **Zone 2** (lateral/perinephric area; may cause injury to the colon and/or genitourinary system). Penetrating injuries to this zone should also be explored in order to check for injuries to the ipsilateral kidney, adrenal gland, ureter, and renal vasculature. It is important to note that even blunt trauma may cause secondary penetrating trauma from fractured ribs. Blunt trauma may safely be managed conservatively. However, if a Zone 2 haematoma is diagnosed during laparotomy, the surgeon must note whether it is expanding or pulsating, and explore if this is the case.

(c) **Zone 3** (pelvic, usually due to pelvic fracture and/or iliofemoral vascular injury). Blunt trauma to this zone requires an external fixation device to compress the haematoma. Selective angio-embolization of bleeding vessels may be required if the patient remains haemodynamically unstable. Surgical exploration is only indicated following penetrating injury.

What Is Damage Control Surgery?

The concept of *damage control* in naval warfare refers to the well-rehearsed, efficient and timely efforts of a crew to keep a damaged ship afloat in order to maintain mission integrity and return to port for more definitive repairs. Along similar lines, damage control surgery (DCS) is a surgical strategy to directly address the physiological stresses of major trauma without the need for definitive restoration of anatomy; to keep the injured soldier alive long enough—like the damaged ship—to return home for definitive 'repairs'. The DCS operative strategy sacrifices the completeness of the immediate surgical repair in order to address the physiological consequences of the combined trauma of injury and subsequent surgery.

Major trauma is characterised by a sudden, severe anatomical insult leading to catastrophic haemorrhage and major imbalance of physiological parameters. Loss of blood volume and subsequent hypothermia stimulate widespread adrenergic vasoconstriction. Clotting factors are depleted, leading to coagulopathy and further bleeding. The resulting haemodynamic compromise and hypoperfusion of organs with tissue injury leads to anaerobic respiration of tissues and metabolic acidosis. This process has been called the 'trauma triad', 'lethal triad' or 'triad of death' of hypothermia, acidosis and coagulopathy [15–17]. It is this physiological cascade that must be mitigated in order for the casualty to remain alive long enough to achieve future definitive care.

Damage Control Versus Primary Surgery

Before the philosophy and practice of DCS, conventional wisdom dictated that a casualty would undergo initial resuscitative measures in the emergency department of a hospital, and when 'stabilised' would be transferred to the operating theatre for definitive repair of their injuries (i.e., primary surgery). The patient may then be transferred to the intensive care unit (ICU) post-operatively for further resuscitation and physiological monitoring.

Such a logical sequence would supposedly negate the requirement for a return to theatre – indeed in such a model the requirement for further surgery might be considered to be an adverse event or complication. The DCS philosophy is different to this traditional model in the respect that surgery is only one part of the overall resuscitation, and that restoration of physiology (rather than anatomy) is the priority. DCS is one part of the overall process of Damage Control Resuscitation (DCR) that focuses on early correction of physiological derangement [18–20]. The introduction of DCR has influenced to practice of DCS as aggressive physiological correction extends surgical options.

Damage Control Sequence

When the term *damage control surgery* was first coined in 1993 by Rotondo and Schwab, the authors first described a classical three-stage approach, which mainly concerned abdominal trauma [21, 22]. Although the general concepts of DCS have remained fairly consistent since this original description, its practice has now evolved, and can be considered in 5 distinct stages [23, 24]. These stages are (i) Patient selection, (ii) Intra-operative, (iii) Critical Care, (iv) Return to theatre; and (v) Formal closure.

I. *Patient selection*

Regardless of physiological and situational parameters used in decision-making, a timely and considered decision is important, and must involve accurate communication between surgical, critical care and anaesthetic teams. This may occur either pre-operatively (before the patient has arrived in the operating room), or within the first minutes of surgical intervention. One formalised approach has been described by Rotondo and Zonies [25], and uses the patient selection factors of *conditions*, *complexes* and *critical factors* (Table 13.6). Additionally some physiological criteria that may indicate that a DCS approach is indicated have been suggested as: Injury severity score >25, systolic blood pressure <70 mmHg, core temperature < 34 °C and pH <7.1.

II. *Intra-operative stage*

The start of the intra-operative stage should be as soon as possible, and the time of surgery should be carefully monitored and kept to a minimum. The surgical team should be mindful of the dynamic changes in the patient's physiology (including acid-base status, coagulation, temperature, blood product requirements). The basic philosophy is that the minimum must be done to stop haemorrhage, limit contamination, and provide temporary closure or cover of abdominal contents before the patient is rapidly transferred to critical

TABLE 13.6 Selection of patients in whom application of damage control principles is likely to be of benefit

Conditions
High energy blunt trauma
Multiple torso penetration
Haemodynamic instability
Presenting coagulopathy and/or hypothermia
Complexes
Major abdominal vascular injury with multiple visceral injuries
Multifocal or multi-cavity exsanguinations with concomitant visceral injuries
Multiregional injury with competing priorities
Critical Factors
Severe metabolic acidosis (pH 7.30)
Hypothermia (temperature <35 °C)
Resuscitation and operative time > 90 min
Coagulopathy as evidenced by the development of non-mechanical bleeding
Massive transfusion (>10 units of PRBC).

Adapted from Rotondo and Zonies [25]

care. Active warming is important and a theatre temperature of 26 °C is normal practice [19].

(a) *Haemorrhage/vascular control*

Although the application of proximal pressure and haemostatic dressings are useful in the initial control of bleeding, only surgical control is considered definitive [26]. The first priority during this operative stage is therefore the control of bleeding. Haemorrhage control may be achieved by ligation, suture, or tamponade (by packing or balloon). Large vascular injuries may also be treated with temporary shunting in order to facilitate subsequent vascular repair in order to preserve a limb. Definitive vascular repair by grafting or anastomosis during this stage is not appropriate, but may be considered in the later stages.

(b) *Limit contamination*

Contamination control is often achieved by stapled or tape closure of the ends of the injured hollow viscus. Anastomoses and stomas are not usually fashioned in DCS. A thorough washout with copious normal saline is also performed to minimize contamination.

(c) *Temporary closure*

Pre-emptive strategies to prevent compartment syndromes such as fasciotomies and laparostomy are employed. Temporary closure or cover is established in order to protect the abdominal contents whilst the patient is moved to a critical care environment. There are various temporary closure techniques used, which are described later in this chapter.

III. *Critical Care Stage*

In the critical care environment attempts continue at correcting the physiological consequences of injury and its associated metabolic failure. These concepts are discussed at length in Chaps. 5, 6, 7 and 8. Early return to the operating theatre is indicated if there is obvious ongoing surgical bleeding or a compartment syndrome develops.

IV. *Return to the operating theatre*

This is dictated by improvement in the patient's physiological status. The following indices are often used to guide re-operation; base deficit >-4 mmol/l, lactate <2.5 mmol/l, core temperature >35 °C and an International Normalised Ratio <1.25 [24]. Before the decision to return to the operating theatre is made, plans to assemble the appropriate surgical team must be put in place to ensure that the optimum repairs of the injuries are performed in the optimum surgical environment. This may require more than one surgical specialty, but with a clearly identified leader to orchestrate the procedures and take a global view of the patient's condition. At this stage anastomoses are fashioned, stomas raised and vascular repairs performed. However, surgical judgment on restoring gastrointestinal continuity should be exercised and in particular the requirements for on going inotropic support.

V. *Formal closure*

This may not be possible at stage IV as there may still be significant oedema or clinical risk of developing a compartment syndrome (abdominal or extremity). Therefore a planned further operative phase for closing or covering the site is made. The balance of risks between leaving the abdomen open as a laparostomy or delayed closure will depend on the injuries sustained and the overall condition of the patient and their abdominal viscera. Component separation or mesh repair may be considered, and are discussed further later in this chapter [27]. If fascial closure has not been possible by day 10 it may be safer to allow the laparostomy to mature and plan a delayed closure many months later rather than risk making an inadvertent enterotomy to get closure earlier.

Vascular Damage Control

Major vascular injuries must be dealt with quickly and urgently in order to stop haemorrhage and potentially enable limb salvage, but cannot wait until transfer to vascular specialist units. Damage control techniques may be utilised during surgery that do not necessarily require vascular specialists to perform. Although most distal vascular injuries can be ligated, an injured proximal portion of an extremity vessel may threaten the viability of that limb. The damage control surgery technique of placing a temporary vascular shunt may make limb salvage possible, and has long-term limb preservation results similar to those where initial revascularisation was attempted [28]. This technique is relatively straightforward, quick, and does not necessarily require specialist vascular support. It enables the preservation of circulatory flow to the threatened limb so that subsequent definitive vascular reconstruction may be performed by an appropriately trained and skilled surgeon. This technique is performed by gaining proximal and distal control of the area of bleeding, followed by proximal and distal thrombec- tomy (using an appropriately sized Fogarty catheter). The tempo- rary shunt is then placed into the vessel lumens creating a 'bridging' temporary pathway for circulatory flow. Where the injuries are so severe that this is technically impossible, or the limb is unsalvageable, amputation is indicated at a level at which viable and vascularised tissue may be preserved.

Military Experience

Damage control surgery is now in routine use for battlefield trauma. Its practice has recently been shown to reduce mor- tality and faecal diversion for abdominal injuries [29], and good limb salvage results following vascular injury [30]. In recent years the experiences of DCS from the deployed mili- tary has had influence on civilian practice [31, 32] but more investigational research is required to demonstrate true translatability. A Cochrane Review found no published or pending randomised evidence that compared DCS with immediate and definitive repair in patients with major abdominal trauma [33], and further evidence-informed con- sensus is required to address this uncertainty [34].

Which Patients Require Acute Operative Intervention Following Abdominal Trauma?

Before the advent of interventional radiology for trauma and detailed cross sectional imaging techniques such as computed tomography (CT), laparotomy was considered mandatory for penetrating trauma and serious blunt trauma with physiological compromise. This was associated with a risk of non-therapeutic laparotomy in some studies ranging from to 9–37 % [35], which can cause potentially preventable complications and morbidity. More recently, non-therapeutic laparotomy has been reported as low as 3.9 % even following battlefield injuries due to the sensitive and specific nature of comprehensive CT imaging and reporting [2]. The management of trauma patients can therefore be divided into (a) surgical; (b) selective non-operative management; and (c) interventional radiology.

Selective Non-operative Management

Selective non-operative management (SNOM) is a management strategy where patients are observed without surgery, by careful and regular examination and clinical assessment. It is preferable that the same examiner or team should regularly assess the patient to detect any deterioration in clinical status that would indicate intervention is required. Such an approach must be tailored to the individual patients' needs on a case-by-case basis. Injuries that may be managed using SNOM include solid organ injuries such as splenic and hepatic lacerations. Indeed SNOM for splenic injury is used as a quality indicator for surgical units that treat children [36]. The subsequent requirement for surgery may increase with the AAST grading of the solid organ injuries, and therefore a higher index of suspicion is warranted the higher the injury grade. Even penetrating injuries to the abdomen do not necessarily require surgery, and can be managed by SNOM. The Eastern Association for the Surgery of Trauma recently published clinical practice guidelines, recommending that "*A routine laparotomy is not indicated in hemodynamically stable patients with abdominal stab wounds without signs of peritonitis or diffuse abdominal tenderness*" [37].

Interventional Radiology

Some solid organ injuries may be suitable for interventional radiological management rather than surgery. Selective angioembolisation following blunt trauma can reduce the non-therapeutic laparotomy rate, and can be used for injury grades IV and V [38]. Inter-disciplinary discussion between radiology and surgical specialists and appropriate imaging techniques are vital for the success of this approach.

Surgical Intervention

Despite advances in diagnostic techniques, there are still some injuries for which laparotomy is mandatory. Hollow viscus injury following trauma with leakage of abdominal contents may only be treated with surgical intervention. Uncontrolled haemorrhage and clinical deterioration are also indications for emergency surgery, and damage control surgery if deemed appropriate. Solid organ injuries which have deteriorated despite SNOM and/or interventional radiology may also require surgical intervention for definitive management.

What Is Abdominal Compartment Syndrome?

Abdominal compartment syndrome is a dangerous complication that may lead to organ failure, diaphragm splinting, compression of the inferior vena cava, and reduction of cardiac return.

Definition

Abdominal Compartment Syndrome (ACS) has been defined by the World Society of the Abdominal Compartment

Syndrome (WSACS) as a sustained intra-abdominal pressure (>20 mmHg) with or without an abdominal perfusion pressure of <60 mmHg that is associated with new organ dysfunction or failure [39].

Diagnosis

Early diagnosis is important, since treatment is urgent. Intra-abdominal pressure is commonly monitored by measuring the intraluminal bladder pressure via urinary catheter. A small volume of water is instilled into the bladder, and the tubing is clamped. A manometer is attached proximal to the clamp, and the pressure reading is given as the number of centimetres above the symphysis pubis (units cmH$_2$O) (Fig. 13.1). However, management decisions should be made on the clinical picture and not solely based on pressure measurements.

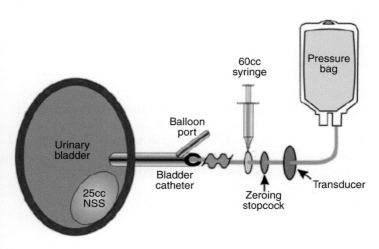

FIGURE 13.1 Intravesicular manometry device (From Gavrilovska-Brzanov et al. [49])

Pathophysiology

ACS can arise for three main reasons: (i) increase in size/volume of intra-abdominal organs; (ii) diminished abdominal wall compliance; and (iii) increase in intra-abdominal fluid through capillary leak or fluid resuscitation. The abdominal organs may increase in size and volume due to inflammation (such as liver dysfunction and acute pancreatitis [40]), ileus and distension, bowel obstruction, malignancy, intra-abdominal collection, or infection. The abdominal wall musculature can decrease in compliance due to the position of the patient (for example if prone), major abdominal wall burns, trauma, and surgical intervention. Fluid leakage into the abdominal cavity can occur during massive fluid resuscitation [41, 42], in particular crystalloid fluid resuscitation [43].

How Should Abdominal Compartment Syndrome Be Managed?

Prevention

The WSACS have recommended that intra-abdominal pressure should be monitored when there are any risk factors for intra-abdominal hypertension or ACS, and that the transbladder technique should be the gold standard [39]. Primary prevention of ACS is preferable to management once it arises. Laparostomy (i.e., leaving an open abdomen) following emergency laparotomy may be indicated if ACS is thought to be likely. Delayed closure may be performed once the oedema and fluid balance have been corrected sufficiently to allow closure.

Treatment

Once ACS is confirmed, urgent decompressive laparotomy is required in order to relieve the pressure [44], and this should be followed with temporary abdominal closure. This may become necessary if the intra-abdominal pressure remains 20–25 mmHg and is causing a deterioration of organ failure. Onward management should include a combination of careful fluid management (to decrease the overall fluid balance), and appropriate utilisation of vasoactive medications.

How Should Critically Injured Patients with Open Abdomens Be Managed?

The primary aims of the management of the open abdomen are to provide temporary cover until a time at which it is appropriate to perform formal closure. Closure should be achieved as soon as feasible (and without causing ACS), since it may lead to fluid and electrolyte imbalance, septic complications (e.g., abscess, systemic infection), formation of fistulae and adhesions, catabolic state, and systemic inflammatory response [45]. The management of the open abdomen therefore has three main priorities: (i) providing cover to the contents, to prevent injury (e.g., bowel) and preventing the introduction of contamination; (ii) control the intra-abdominal fluid volumes (i.e., from ascites and resuscitative fluid leakage); and (iii) to enable future wound closure by preventing the formation of adhesions and lateral recession of the abdominal musculature [46]. Concurrent attention should be paid to nutrition [44] and fluid maintenance to ensure the patient has appropriate nutritional supplementation via the best route, and electrolyte balance. Antibiotic coverage (both antibacterial and antifungal) should be considered in close collaboration with microbiology specialists.

Temporary Covering of the Open Abdomen

Before fascial closure is performed, the open abdomen requires temporary closure to minimise the complications listed above. Adequate temporary closure of the abdomen must take into account the fact that there will be considerable amounts of fluid accumulated in the abdomen, which requires either frequent dressings changes or a system that can adequately collect and drain the fluid. The simplest version of temporary closure may be in the form of simple packing, such as non-adherent wet gauze. Although such an approach may be suitable for severe sepsis, it is not commonly performed for trauma. Skin may be closed without closure of the fascia, but this also carries a high risk of dehiscence and loss of skin. More common techniques in usage include the Bogotoa bag, mesh, and vacuum assisted (negative pressure) drainage. The necessity of siting stomas and minimising potential contamination is an important consideration.

(a) *Bogota bag* (Fig. 13.2)

A large IV bag may be fashioned into a shape suitable for coverage of the abdominal defect, and sutured or stapled to the skin edges [47]. This can then be covered by antibiotic-covered dressings and drapes. The whole dressing may be replaced at the bedside without requirement for further trips to theatre.

(b) *Mesh*

Non-absorbable mesh may be loosely fixed by suture to fascia on either side of the abdominal defect. As the swelling reduces, the central portion of mesh can be excised and the two edges re-sutured, or the central portion can be plicated (Fig. 13.3). This process can be repeated until the point at which the fascial edges can be brought together for definitive closure.

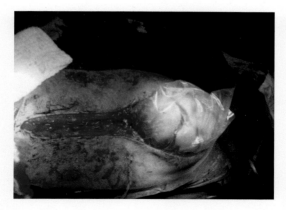

FIGURE 13.2 Bogota bag temorpary closure of the abdomen (von Ruden et al. [50])

(c) *Negative pressure dressings* (Fig. 13.4)

Negative pressure therapy has the advantage of being suitable for fluid drainage (reducing the risk of intra-abdominal sepsis), as well as promoting angiogenesis, tissue perfusion, granulation, and bringing the skin edges closer together [48]. This is the approach recommended by the WSACS for the management of open abdomens [39]. The most common negative pressure dressings are the VAC Abdominal Dressing and ABThera Systems. Both of these systems are designed with individual layers: first a layer to protect the viscera, then a sponge fashioned into the shape of the defect, which is then covered with an adhesive occlusive (airtight) dressing. A vacuum is then created by connecting the perforated centre of the dressing to a negative pressure system. Such systems may allow definitive closure to be delayed.

Definitive Closure of the Abdomen

Fascial closure must be tension-free in order to prevent increased abdominal pressure, dehiscence, and ventral herni-

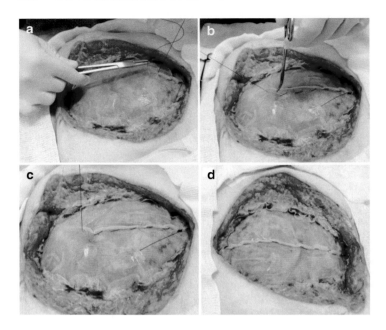

FIGURE 13.3 Mesh temporary closure of the open abdomen: plication of the central part at the bedside. (**a**) A suture is tied at one end of the mesh. (**b**) The mesh is pinched in the central portion, and plicated with a running suture. (**c**) The suture continues to the opposite end of the wound. (**d**) The suture is now tied so that it has been plicated along its entire length (From Correa et al. [51])

ation. If the fascial edges do not come together without tension, then the options for closure include: intentional ventral hernia, component separation, or utilisation of bridging mesh between the fascial edges. The exact timing and technique for definitive abdominal closure should be decided on a case-by-case basis depending on the clinical status of the patient in terms of their anatomical and physiological suitability for further surgery.

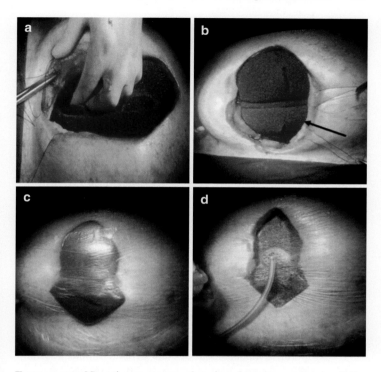

FIGURE 13.4 Negative pressure dressing for management of the open abdomen. (**a**) The edges of the fascia are placed under tension using interrupted sutures. (**b**) Sutures are spaced approximately 5 cm apart circumferentially. (**c**) A second sponge is positioned and sealed with an airtight plastic sheet. (**d**) The sponge is connected to a suction system (pressure between 50 and 150 mm Hg) (From Pliakos et al. [52] with permission)

References

1. Huber-Wagner S, Lefering R, Qvick LM, Korner M, Kay MV, Pfeifer KJ, et al. Effect of whole-body CT during trauma resuscitation on survival: a retrospective, multicentre study. Lancet. 2009;373(9673):1455–61.

2. Smith IM, Naumann DN, Marsden ME, Ballard M, Bowley DM. Scanning and war: utility of FAST and CT in the assessment of battlefield abdominal trauma. Ann Surg. 2015;262(2): 389–96.

3. Arumugam S, Al-Hassani A, El-Menyar A, Abdelrahman H, Parchani A, Peralta R, et al. Frequency, causes and pattern of abdominal trauma: a 4-year descriptive analysis. J Emerg Trauma Shock. 2015;8(4):193–8.

4. Moore EE, Cogbill TH, Jurkovich GJ, Shackford SR, Malangoni MA, Champion HR. Organ injury scaling: spleen and liver (1994 revision). J Trauma. 1995;38(3):323–4.

5. Moore EE, Shackford SR, Pachter HL, McAninch JW, Browner BD, Champion HR, et al. Organ injury scaling: spleen, liver, and kidney. J Trauma. 1989;29(12):1664–6.

6. Brilliantine A, Iacobellis F, Robustelli U, Villamaina E, Maglione F, Colletti O, et al. Non operative management of blunt splenic trauma: a prospective evaluation of a standardized treatment protocol. Eur J Trauma Emerg Surg. 2015. [Epub ahead of print] DOI 10.1007/s00068-015-0575-z.

7. Berg RJ, Inaba K, Okoye O, Pasley J, Teixeira PG, Esparza M, et al. The contemporary management of penetrating splenic injury. Injury. 2014;45(9):1394–400.

8. Boese CK, Hackl M, Muller LP, Ruchholtz S, Frink M, Lechler P. Nonoperative management of blunt hepatic trauma: a systematic review. J Trauma Acute Care Surg. 2015;79(4):654–60.

9. Stassen NA, Bhullar I, Cheng JD, Crandall M, Friese R, Guillamondegui O, et al. Nonoperative management of blunt hepatic injury: an Eastern Association for the Surgery of Trauma practice management guideline. J Trauma Acute Care Surg. 2012;73(5 Suppl 4):S288–93.

10. MacGoey P, Navarro A, Beckingham IJ, Cameron IC, Brooks AJ. Selective non-operative management of penetrating liver injuries at a UK tertiary referral centre. Ann R Coll Surg Engl. 2014;96(6):423–6.

11. McCombie SP, Thyer I, Corcoran NM, Rowling C, Dyer J, Le Roux A, et al. The conservative management of renal trauma: a literature review and practical clinical guideline from Australia and New Zealand. BJU Int. 2014;114 Suppl 1:13–21.

12. Watts DD, Fakhry SM. Incidence of hollow viscus injury in blunt trauma: an analysis from 275,557 trauma admissions from the East multi-institutional trial. J Trauma. 2003;54(2):289–94.

13. Swaid F, Peleg K, Alfici R, Matter I, Olsha O, Ashkenazi I, et al. Concomitant hollow viscus injuries in patients with blunt hepatic and splenic injuries: an analysis of a National Trauma Registry database. Injury. 2014;45(9):1409–12.

14. Moore EE, Cogbill TH, Malangoni MA, Jurkovich GJ, Champion HR, Gennarelli TA, et al. Organ injury scaling, II: pancreas, duodenum, small bowel, colon, and rectum. J Trauma. 1990;30(11):1427–9.

15. Mikhail J. The trauma triad of death: hypothermia, acidosis, and coagulopathy. AACN Clin Issues. 1999;10(1):85–94.

16. De Waele JJ, Vermassen FE. Coagulopathy, hypothermia and acidosis in trauma patients: the rationale for damage control surgery. Acta Chir Belg. 2002;102(5):313–6.

17. Mitra B, Tullio F, Cameron PA, Fitzgerald M. Trauma patients with the 'triad of death'. Emerg Med J. 2012;29(8):622–5.

18. Lamb CM, MacGoey P, Navarro AP, Brooks AJ. Damage control surgery in the era of damage control resuscitation. Br J Anaesth. 2014;113(2):242–9.

19. Morrison JJ, Ross JD, Poon H, Midwinter MJ, Jansen JO. Intraoperative correction of acidosis, coagulopathy and hypothermia in combat casualties with severe haemorrhagic shock. Anaesthesia. 2013;68(8):846–50.

20. Midwinter MJ, Woolley T. Resuscitation and coagulation in the severely injured trauma patient. Philos Trans R Soc Lond B Biol Sci. 2011;366(1562):192–203.

21. Rotondo MF, Schwab CW, McGonigal MD, Phillips 3rd GR, Fruchterman TM, Kauder DR, et al. 'Damage control': an approach for improved survival in exsanguinating penetrating abdominal injury. J Trauma. 1993;35(3):375–82; discussion 382–3.

22. Waibel BH, Rotondo MM. Damage control surgery: it's evolution over the last 20 years. Rev Col Bras Cir. 2012;39(4):314–21.

23. Moore EE, Burch JM, Franciose RJ, Offner PJ, Biffl WL. Staged physiologic restoration and damage control surgery. World J Surg. 1998;22(12):1184–90; discussion 1190–1.

24. Midwinter MJ. Damage control surgery in the era of damage control resuscitation. J R Army Med Corps. 2009;155(4):323–6.

25. Rotondo MF, Zonies DH. The damage control sequence and underlying logic. Surg Clin North Am. 1997;77(4):761–77.

26. Parker P. Consensus statement on decision making in junctional trauma care. J R Army Med Corps. 2011;157(3 Suppl 1):S293–5.

27. Sharrock AE, Barker T, Yuen HM, Rickard R, Tai N. Management and closure of the open abdomen after damage control laparotomy for trauma. A systematic review and meta-analysis. Injury. 2016;47:296–306.

28. Hornez E, Boddaert G, Ngabou UD, Aguir S, Baudoin Y, Mocellin N, et al. Temporary vascular shunt for damage control of extremity vascular injury: a toolbox for trauma surgeons. J Visc Surg. 2015;152(6):363–8.

29. Smith IM, Beech ZK, Lundy JB, Bowley DM. A prospective observational study of abdominal injury management in contemporary military operations: damage control laparotomy is associated with high survivability and low rates of fecal diversion. Ann Surg. 2015;261(4):765–73.

30. Dua A, Patel B, Kragh Jr JF, Holcomb JB, Fox CJ. Long-term follow-up and amputation-free survival in 497 casualties with combat-related vascular injuries and damage-control resuscitation. J Trauma Acute Care Surg. 2012;73(6):1517–24.

31. Haider AH, Piper LC, Zogg CK, Schneider EB, Orman JA, Butler FK, et al. Military-to-civilian translation of battlefield innovations in operative trauma care. Surgery. 2015;158(6):1686–95.

32. Blackbourne LH, Baer DG, Eastridge BJ, Renz EM, Chung KK, Dubose J, et al. Military medical revolution: deployed hospital and en route care. J Trauma Acute Care Surg. 2012;73(6 Suppl 5):S378–87.

33. Cirocchi R, Montedori A, Farinella E, Bonacini I, Tagliabue L, Abraha I. Damage control surgery for abdominal trauma. Cochrane Database Syst Rev. 2013;(3):CD007438.

34. Roberts DJ, Bobrovitz N, Zygun DA, Ball CG, Kirkpatrick AW, Faris PD, et al. Indications for use of damage control surgery and damage control interventions in civilian trauma patients: A scoping review. J Trauma Acute Care Surg. 2015;78(6):1187–96.

35. Ertekin C, Yanar H, Taviloglu K, Guloglu R, Alimoglu O. Unnecessary laparotomy by using physical examination and different diagnostic modalities for penetrating abdominal stab wounds. Emerg Med J. 2005;22(11):790–4.

36. Safavi A, Skarsgard ED, Rhee P, Zangbar B, Kulvatunyou N, Tang A, et al. Trauma center variation in the management of pediatric patients with blunt abdominal solid organ injury: a national trauma data bank analysis. J Pediatr Surg. 2016;51:499–502.

37. Como JJ, Bokhari F, Chiu WC, Duane TM, Holevar MR, Tandoh MA, et al. Practice management guidelines for selective nonoperative management of penetrating abdominal trauma. J Trauma. 2010;68(3):721–33.

38. Bhullar IS, Frykberg ER, Siragusa D, Chesire D, Paul J, Tepas 3rd JJ, et al. Selective angiographic embolization of blunt splenic traumatic injuries in adults decreases failure rate of nonoperative management. J Trauma Acute Care Surg. 2012;72(5):1127–34.

39. Kirkpatrick AW, Roberts DJ, De Waele J, Jaeschke R, Malbrain ML, De Keulenaer B, et al. Intra-abdominal hypertension and the abdominal compartment syndrome: updated consensus definitions and clinical practice guidelines from the World Society of the Abdominal Compartment Syndrome. Intensive Care Med. 2013;39(7):1190–206.

40. Reintam Blaser A, Parm P, Kitus R, Starkopf J. Risk factors for intra-abdominal hypertension in mechanically ventilated patients. Acta Anaesthesiol Scand. 2011;55(5):607–14.

41. Dalfino L, Tullo L, Donadio I, Malcangi V, Brienza N. Intra-abdominal hypertension and acute renal failure in critically ill patients. Intensive Care Med. 2008;34(4):707–13.

42. Madigan MC, Kemp CD, Johnson JC, Cotton BA. Secondary abdominal compartment syndrome after severe extremity injury: are early, aggressive fluid resuscitation strategies to blame? J Trauma. 2008;64(2):280–5.

43. Balogh Z, McKinley BA, Holcomb JB, Miller CC, Cocanour CS, Kozar RA, et al. Both primary and secondary abdominal compartment syndrome can be predicted early and are harbingers of multiple organ failure. J Trauma. 2003;54(5):848–59; discussion 859–61.

44. Diaz Jr JJ, Cullinane DC, Dutton WD, Jerome R, Bagdonas R, Bilaniuk JW, et al. The management of the open abdomen in trauma and emergency general surgery: part 1-damage control. J Trauma. 2010;68(6):1425–38.

45. Huang Q, Li J, Lau WY. Techniques for abdominal wall closure after damage control laparotomy: from temporary abdominal closure to early/delayed fascial closure-a review. Gastroenterol Res Pract. 2016;2016:2073260.

46. De Waele JJ, Kaplan M, Sugrue M, Sibaja P, Bjorck M. How to deal with an open abdomen? Anaesthesiol Intensive Ther. 2015;47(4):372–8.

47. Fernandez L, Norwood S, Roettger R, Wilkins 3rd HE. Temporary intravenous bag silo closure in severe abdominal trauma. J Trauma. 1996;40(2):258–60.
48. Moues CM, Heule F, Hovius SE. A review of topical negative pressure therapy in wound healing: sufficient evidence? Am J Surg. 2011;201(4):544–56.
49. Gavrilovska-Brzanov A, Nikolova Z, Jankulovski N, Sosolceva M, Taleska G, Mojsova-Mijovska M, et al. Evaluation of the effects of elevated intra-abdominal pressure on the respiratory mechanics in mechanically ventilated patients. Macedonian J Med Sci. 2013;6:261.
50. von Ruden C, Benninger E, Mayer D, Trentz O, Labler L, Bogota VAC. A newly modified temporary abdominal closure technique. Eur J Trauma Emerg Surg. 2008;34(6):582.
51. Correa JC, Mejia DA, Duque N, J MM, Uribe CM. Managing the open abdomen: negative pressure closure versus mesh-mediated fascial traction closure: a randomized trial. Hernia. 2016; 20:221–9.
52. Pliakos I, Papavramidis TS, Mihalopoulos N, Koulouris H, Kesisoglou I, Sapalidis K, et al. Vacuum-assisted closure in severe abdominal sepsis with or without retention sutured sequential fascial closure: a clinical trial. Surgery. 2010;148(5):947–53.

Chapter 14
Orthopaedic Problems in the Critically Injured Patient

Edward Spurrier and Sarah A. Stapley

Abstract Polytrauma patients present significant challenges to intensivists and orthopaedic surgeons and benefit from a team approach to management. The challenges of identifying missed injuries, mitigating the risks of spinal injury, and the timing of multiple operations can only be overcome by careful and thorough shared care.

Once a patient is established on a treatment pathway, there are several avoidable and unavoidable complications, which ideally should be spotted early and treated urgently to avoid undesirable outcomes. Compartment syndrome remains one

E. Spurrier, BM MD (Res) MRCS FRCS (Tr&Orth) (✉)
Academic Department of Military Surgery and Trauma,
Royal Centre for Defence Medical, Birmingham, UK
e-mail: edward@edspurrier.co.uk

S.A. Stapley, MB ChB FRCS FRCS (Tr&Orth) DM
Trauma and Orthopaedics Portsmouth NHS Trust, Academic
Department of Military Surgery and Trauma, Royal Centre for
Defence Medicine (Research and Academia), Birmingham, UK

S.D. Hutchings (ed.), *Trauma and Combat Critical Care
in Clinical Practice*, In Clinical Practice,
DOI 10.1007/978-3-319-28758-4_14,
© Crown Copyright 2016

of the commonest and most challenging complications to detect, particularly in obtunded patients. Clinicians must maintain a high index of suspicion and be prepared to institute compartment pressure monitoring early. Rhabdomyolysis and fat embolism syndrome can also complicate management of the polytrauma patient.

Keywords   Major trauma • Long bone injury • Pelvic injury • Spinal injury • External fixation • Internal fixation • Spinal immobilisation • Compartment syndrome • Fat embolism • Heterotopic calcification

Introduction

Patients admitted to intensive care following trauma may have a spectrum of orthopaedic injuries and complications that must be identified and managed. Significant problems can arise where pitfalls are not anticipated and avoided. The trauma patient may have known issues, have missed injuries, or develop complications during their admission. This chapter therefore provides an overview of the most common and significant conditions that are likely to face intensive care teams when managing patients with orthopaedic injuries.

What Is a Tertiary Survey and When Should It Be Performed?

In the modern trauma system, most patients will have received a thorough assessment before presentation to intensive care. However, a proportion will have been partly assessed before urgent surgery or transfer to the critical care unit and there is always a risk of injuries having been missed. One case series from Australia noted 12 significant missed injuries in 10 out of 65 patients admitted to critical care following trauma [1]. A Dutch series identified missed injuries in 8.2 % of trauma patients in critical care [2]. Such injuries are much easier to miss in critically injured patients with a reduced level of consciousness [2, 3]. As a consequence, patients admitted to critical care following trauma should be assessed with a thorough tertiary survey.

The timing of such a survey is controversial [4]. Generally, a tertiary survey should take place after the initial fast-paced resuscitative and surgical management has settled down. This tertiary survey should include clinical examination alongside radiographs of limbs that may be injured, based on examination or mechanism of injury, and that were not visualised on initial imaging. Where patients remain obtunded or intubated, the threshold for imaging may be lower. Repeat examination is always advisable, especially once a patient has regained consciousness.

Most trauma patients will have had a comprehensive trauma CT series prior to admission to intensive care. Admission imaging studies should be re-assessed in concert with radiologist reports, the findings at surgery and repeat clinical assessment. It has been suggested that almost 20 % of errors in diagnosis and management are caused by mistakes in interpreting initial diagnostic studies which may have been hurried before resuscitative surgery [4].

How Should the Unconscious Patient with Potential Spinal Fractures Be Managed in the Intensive Care Unit?

A substantial number of missed injuries are spinal fractures, which potentially have significant consequences [4]. However, there are risks to taking an over-cautious approach to protecting the spine; cervical collars have their own risks and require a great deal of nursing input [5].

Patients with a diagnosed spinal injury should be managed with advice from a specialist spinal surgeon and with reference to national and local guidelines. Those with a spinal cord injury should be referred to a spinal injuries centre within 24 h of injury and their management should proceed with advice from the specialist centre.

Advanced Trauma Life Support (ATLS) doctrine mandates the assumption that trauma patients have a spinal
injury, and in particular a cervical spine injury, until proven
otherwise. This doctrine aims to avoid causing complications
in the presence of an undiagnosed unstable fracture or ligamentous spinal injury. It is supported by the principle that
patients should be kept in a cervical spine collar, kept flat,
and log rolled until an injury is excluded; the principle of
"spinal clearance". While it is wise to assume that there may
be a spinal injury, collars can offer a false sense of security,
and thus may not be advisable in all cases. Rigid collars have
been shown to increase intracranial pressure [6] and to cause
pressure sores [7], which may be exacerbated by spinal injury.
In the absence of injury, patients with ankylosing spondylitis
and rheumatoid disease are at risk of injury from the application of a collar alone [8]. The effectiveness of cervical spine
immobilisation utilising a collar remains controversial at
present. Recent guidelines for pre-hospital trauma care
increasingly suggest avoiding the use of rigid collars as they
are felt to be ineffective, especially in conscious patients, and
have significant risks. There is evidence that collars alone do
not immobilise the spine [9], and that immobilising with
sandbags but no collar is more effective than a rigid collar
[10]. One analysis of pre-hospital care practice comparing
one nation where cervical spine collars are not used at all
with one where they are used routinely found no evidence of
a difference in the risk of neurological injury in blunt spinal
trauma [11].

Most patients will have had a cervical spine CT scan prior
to admission to critical care. This scan has high sensitivity
and specificity for an unstable injury. There may be a role
for secondary imaging such as MRI, to identify associated
cervical disc trauma, and the extent of the cord oedema and
contusions. However, this must be weighed against the hazards of moving each individual patient from the critical care
unit. For example, placing a head injured patient in the
supine position is associated with raised ICP, which may

further compromise cerebral perfusion. Each case must be assessed individually to determine the risk of undertaking the scan against the benefit provided by the additional information [12].

The British Orthopaedic Association has published guidelines for spinal clearance in the trauma patient [13]. This policy recommends that spinal immobilisation should not continue for more than 48 h. It acknowledges that there is a risk of ligamentous instability in the neck without fracture, but that CT scanning has high sensitivity and specificity for spinal injuries. It therefore recommends that a fine-slice CT scan is undertaken with the first CT brain scan in head injured patients, and that the thoracic and lumbar spine be imaged with plain films or with reconstructed CT scans from thoracic and abdominal series. MRI is considered the investigation of choice for spinal cord injury.

We suggest that all trauma patients should have CT scans as part of their initial imaging, and that these scans are reviewed to exclude spinal injury. The incidence of unstable injury – defined as failure of the bony and/or ligamentous structures of the spinal complex to withstand normal physiological loads leading to potential deformity, neurological deficit and pain – following blunt trauma is approximately 2 %, and this increases to 34 % in the unconscious patient. Fifty percent of spinal injuries occur in the thoracic spine, and 20 % have 2 levels of injury [13]. While a suspicion of spinal injury remains, the patient should be kept immobilised in an appropriate posture based on their known injuries. Head blocks should provide adequate immobilisation. Patients should be log rolled until the spine is cleared. Rigid collars are not recommended unless advised for a specific injury. Spinal clearance should only be undertaken following the reporting of normal spinal CT images by a senior radiologist. Spinal column and spinal cord injuries, where identified, should be managed by orthopaedic or neurosurgical specialists as appropriate to the institution. Figure 14.1 summarises the advice given in this section.

340   E. Spurrier and S.A. Stapley

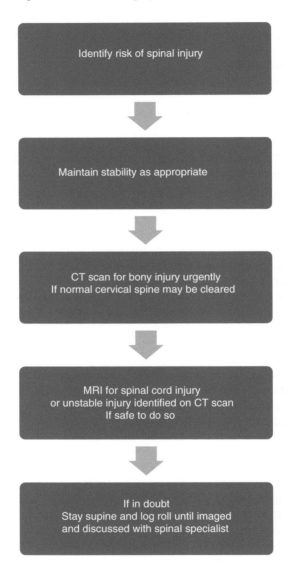

FIGURE 14.1 Suggested process for spinal imaging and clearance

What Are the Treatment Options for Long Bone Fractures in the Critically Injured Patient?

Long bone fractures are associated with haemorrhage, pain and fat embolus. It is desirable to stabilise such injuries early to reduce the incidence of these complications. There are a variety of options for long bone stabilisation which may be used by the orthopaedic team. This section will briefly discuss the options available.

The first decision to make will be whether to definitively stabilise long bone fractures during initial resuscitative surgery, or to perform a stabilisation procedure and delay definitive surgery.

Traditionally, polytrauma victims could expect long primary surgery as all their long bone fractures were stabilised definitively. It was understood that early fracture stabilisation led to a reduced risk of fat embolism and sepsis, and it was believed that ARDS was less likely if all fractures were fixed as soon as possible. It was also believed that these patients were too sick for their surgery to be delayed, as prolonged immobility had been shown to have negative effects [14]. However, a picture began to emerge of a high price for aggressive early surgery with multi-organ failure, ARDS and death. The concept of damage control surgery therefore emerged, with the simplest possible operation to stabilise the patient as fast as possible, reducing the physiological hit from surgery.

As understanding of the inflammatory response to trauma evolved, the concept of the "2 hit phenomenon" arose [15]. It was suggested that the physiological insult of trauma primes the immune system for an inappropriate and exaggerated response, which may lead to ARDS and organ failure when the second hit of surgery is poorly timed or excessive. This led to the concept of damage control orthopaedics, with the primary surgery being made as simple and fast as possible to stabilise long bones and avoid the complications of immobility, but without a stimulating second hit. It eventually became apparent that the second hit phenomenon has significant individual variability and that surgery that would harm some individuals would be safe in others despite a similar injury burden [14].

"Early Appropriate Care" is a recent term described by Nahm et al. [16]. This recognises that there are advantages to early definitive fixation which may outweigh the risks of a more invasive procedure; neither damage control surgery or early total care are necessarily appropriate in any given patient. The timing and extent of individual surgery must be planned with regard to the overall injury burden and physiological status, and the risks and benefits of each surgical modality for each injury. Stable patients may be amenable to early definitive fixation while extremely unstable patients do require damage control surgery. The majority of patients lie in between the extremes, and benefit from a mixture of approaches.

Much of the current literature focuses on the timing of femoral fracture fixation [14]. The femur is not amenable to splinting without the patient being left recumbent, so there are advantages to early fixation. Femoral fractures are commonly definitively fixed with an intramedullary nail. Reamed femoral nailing has been associated with increased lung capillary permeability and increased pulmonary arterial pressures, so femoral nailing may not be suitable in the early stages.

A staged approach to surgery is therefore recommended in most cases. Initial surgery includes stabilising injuries which pose a haemorrhage risk or would otherwise increase immobilisation; these include pelvic and long bone fractures. The initial stabilisation may include internal or external fixation or perhaps simple plaster application depending on the patient's overall condition and the configuration of individual injuries. Once the patient's condition improves, temporary measures may be replaced with definitive fixation.

The resuscitative and metabolic status of the patient are the primary decision tool when selecting temporary or definitive initial fixation. The best way to measure this remains the subject of ongoing research. Simple measures of organ perfusion, such as urine output, make a useful contribution as do measurements of lactate and base deficit. Lactate is currently considered the best measurement of resuscitation to guide surgical decision making [17] with a lactate of 2.5 mmol/l suggested as indicating adequate resuscitation [14, 18]. Interleukin IL-6 is a useful measure and has been shown to be effective [19], but is not available in all units. Where there is doubt over the best approach to take, it is probably safer to tend towards damage control surgery in favour of definitive fixation [20].

Options for stabilising long bone injuries are numerous, and many differing opinions will exist as to the best option. Individual techniques include plaster, external fixation, internal fixation with plates, and intramedullary nails. The benefits of each are beyond the scope of this chapter, as there is great variability in the stability and nature of fractures of any given long bone which may favour a particular technique. However, each method has specific features that merit a brief discussion. In the more austere setting, such as military deployment or humanitarian operations, insertion of metalwork at initial stabilisation is kept to a minimum. This is mainly due to the nature of the operating environment which generally does not have the infection control considerations which we take for granted in a westernised hospital, but also the simple lack of availability of complex operative sets and equipment.

Simple Splints

Simple splints, including the Thomas splint, are satisfactory ways of temporarily and rapidly immobilising a limb. The Thomas splint, and some more modern devices, allow the application of traction to help reduce a femoral fracture into a more anatomical position. However, these devices are bulky, limit patient mobility and positioning, essential in the critically ill patient, and apply traction against part of the patient, thus potentially introducing the risk of pressure sores. They may be used initially, but consideration for further stabilisation should be undertaken in a timely fashion, with splints used for no longer than is necessary.

Plaster Stabilisation

The simplest method of stabilising a fracture is plaster of Paris. The fracture is reduced and the limb stabilised with a plaster splint. This is a quick and simple solution and hence is effective in austere environments; the Red Cross recommends it for most injuries in field hospitals. However, it can be difficult to maintain perfect reduction and the constrictive dressings bring an increased risk of compartment syndrome. In UK practice, plaster is therefore more likely to be a temporary measure in polytrauma depending on the fracture pattern. Patients with a plaster in situ demand monitoring for evidence of compartment syndrome, especially if sedated; if there is a concern of evolving compartment syndrome the plaster must *immediately* be split to the skin.

External Fixation

External fixators use a combination of pins inserted into bone and bars to stabilise an injury. This may be a temporary or definitive treatment. In either case, close attention must be paid to care of the pin sites to prevent infection. The stability of the construct, and therefore what effect the fixator has on patient handling, depends on the fracture configuration so the critical care team must liaise with the surgical team with respect to moving the patient. If an external fixator is a temporary device, it will generally be replaced with definitive fixation within 2 weeks.

Internal Fixation

Internal fixation with plates and screws or nails, is likely to be a definitive treatment modality and may take place at initial or late surgery. Depending on what plates or nails are used, the procedure may be open – with an incision directly to the fracture site and over the hardware – or minimally invasive, with incisions as required to insert hardware and reduce the fracture. In most cases, mobility will be minimally restricted once the fracture is definitively fixed but this is not always the case and operation notes must be reviewed. Whilst this method of fixation appears to provide the definitive answer to fracture management, fracture patterns are not always straightforward and may require the acquisition of particular hardware from differing manufacturers, which is not immediately available within the hospital. Thus a time delay may ensue. A delay of 2–3 weeks will not have a deleterious effect on the overall fracture outcome, but may be deleterious to the physiological status of the patient, particularly if it prevents early mobilisation. Therefore, continuous multidisciplinary discussions between orthopaedic and ICU teams are required.

What Are the Principals of Management for Patients with Pelvic Fractures?

Fractures of the pelvic ring are a common injury following polytrauma. Such patients are at risk of death from haemorrhage, particularly from bleeding sacral veins in certain patterns of fracture. Precautions must be taken to support pelvic injuries in order to reduce bleeding as much as possible, and it is now routine practice to bind the pelvis as early as possible on the assumption that a fracture is present. Open pelvic fractures/disruptions of the pelvic ring demonstrate an overall mortality rate of 50 %.

Pelvic binders have been introduced which can be rapidly applied in the pre hospital environment. They are designed to compress the iliac wings together and reduce the volume within the pelvic cavity, thus reducing the available volume for haemorrhage and providing a tamponade. They have been proven to effectively stabilise certain fracture patterns, but are not entirely without risk. In certain fracture patterns, there is a risk of over-reducing the pelvis if applied too tightly, consequently injuring the structures within. It is easy to place the binder incorrectly, which markedly reduces its efficacy [21]. Binders also apply high pressure to the skin over the greater trochanters, and therefore have a significant risk of skin breakdown and wound complications.

In the presence of a suspected pelvic fracture, it is suggested that the best means of providing stability is to apply a proprietary binder at the correct tension and to obtain imaging as soon as possible. This would normally be undertaken before transfer to critical care. Clinical examination must include assessment of deformity, groin and scrotal swelling and haematoma, urethral bleeding and rectal and vaginal examination to exclude an open fracture. There is no role in any circumstances for "springing the pelvis"; this will destabilise any bleeding vessels around the sacrum and may cause significant blood loss.

Where a pelvic fracture is associated with hypovolaemic shock, it is likely that the bleeding originates from sacral venous plexi. Fractures of the iliac wing and sacrum, and fracture patterns with pubic symphysis diastasis, are more prone to fatal haemorrhage [22]. Some controversy exists regarding the optimal method for controlling haemorrhage, but local resources will likely dictate the best path. Options for haemorrhage control include external fixation and packing, or radiological embolization of bleeding vessels. Embolization is effective in around 85 % of cases [23] but there is a risk of failure to control bleeding and of recurrent haemorrhage. Where a patient is in extremis and interventional radiology is not available, urgent surgery to pack the pelvis is usually effective. If interventional radiology is available and haemorrhage control is successful, this is usually a better option as it is less invasive. Early stabilisation of pelvic fractures by a suitable specialist surgeon will allow easier nursing care. However, this requires sub-specialty care and may therefore require transfer of the patient to a suitably equipped unit, with consequent delay. The development of major trauma networks within the UK, will hopefully reduce the requirement for such transfers, with all suitable sub-specialty management available in one institution.

If a patient is to be transferred to another facility, a pelvic fracture should be stabilised by a suitable means in discussion with the receiving surgeon. Pelvic binders are suitable for transfer provided that their position is checked and re-checked, and that adequate care is taken of the skin. External fixators may be more stable, but are awkward when transferring a patient by ambulance and especially by air.

How Should Hand Injuries Be Managed in the Polytrauma Patient?

Hand fractures are common in polytrauma and may be managed by a combination of orthopaedic and plastic surgeons. Fractures of the hand are commonly missed, with reported incidences of 4–33 % [24], often because they are considered less important than other more dramatic long bone injuries. Poor management of hand injuries is associated with significant loss of function and morbidity, and litigation is not uncommon. Whilst these injuries are clearly not life threatening, patients who develop severe disabilities as a result of polytrauma injuries, require the full use of hands and digits in order to perform activities of daily living. Thus hand and wrist injuries must be identified and appropriate subspecialty management undertaken. Experience has shown that once all the other injuries have recovered it remains the hand injury that causes long term disability and frustration. Therefore, all possible steps must be taken to ensure that the hand is not allowed to become stiff and non-functional and consistent multidisciplinary approach is required.

The spectrum of hand injuries is broad and many can be managed non-operatively. Where surgery is likely to be helpful, it is usually best to operate early, within 14 days – the hand heals quickly and outcomes rapidly worsen if surgery is delayed beyond this.

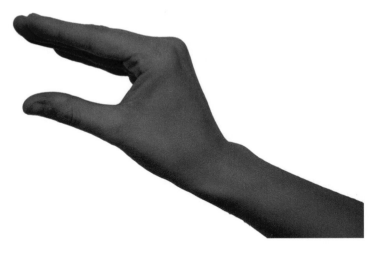

FIGURE 14.2 Position of safe immobilisation for the hand

Where the hand is to be rested immobile, it is essential that it is immobilised in the correct position. The metacarpophalangeal joints have strong collateral ligaments which are tightest when the joint is at 90°. The interphalangeal joint collateral ligaments are tightest when the joint is straight. These ligaments contract rapidly when not allowed to move. If a hand is plastered, it must be immobilised with the collaterals at their tightest – otherwise they will contract, leaving the hand stiff. The hand should therefore be plastered or splinted with the metacarpophalangeal joints at 90° and the fingers straight; this is most comfortable if the wrist is in slight extension. This is known as "position of safe immobilisation" (POSI) splinting or Edinburgh splinting and is shown in Fig. 14.2.

Ideally, the hand should be allowed to move as much as possible. Surgeons will aim to select surgery which allows early movement where possible. If the patient is unconscious, hand therapists should provide daily passive exercises to prevent stiffening.

Which Patients Are at Risk of Limb Compartment Syndrome and How Should They Be Managed?

Compartment syndrome is a condition in which a constricted fascial compartment experiences a rise in pressure, leading to compromised microvascular perfusion and eventual tissue death. It is a difficult condition to diagnose in the obtunded patient, requiring a high index of suspicion [25]. Mortality of critically ill patients with acute limb compartment syndrome is reported to be as high as 67 % [26]. There are many causes, including fractures and soft tissue injury but other causes must be considered including extravascular injection and ischaemic tissue injury. Extracorporeal membrane oxygenation has also been reported as a cause [27]. A full list of causes and incidences is shown in Table 14.1.

After an initial trigger injury, local inflammation and oedema within an enclosed compartment will result in a rise in pressure. Although a significant rise would be needed to cause a loss of arterial circulation, capillary flow will be reduced much faster and this leads to increased local injury, oedema and a vicious cycle of increasing compartment pressures. Eventually, the arterial inflow will fall but, by this stage, the muscular tissue in the compartment may already be dead.

In conscious patients, symptoms of compartment syndrome include pain, pallor, paraesthesia and pulselessness. Other than pain, all of these occur late and if they are present it may be too late to prevent significant tissue death. The most useful early symptom is pain out of proportion to that expected from the injury. The best sign is pain on passive stretch of the involved muscle compartment. Either of these may be absent in sedated or unconscious patients. Affected compartments may be clinically swollen and tense, but this is an unreliable sign to exclude compartment syndrome.

Where there is a risk of compartment syndrome evolving, and clinical signs will be absent, it is possible to monitor the relevant compartments with an indwelling catheter, as shown

TABLE 14.1 Causes and incidence of limb compartment syndrome [28] with permission

Causes of compartment syndrome	Incidence %
Closed tibial shaft fractures	33
Radius and ulna fractures	20
Other fractures including tight casts	7
Foot injuries	6
Blunt and crushed soft tissue limb trauma	25
Total other causes	9

Other surgical causes

Burns

Blast injury

High energy gun shot wounds

Prolonged lithotomy position during surgery

Arterial and venous injury/revascularisation/reperfusion injury

Use of pulsatile lavage

Use of pneumatic anti-shock garment

Other accidental causes

Excessive exercise in athletes

Non routine/overuse in non athletes

Non- accidental causes

Nephrotic syndrome

Viral myositis

Hypothyroidism

Bleeding disorders/anticoagulation

Malignancies

Diabetes-associated muscle infarction

Ruptured bakers cyst

Snake bite

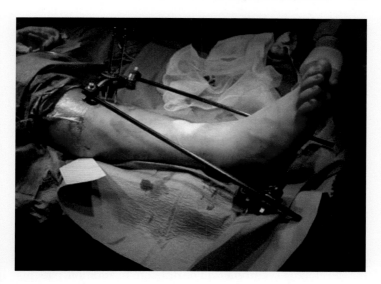

FIGURE 14.3 External fixation used to treat a lower limb fracture. A catheter has been inserted in order to measure compartment pressure and provide an early warning of impending compartment syndrome

in Fig. 14.3, or intermittent aspiration. The diagnostic criterion for compartment syndrome is a pressure difference (Delta P) of less than 30 mmHg between diastolic blood pressure and compartment pressure, which indicates a risk of circulation compromise [26].

$$\delta P = Diastolic\ blood\ pressure - Compartment\ Pressure$$

Other measures, such as intra-compartment pH, remain controversial, but may become established in the future. Compartment syndrome should also be considered in the obtunded patient where there is concern of ongoing progressive tissue necrosis or inflammation and no other cause has been found. Other, more subtle, physiological changes can be identified if patients are continually monitored. Even in the unconscious patient, trends in oxygen consumption, increased heart rate and increased sedation requirements may all be indicators of evolving compartment pressure rises, prompting the clinician to be suspicious of this developing condition.

Established compartment syndrome is a surgical emergency. Initial management is to release constrictive dressings and ensure that the limb is not below the level of the heart. The definitive management of compartment syndrome is surgical release along with debridement of any necrotic tissue. This will normally be accompanied by stabilising any underlying fracture to halt the cycle of worsening tissue injury. Male patients aged 15–30 years with a high energy closed tibial fracture are at extremely high risk with 1 in 4 developing compartment syndrome, requiring decompression. Therefore, in the polytraumatised, obtunded patient within this age group and with this injury pattern, consideration may be given to pre-emptively perform surgical decompression as diagnosis of the developing syndrome will be difficult. In addition, patients requiring prolonged transfer to another health care facility, particularly by air, with lower limb fractures, blast injuries or reperfusion/vascular injuries should have decompression performed pre-emptively before transfer.

Which Patients Are at Risk of Rhabdomyolysis and How Should They Be Managed?

Where significant volumes of muscle are injured, as may happen following crush or compartment syndrome, rhabdomylosis is likely to follow. The release of intracellular muscle components such as myoglobin and creatine kinase (CK) into the circulation may lead to acute renal failure, disseminated intravascular coagulation and significant electrolyte imbalance [29].

Most cases of rhabdomyolysis follow direct trauma, but other causes include infections of muscle tissue, compartment syndrome and ischemia, drugs and toxins. The common denominator of all causes is massive muscle BREAKDOWN. Once muscle cellular breakdown starts, as in compartment syndrome, a self-sustaining cascade of necrosis arises and muscle contents are released to the circulation.

Clinical manifestations of rhabdomyolysis include myalgia, weakness and myoglobinuria but this classical triad is rarely present. The most sensitive laboratory test is elevated serum CK.

Once rhabdomyolysis is suspected, the causative pathology – such as compartment syndrome – must be addressed. The key complication is acute renal failure and fluid management is therefore critical. Aggressive hydration is generally recommended along with alkalinising the urine. However, excessive volume administration in the context of established critical illness can de deleterious and some patients may require early institution of renal replacement therapy.

What Is Fat Embolism Syndrome?

Fat embolus occurs in patients with long bone fractures, although few develop systemic dysfunction. The classical triad of skin, brain and lung dysfunction is uncommon but serious [30].

In fat embolism syndrome, circulating microglobules of fat lead to multisystem dysfunction. It is commonly associated with long bone fractures, especially after intramedullary nailing, but it has also been reported following burns, marrow biopsy and liposuction. Non-traumatic causes are very uncommon and include pancreatitis, fat emulsion infusion and haemoglobinopathies [30].

There are two causative theories. Gossling et al. suggest a mechanical theory in which fat is forced INTO the circulation, perhaps by the force of intramedullary instrumentation causing a rise in pressure within the intramedullary canal, and is deposited in capillary beds [31]. Local tissue inflammation results leading to systemic effects. Alternatively, the response to trauma may lead to systemic release of chylomicrons,

which coalesce under the influence of inflammatory mediators leading to the same effects [32].

The key features of fat embolus syndrome are respiratory
failure, cerebral dysfunction, and skin petechiae. Manifestations
may develop 24–72 h following trauma [30]. The vascular
occlusion in fat embolus is often temporary or incomplete as
deformable fat globules do not completely obstruct flow.

The skin manifestations include a petechial rash, typically
around the chest and axilla. Signs of respiratory and cerebral
dysfunction are nonspecific and include tachypnoea and
confusion.

Diagnosis is based on excluding other causes in the presence of clinical features of fat embolism [30]. Specific diagnostic criteria have been proposed by Schonfeld [33] and
Lindeque [34] and are shown in Table 14.2.

Management is supportive and focuses on maintaining
oxygenation and circulating volume. Stabilising long bone
fractures early is essential, as delayed stabilisation increases
the risk [36], though this must be balanced against the disadvantages of early surgery. Specific medical treatments for fat
embolism syndrome have not been shown to be effective.

What Is Heterotopic Ossification and Which Patients Are at Risk?

Heterotopic ossification (HO) is the formation of bone in
soft tissues. In patients with traumatic brain injury, the
reported incidence of HO is between 10 and 20 % and it can
have a significant impact on mobility and function [37].

HO generally forms in neurologically impaired limbs and
in these patients is often found in muscle planes surrounding
joints, as shown in Fig. 14.4. It may not necessarily occur in an
injured limb. In other patients, such as those with traumatic
amputations, HO may invade muscle compartments [38].

Unfortunately, there is little evidence to support any
effective therapy in preventing or slowing the formation of

TABLE 14.2 Two scoring systems developed to diagnose fat embolism syndrome

Schonfeld et al. [33] scoring system	**A score of 5 or more equals a diagnosis of fat embolism syndrome**
Sign/Symptom	Score
Petechial Rash	5
Diffuse infiltrates on CXR	4
Hypoxemia	3
Raised Temperature	1
Tachycardia	1
Confusion	1
Lindeque et al. [34] **specific diagnostic criteria**	
Sustained PaO_2	<60 mmHg/8 Kpa
Sustained $PaCO_2$	>55 mmHg/7.3 Kpa (pH<7.3)
Respiratory Rate	>35 bpm
Increased work of breathing	Dyspnoea
	Use of accessory muscles of respiration
	Tachycardia
	Anxiety

Although both systems were developed in the early 1980's they are still utilized [35]

HO. Diphosphonates have been shown to have some efficacy. A 6 week course of indomethacin may be effective at reducing HO, but evidence is limited. Radiation therapy may be effective, but the risk of radiation induced sarcoma is significant [37]. Physiotherapy has not been shown to prevent HO.

Once established, the only effective therapy is surgery. However, this may be invasive and carries its own morbidity.

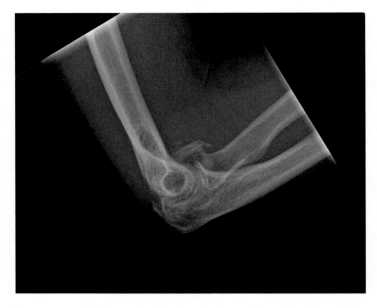

FIGURE 14.4 Radiograph showing heterotopic ossification of the anterior capsule of the elbow joint

References

1. Brooks A, Holroyd B, Riley B. Missed injury in major trauma patients. Injury. 2004;35(4):407–10.
2. Giannakopoulos GF et al. Missed injuries during the initial assessment in a cohort of 1124 level-1 trauma patients. Injury. 2012;43(9):1517–21.
3. Chen C-W et al. Incidence rate and risk factors of missed injuries in major trauma patients. Accid Anal Prev. 2011;43(3):823–8.
4. Thomson CB, Greaves I. Missed injury and the tertiary trauma survey. Injury. 2008;39(1):107–14.
5. Webber-Jones JE, Thomas CA, Bordeaux Jr RE. The management and prevention of rigid cervical collar complications. Orthop Nurs. 2002;21(4):19–25; quiz 25–7.
6. Mobbs RJ, Stoodley MA, Fuller J. Effect of cervical hard collar on intracranial pressure after head injury. ANZ J Surg. 2002;72(6):389–91.

7. Sundstrom T et al. Prehospital use of cervical collars in trauma patients: a critical review. J Neurotrauma. 2014;31(6):531–40.
8. Benger J, Blackham J. Why do we put cervical collars on conscious trauma patients? Scand J Trauma Resusc Emerg Med. 2009;17:44.
9. James CY et al. Comparison of cervical spine motion during application among 4 rigid immobilization collars. J Athl Train. 2004;39(2):138–45.
10. Podolsky S et al. Efficacy of cervical spine immobilization methods. J Trauma. 1983;23(6):461–5.
11. Hauswald M et al. Out-of-hospital spinal immobilization: its effect on neurologic injury. Acad Emerg Med. 1998;5(3):214–9.
12. Dunham CM et al. Risks associated with magnetic resonance imaging and cervical collar in comatose, blunt trauma patients with negative comprehensive cervical spine computed tomography and no apparent spinal deficit. Crit Care. 2008;12(4):R89.
13. BOA, BOAST 2 version 2: Spinal clearance in the trauma patient, in British Orthopaedic Association Standards for Trauma. London: British Orthopaedic Association; 2015.
14. D'Alleyrand J-CG, O'Toole RV. The evolution of damage control orthopedics. Orthop Clin. North Am. 2013;44(4):499–507.
15. Faist E et al. Multiple organ failure in polytrauma patients. J Trauma. 1983;23(9):775–87.
16. Nahm NJ et al. Early appropriate care: definitive stabilization of femoral fractures within 24 hours of injury is safe in most patients with multiple injuries. J Trauma. 2011;71(1):175–85.
17. Giannoudis PV. Surgical priorities in damage control in polytrauma. J Bone Joint Surg Br. 2003;85(4):478–83.
18. O'Toole RV et al. Resuscitation before stabilization of femoral fractures limits acute respiratory distress syndrome in patients with multiple traumatic injuries despite low use of damage control orthopedics. J Trauma. 2009;67(5):1013–21.
19. Pape HC et al. Major secondary surgery in blunt trauma patients and perioperative cytokine liberation: determination of the clinical relevance of biochemical markers. J Trauma. 2001;50(6):989–1000.
20. Tuttle MS et al. Safety and efficacy of damage control external fixation versus early definitive stabilization for femoral shaft fractures in the multiple-injured patient. J Trauma. 2009;67(3):602–5.
21. Bonner TJ et al. Accurate placement of a pelvic binder improves reduction of unstable fractures of the pelvic ring. J Bone Joint Surg Br Vol. 2011;93-B(11):1524–8.

22. Ruatti S et al. Which pelvic ring fractures are potentially lethal? Injury. 2015;46(6):1059–63.
23. Ierardi A, et al. The role of endovascular treatment of pelvic fracture bleeding in emergency settings. Eur Radiol. 2015:1–11.
24. Pfeifer R, Pape H-C. Missed injuries in trauma patients: a literature review. Patient Saf Surg. 2008;2:20.
25. Farrow C, Bodenham A, Troxler M. Acute limb compartment syndromes. Contin Educ Anaesth Crit Care Pain. 2011;11(1):24–8.
26. Kosir R et al. Acute lower extremity compartment syndrome (ALECS) screening protocol in critically ill trauma patients. J Trauma. 2007;63(2):268–75.
27. Wall CJ, Santamaria J. Extracorporeal membrane oxygenation: an unusual cause of acute limb compartment syndrome. Anaesth Intensive Care. 2010;38(3):560–2.
28. Köstler W, Strohm PC, Südkamp NP. Acute compartment syndrome of the limb. Injury. 2005;36(8):992–8.
29. Torres PA et al. Rhabdomyolysis: pathogenesis, diagnosis, and treatment. Ochsner J. 2015;15(1):58–69.
30. Shaikh N. Emergency management of fat embolism syndrome. J Emerg Trauma Shock. 2009;2(1):29–33.
31. Gossling HR, Pellegrini Jr VD. Fat embolism syndrome: a review of the pathophysiology and physiological basis of treatment. Clin Orthop Relat Res. 1982;165:68–82.
32. Baker PL, Pazell JA, Peltier LF. Free fatty acids, catecholamines, and arterial hypoxia in patients with fat embolism. J Trauma. 1971;11(12):1026–30.
33. Schonfeld SA et al. Fat embolism prophylaxis with corticosteroids. A prospective study in high-risk patients. Ann Intern Med. 1983;99(4):438–43.
34. Lindeque BG et al. Fat embolism and the fat embolism syndrome. A double-blind therapeutic study. J Bone Joint Surg Br. 1987;69(1):128–31.
35. Kwiatt ME, Seamon MJ. Fat embolism syndrome. Int J Crit Illness Injury Sci. 2013;3(1):64–8.
36. Behrman SW et al. Improved outcome with femur fractures: early vs. delayed fixation. J Trauma. 1990;30(7):792–7; discussion 797–8.
37. Cipriano CA, Pill SG, Keenan MA. Heterotopic ossification following traumatic brain injury and spinal cord injury. J Am Acad Orthop Surg. 2009;17(11):689–97.
38. Edwards DS, Clasper JC, Patel HD. Heterotopic ossification in victims of the London 7/7 bombings. J R Army Med Corps. 2015;161(4):345–7.

Chapter 15
Imaging the Critically Injured Patient

David A.T. Gay and Jonathan Crighton

Abstract Critically injured patients will often require the full range of radiological investigations. Most patients with major traumatic injury will undergo an initial trauma series CT scan which provides images of the head, cervical spine, thorax abdomen and pelvis. The brain can be imaged using CT or MRI; different patterns of intra cranial bleeding are illustrated. Recognition of unstable spinal injuries is vital and the pattern of injury is compared with the type of fractures typically seen. Although initial thoracic imaging is usually undertaken with CT, plain films are used routinely thereafter to detect complications or to investigate changes in the clinical picture. Plain films are particularly useful to confirm correct placement of devices, such as intravascular lines. Various intra abdominal injuries have typical CT appearances which are described. Pelvic fractures can be stable or

D.A.T. Gay, MBBS, FRCR, PGCE (✉)
Peninsular Radiology Academy, Plymouth, Devon PL6 5WR, UK
e-mail: davegay@nhs.net

J. Crighton, LLB, MBBS, MRCS, FRCR, PgCertCE
Derriford Hospital, Plymouth, PL6 8DH, UK

S.D. Hutchings (ed.), *Trauma and Combat Critical Care in Clinical Practice*, In Clinical Practice,
DOI 10.1007/978-3-319-28758-4_15,
359

unstable and CT imaging is vitally important to determine the correct management.

Keywords Trauma CT • Spinal fractures • Pelvic fractures • Head CT • Thoracic CT • Abdominal CT • Chest X Ray

Introduction

Critically injured patients often require the full range of radiology investigations. It can be challenging to select the right investigation and even harder to interpret the results. This chapter aims to clarify the most useful investigations and provide examples of some of the more common diagnoses and pitfalls.

What Is a 'Trauma CT'?

A recent systematic review showed that early whole body or Trauma CT is associated with decreased mortality [1] although the mechanism of this effect is uncertain and is highly likely to be based on multiple factors. A polytrauma patient is potentially physiologically unstable and in order to reduce the length of time that a trauma patient spends in the CT scanner a Trauma CT protocol is used to reduce scanning preparation and acquisition time. Two sequential contrast boluses are injected intravenously and the entire scan is completed in one acquisition or 'run'. This produces an arterial phase head, cervical spine and thorax and arterial and portal venous phase abdomen and pelvis.

Part One: Head Imaging

Do Plain Films Have a Role?

The current investigation of choice for the detection of clinically important acute brain injuries is CT imaging [2]. Plain radiography is used to assess facial fractures in the absence of concern of an intracranial injury. The most common protocol is two views – occipitomental (OM) (frontal radiograph with upwards beam angle) and an OM 30° (an OM with 30° up-tilt). Additionally an orthopantomogram (OPG) is used to visualise the 'straightened' mandible. These views require the patient to be concordant and have a mobile cervical spine and mandible which largely precludes their use in the critically injured patient. Additionally, CT is excellent at visualising complex facial fractures.

When Is it Appropriate to Obtain a CT Head?

Any patient presentation that fulfils NICE Head Injury Guidelines [2] should have a CT Head prior to transfer to Critical Care. This is essential to identify any underlying potentially life threatening acute injuries and acts as a baseline for comparison with subsequent studies. The majority of polytruama patients with a significant mechanism of injury will have a head CT performed as part of the initial trauma CT series.

When Is it Appropriate to Request a Repeat CT Head?

Any of the following examples of neurological deterioration should prompt urgent reappraisal by the supervising doctor and consideration of repeat CT:

- Development of agitation or abnormal behaviour.
- A sustained (that is, for at least 30 min) drop of 1 point in GCS score (greater weight should be given to a drop of 1 point in the motor response score of the GCS).
- Any drop of 3 or more points in the eye-opening or verbal response scores of the GCS, or 2 or more points in the motor response score.
- Development of severe or increasing headache or persisting vomiting.
- New or evolving neurological symptoms or signs such as pupil inequality or asymmetry of limb or facial movement.

- Patients who are sedated and ventilated can be difficult to assess using these criteria. Repeat imaging of ventilated patients with severe head trauma is covered in more detail in Chap. 11.

Does MRI Have Role in Imaging Following Traumatic Brain Injury?

CT is neither sensitive nor specific for subtle parenchymal changes, such as micro-haemorrhage and diffuse axonal injury (DAI), found in traumatic brain injury. DAI is suggested in any patient who demonstrates clinical symptoms disproportionate to their CT findings. Whilst MRI is the preferred examination for DAI it is contraindicated in patients who have metallic foreign bodies, such as shrapnel or bullet fragments, in their head or neck or near important vascular structures. In addition, MRI is logistically more challenging in ventilated, critically injured patients. It should reserved as a second line investigation for those patients whose anatomical abnormalities on CT are out of keeping with their neurological examination.

What Does Raised Intracranial Pressure Look Like on CT Imaging?

CT image appearances associated with intra cranial hypertension are discussed in more detail in Chap. 11 which describes the use of CT imaging in the management of severe TBI.

Are There Different Types of Cranial Herniation and Is it Important to Differentiate Between Them?

The brain is essentially divided into discrete volumes by the falx cerebri and tentorium cerebelli. A SOL in one or more of these volumes will force brain parenchyma to herniate from one compartment to another. Understanding the type of herniation allows the prediction of associated structures that may be compromised e.g. cranial nerves, arteries and veins. Brain herniation can be divided anatomically into;

- Supratentorial herniation
    - **Uncal** (transtentorial) – the uncus hippocampus becomes compressed against the free edge of the tentorium cerebelli, frequently leading to brainstem compression.
    - **Central** (transtentorial) – the diencephalon and parts of the temporal lobes of both of the cerebral hemispheres are squeezed through a notch in the tentorium cerebelli.
    - **Cingulate** (subfalcine) – the medial part of the frontal lobe is forced under the falx cerebri. The easiest method of evaluating for subfalcine shift is a straight line drawn in the expected location of the septum pellucidum from the posterior most aspects to the falx on axial images. Shift of the septum pellucidum from this midline can be measured in mm and compared over time to determine any change. Note that the midline structures rather than the midline move. Figure 10.4 demonstrates subfalcine herniation associated with a subdural haematoma.
    - **Transcalvarial** – the brain herniates through a fracture or a surgical site in the skull.

- Infratentorial herniation
    - **Upward cerebellar** (transtentorial) – The midbrain is pushed through the tentorial notch.
    - **Downward cerebellar/Tonsillar** (transforaminal) – The cerebellar tonsils move downward through the foramen magnum possibly causing compression of the lower brainstem and upper cervical spinal cord. Increased pressure on the brainstem can result in dysfunction of the centres in the brain responsible for controlling cardiorespiratory function.

What Do Different Types of Intracranial Bleeding Look Like?

Intracranial haemorrhage is a collective term encompassing many different conditions characterised by the extravascular accumulation of blood within different intracranial spaces. Categorising the type of bleed helps to predict associated complications. A simple categorisation is based on location:

- Intra-axial Haemorrhage
    - **Intra-cerebral** (parenchymal) – This can encompass a number of entities that share the acute accumulation of blood in the parenchyma of the brain. The aetiology, demographics, treatment and prognosis vary widely depending on the type and location of haemorrhage (Fig. 15.1).

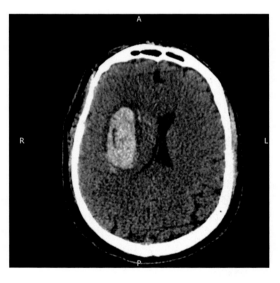

FIGURE 15.1 Intraparenchymal Haemorrhage. Axial section of a non-contrast enhanced head CT study demonstrating a large hyperdense left hemisphere intraparenchymal haemorrhage with associated peripheral oedema and mass effect.

- **Intra-ventricular** – responsible for significant morbidity due to the development of obstructive hydrocephalus. It can be divided into primary (little or no parenchymal blood) or secondary (where the haemorrhage has migrated to the ventricles from a parenchymal or subarachnoid haemorrhage). Primary intra-ventricular haemorrhage is very rare in adults. On CT blood in the ventricles appears as hyper-dense material, and being heavier than CSF tends to pool dependently – commonly in the occipital horns of the lateral ventricles. MRI is more sensitive than CT to very small amounts of blood, especially in the posterior fossa, where CT remains marred by artifact. A common mistake is to confuse a normal calcified choroid plexus with blood (Fig. 15.2).

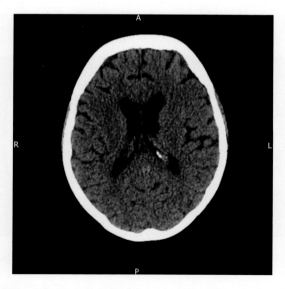

FIGURE 15.2 Calcified choroid plexus. Axial non-contrast enhanced section of a normal CT head demonstrating normal calcified choroid plexus within the left posterior horn.

- Extra-axial Haemorrhage
  - **Extradural** – forms between the inner surface of the skull and outer layer of dura. They are commonly associated with a history of trauma and in 75 % of cases an associated skull fracture. The source of bleeding is usually a torn meningeal artery. Extradural haemorrhage (EDH) is classically biconvex in shape and can cause mass effect. They are limited by cranial sutures, but generally not by venous sinuses. Both CT and MRI are suitable to evaluate EDHs. When the blood clot is evacuated promptly (or treated conservatively when small), the prognosis of EDHs is generally good (Fig. 15.3a, b).
  - **Subdural** – Subdural haematomas are interposed between the dura and arachnoid. Typically crescent-shaped, they are usually more extensive than extradural hematomas. In contrast to extradural haemorrhage,

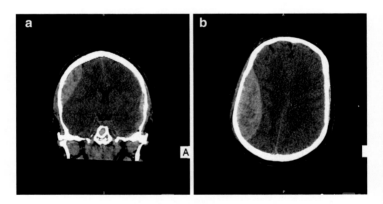

FIGURE 15.3 (**a, b**) Extradural haemorrhage. Coronal (**a**) and axial (**b**) non-contrast CT head demonstrating bi-convex heterogeneous hyperdense right extradural haemorrhage causing mass effect but little parenchymal oedema. Note is made of the contralateral hyperdense subdural haemorrhage seen on the coronal view.

SDH is not limited by sutures but are limited by dural reflections – such as the falx cerebri, tentorium and the falx cerebelli. The appearance of SDHs on CT varies with clot age and organization (Fig. 15.4a, b).

- **Subarachnoid** – Presence of blood within the subarachnoid space. Although MRI is thought to be more sensitive to the presence of subarachnoid blood than CT, as well as having greater sensitivity to the wide range of causative lesions, logistics and limited access mean that in the vast majority of cases a CT of the brain is obtained as the first investigation. The sensitivity of CT to the presence of subarachnoid blood is strongly influenced by both the amount of blood and the time since the haemorrhage. Complications depend on the volume and location of haemorrhage but include elevated intracranial pressure, hydrocephalus and cerebral vasospasm (Fig. 15.5).

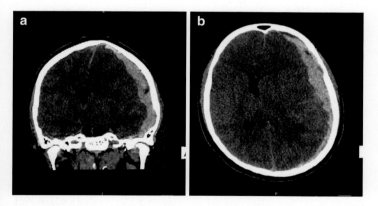

FIGURE 15.4 (**a, b**) Subdural haemorrhage with associated Cingulate (subfalcine) herniation. Axial (**a**) and coronal (**b**) non-contrast enhanced CT head demonstrating a large hyper-dense left sub-dural haemorrhage and left hemisphere parenchymal oedema that are together causing significant mass effect and shift of the midline structures to the right with additional subfalcine herniation

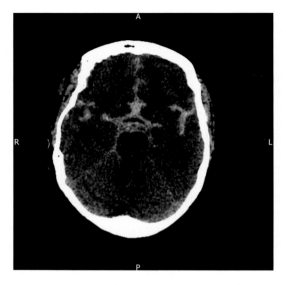

FIGURE   15.5 Subarachnoid   haemorrhage.   Axial   non-contrast
enhanced CT head showing hyperdense acute subarachnoid haemorrhage within the subarachnoid space surrounding the cerebral
hemispheres and brainstem

Part Two: Spinal Imaging

Is a Spinal Fracture Stable?

Spine fractures can occur secondary to flexion, extension,
axial loading or direct trauma. There are many types of
spine fracture, some of which are unstable. The cervical
spine is particularly susceptible to injuries due to its relatively high mobility, small vertebral bodies and weight of
the head.

The three-column concept of spinal fractures is a useful
way of approaching spinal injuries. Whilst primarily used to
classify of thoracolumbar spinal fractures, it can also be used
in the lower cervical spine. The vertebral column can be

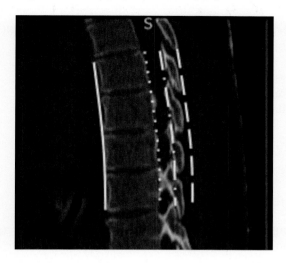

FIGURE 15.6 Three column schematic. Sagittal section of a CT tho-racolumbar spine. Anterior Longitudinal Ligament – solid line, Posterior Longitudinal Ligament – dotted line, Ligamentum Flavum – dot/dash line, Interconnecting Ligaments – dashed line

divided into three parts. Instability occurs when injuries involve two contiguous columns.

What Are the Three Columns?

- Anterior column – anterior longitudinal ligament (ALL), anterior two-thirds of the vertebral body/intervertebral disc.
- Middle column – posterior one-third of the vertebral body/intervertebral disc, posterior longitudinal ligament (PLL).
- Posterior column – neural arch, ligamentum flavum (LF), facet joints and articular processes and interconnecting ligaments (IL) (Fig. 15.6).

Are There Additional Indicators of Spinal Fracture Instability?

- Increased distance between the spinous processes.
- Increased or reduced intervertebral disc space.
- Unilateral or bilateral facet joint widening.

How Do the Different Mechanisms of Injury Relate to Fracture Patterns?

Hyperextension

- **Hangman fracture – unstable**. Hyperextension or lateral hyperflexion – commonly high-speed road traffic collisions (RTC).
    - Bilateral lamina and pedicle fracture at C2
    - Anterolisthesis of C2 on C3 (Fig. 15.7a–c).
- **Extension teardrop fracture – potentially unstable**. Forced extension of the neck. Stable in flexion, unstable in extension as the anterior longitudinal ligament is disrupted.

    - 'Tear-drop' avulsion fracture of the attachment of the anterior longitudinal ligament to the anteroinferior corner of the vertebral body.
    - Anterior disc space widening.

Hyperflexion

- **Flexion teardrop fracture – unstable**. Occurs from flexion and compression, most commonly at C5/C6 e.g. diving impact, RTC deceleration. Often associated with anterior cervical cord syndrome and quadriplegia. The 'teardrop' fragment appears similar to that in extension teardrop fractures however the flexion teardrop is a more severe injury as the vertebral body is displaced.
    - Teardrop fracture of antero-inferior vertebral body.
    - Intervertebral disc space narrowing – contrast with widening in Extension Teardrop fractures.

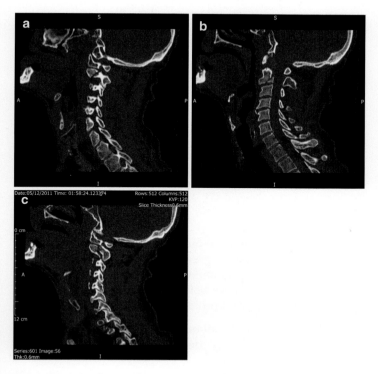

FIGURE 15.7 (**a–c**) Hangman fracture. Sagittal non-contrast enhanced CT of the cervical spine demonstrating fractures of both pedicles (**a, c**) and the vertebral body (**b**). There is incidental degenerative change at the C4/C5 level

- Anterior dislocation of the facet joints.
- Loss of anterior height of the vertebral body causing kyphosis.
- Increased distance between the spinous processes on plain film lateral projection.
- Sagittal fracture through the vertebral body (Fig. 15.8a, b).

• **Bilateral facet dislocation – unstable**. Hyperflexion injury. The inferior articular facet of the cephalad vertebra moves over the superior facet of the vertebra below.

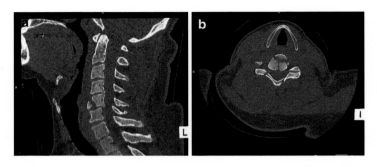

FIGURE 15.8 (**a**, **b**) Flexion teardrop fracture. Sagittal (**a**) and axial (**b**) non-contrast enhanced CT cervical spine demonstrating a C5 flexion teardrop fracture

- – Facet joints may be either perched or locked.
- – Anterolisthesis of greater than 50 % – in contrast to less than 25 % in unilateral facet dislocation.
- – Increased distance between the spinous processes on plain film lateral projection.

- **Unilateral facet dislocation – stable**. Flexion, distraction and rotation injury that commonly involves C4/C5 or C5/C6.
  - – Misalignment of spinous processes on plain film AP projection.
  - – Increased distance between the spinous processes on plain film lateral projection.
  - – Anterolisthesis of less than 25 % – in contrast to greater than 50 % in bilateral facet dislocation.

- **Hyperflexion fracture-dislocation – unstable**. Often associated with marked neurologic deficit e.g. cord transection or central cord syndrome.

  - – Pre-vertebral soft tissue swelling with normal alignment of C-spine on plain film lateral projection.
  - – Avulsion fragment from antero-inferior end plate of dislocated body.
  - – Widening of the intervertebral disc space on plain film lateral projection (Fig. 15.9a, b).

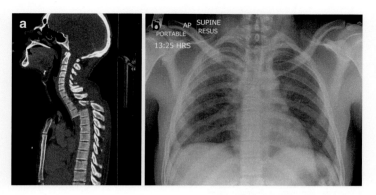

FIGURE 15.9 (**a, b**) Hyperflexion fracture-dislocation. Sagittal non-contrast enhanced CT cervicothoracic spine (**a**) demonstrating fracture dislocation at the T3/T4 level. Sagittal non-contrast enhanced T2 weighted MRI showed the spinal cord transection. The plain radiograph (**b**) acquired in the Emergency Department highlights the pitfalls of relying on single plane imaging as this catastrophic and unstable injury is very difficult to discern

Axial Compression

- **Jefferson fracture – unstable**. Axial loading drives the occipital condyles into the C1 lateral masses causing a ring burst fracture. Neurological deficit may be caused by fragment retropulsion in to the spinal canal. The nature of the mechanism means there is a high incidence of associated cervical spine fractures and head injuries.
- **Burst fracture – potentially unstable**. Disruption of the posterior vertebral body cortex due to compression through axial loading.
    - Loss of posterior vertebral height.
    - Retropulsion of fragments into the spinal canal with potential cord/cauda equine compression.
    - Commonly affecting the lower thoracic and lumbar spine (Fig. 15.10a–c).

- **Wedge fracture – usually stable**. Hyperflexion injuries with axial loading. Usually affecting the thoracolumbar junction

374   D.A.T. Gay and J. Crighton

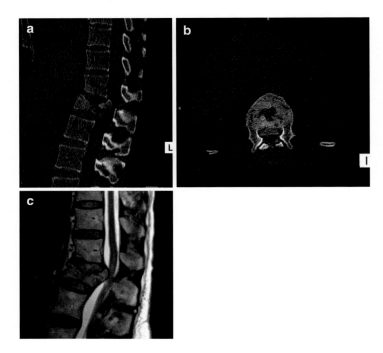

Figure 15.10 (**a–c**) Burst fracture. Sagittal thoracolumbar spine CT (**a**) demonstrating an L1 burst fracture with retropulsed fragment. There is an associated T12 anterior wedge fracture. Axial CT (**b**) illustrates the degree of spinal canal stenosis due to retropulsed fragment. As with most spinal injuries an MRI is required to evaluate the spinal cord and corda equine. T2 weighted MRI (**c**) shows more elegantly the cord compression at the fracture site and increased signal in the conus medullaris consistent with an acute injury

with disruption of the anterior column and preservation of the middle and posterior columns.

Complex Injuries

- **Odontoid process fracture – potentially unstable**. Mechanism includes both flexion and extension injuries.

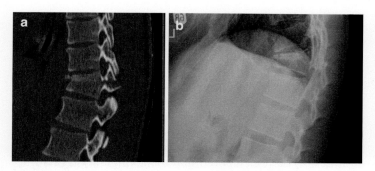

FIGURE 15.11 (**a**, **b**) Chance fracture. Sagittal thoracolumbar CT demonstrating three column disruption at the T12 level. Comparison is made with the lateral radiograph (**b**)

- **Chance fracture – potentially unstable.** Transverse fracture through all three columns of the thoracolumbar spine. The fracture line can pass through non-bony elements and so if un-displaced can be difficult to see. Flexion-distraction injury commonly caused by lap belts in RTCs.
  - High incidence of associated intra-abdominal injuries due to mechanism.
  - Widening of the facet joints.
  - Increased distance between the spinous processes on plain film lateral projection (Fig. 15.11a, b).

- **Atlanto-occipital dissociation (AOD) – unstable.** Includes dislocations and subluxations. CT is not sensitive for the soft tissue injuries that are sustained AOD. MRI will demonstrate damage to the anterior atlanto-occipital membrane (a continuation of the anterior longitudinal ligament) and posterior atlanto-occipital membrane (connecting the posterior foramen magnum to the superior aspect of the posterior atlantal arch). CT can demonstrate gross disruption of the normal alignment of the atlanto-occipital joints by using a number of lines on the reconstructed sagittal lateral (or lateral cervical spine plain film).

Is There a Spinal Cord Injury or Is the Cord Threatened?

Traumatic spinal cord injury is caused by either mechanical or vascular insult. The former is far more common and can be secondary to spinal column injury, penetrating injury or spinal canal haematoma. CT is excellent at demonstrating bony injury but poor at visualising the contents of the spinal canal. It must also be remembered that the configuration of a fracture post injury will not reflect the extreme limit of deformation achieved during the trauma. In the context of trauma with symptoms of cord or cauda equina compression syndrome out of proportion to any spinal column bony injury there should be a high index of suspicion of a spinal canal haematoma and urgent neurosurgical review sought. MRI is the appropriate imaging modality to visualise the canal and neural axis.

Part Three: Thoracic Imaging

Is the Chest Radiograph (CXR) Technically Adequate?

Chest radiograph interpretation can be daunting. There are a myriad of causes for opacification. A good starting point is to check if the film is rotated. Positioning of the patient in Critical Care can be very problematic for radiographers and rotated or lordotic films are quite common. The best method is to ensure the medial clavicles are equidistant from the spinous process.

Chest radiographs on Critical Care are invariably anteroposterior (AP) projections. This means that the heart size is artificially large due to the magnifying effect of the x ray. If the heart is not enlarged on an AP view then there is no cardiomegaly. If the heart is enlarged on an AP there is not necessarily cardiomegaly.

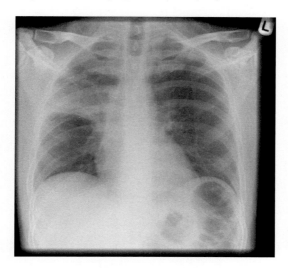

FIGURE 15.12 Right upper lobe consolidation. PA chest radiograph demonstrating right upper lobe consolidation

There Is Opacification on the Chest X Ray: What Does it Mean?

Often focal opacification on the radiograph is caused by consolidation. Any disease process that can fill the alveoli can cause this appearance. The more common causes are pus, blood, fluid, tumour cells and protein. The nature of the consolidation will be context dependent and may change over the course of a patient's admission (Fig. 15.12).

Hazier opacification, particularly at the bases, can result from pleural fluid. Whether the fluid is an exudate, transudate, haemothorax or chylothorax cannot be determined by plain film and the clinical picture is of paramount importance. If the diagnosis of pleural fluid is in doubt an ultrasound of the chest should differentiate consolidation and pleural fluid (Fig. 15.13).

Pulmonary oedema can normally be seen with plain film alone. The classic appearance is the perihilar bat wing consolidation but more subtle interstitial changes can be very

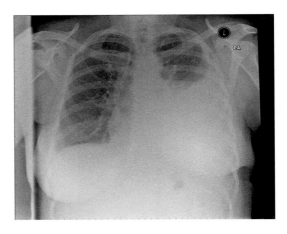

FIGURE 15.13 Pleural effusion

hard to identify. Often the key to diagnosing pulmonary oedema on plain film is the pattern of changes compared to previous films. A rapid onset of consolidation is often due to failure rather than infection. It is also worth noting that there is often a significant lag between radiograph appearances and clinically picture – especially when a patient is improving.

Pulmonary oedema does not always follow the classic appearance especially if the patient has been nursed on their side or prone for a significant period.

Is There a Pneumothorax?

Pneumothoraces can be difficult to see when they are small. They are most commonly seen at the apices. They are sometimes easier to detect when the grey white inversion setting is used on a workstation. Ultrasound detection of a pneumothorax is well described but can be difficult in practice (Fig. 15.14).

Where Are My Lines?

A crucial part of any Critical Care CXR is identifying the position of any lines and tubes. Reporting Critical Care

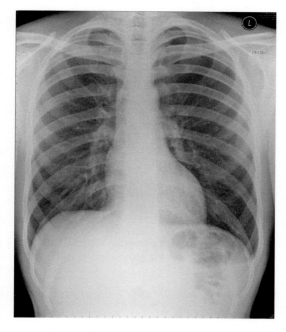

FIGURE 15.14 Chest radiograph demonstrating a pneumothorax

CXRs with a radiologist and Critical Care team together is very helpful in determining which line is where and for what.

- An endotracheal tube (ETT) – should be seen midway between the vocal cord and the carina. It is important to remember that the tip moves with neck flexion and rotation. A safe position for the tip to lie is between the medial ends of the clavicles (Fig. 15.15).
- Nasogastric Tube (NGT) – should traverse the mediastinum, cross the diaphragm in the midline and the tip should lie at least 10 cm beyond the gastro-oesophageal junction (Fig. 15.16).
- Central Venous Lines – the catheter should conform to the line of vessel (with no unexplained loops or deviations) and the tip should lie within the SVC not the right atrium or beyond (Fig. 15.17).

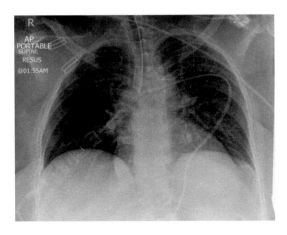

FIGURE 15.15 Chest radiograph demonstrating incorrect ETT placement – the tip of the ETT is within the right main bronchus

What Does Acute Respiratory Distress Syndrome (ARDS) Look Like?

There are multiple causes for ARDS but the common result is fluid and protein filling the alveoli. This is demonstrated as diffuse, bilateral, symmetrical opacification that involves the whole of the lungs. Radiographic appearances lag behind the clinical picture by up to 3 days. Pleural effusions are not a direct result of ARDS, in contrast with non cardiogenic pulmonary oedema, but they very often co-exist.

What Role Does Plain Radiography Have in Diagnosing a Pulmonary Embolus (PE)?

CT Pulmonary Angiogram (CTPA) is the gold standard for diagnosing PE however the CXR can be useful in ruling out other causes for the patient's symptoms. Marked lung field oligaemia can be present in large PEs (Fig. 15.18).

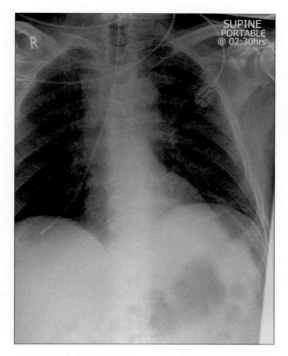

FIGURE 15.16 Chest radiograph demonstrating incorrect NGT placement – the NGT is positioned within the right main bronchus

What Information Can Be Gained from Thoracic CT in Critically Injured Patients?

CT is used in the trauma setting to diagnose acute injuries. Plain CXR is usually adequate for subsequent imaging to demonstrate progression or resolution of acute parenchymal and pleural space lung pathology. CT PA is the gold standard for diagnosing a PE. In order to reduce radiation burden, or dose, the apices and lung bases are excluded from the study.

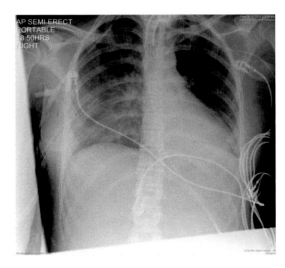

FIGURE 15.17 Chest radiograph demonstrating incorrect PICC placement – the line is too distal and is situated within the right atrium

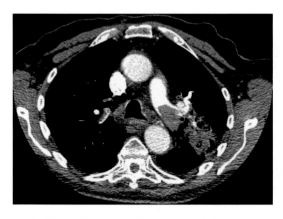

FIGURE 15.18 CTPA demonstrating a large left pulmonary artery thrombus

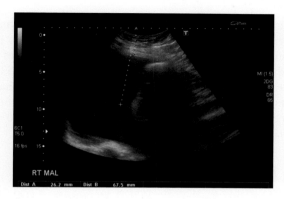

FIGURE 15.19 USS demonstrating a simple pleural effusion

How Can I Differentiate a Pleural Effusion from Consolidated Lung?

The quality of CXR in Critical Care patients often makes this difficult. In a patient requiring increasing ventilatory support this distinction can be important. US of the thorax can help to identify the presence of an effusion, it's complexity and also mark an appropriate site for a drain insertion. The drain should be inserted at the marked point with the patient in exactly the same position as when the mark was made (Fig. 15.19).

Part Four: Abdominal Imaging

The solid abdominal organs are more frequently injured than hollow viscus. Ultrasound has a limited role in diagnosing abdominal injuries as CT is far more sensitive and specific. Extended Focused Assessment with Sonography for Trauma (EFAST) is a limited examination directed solely at identifying the presence or absence of free intraperitoneal, pericardial or pleural fluid and is an adjunct to the Advanced Trauma Life Support primary survey. In the context of traumatic injury free fluid is assumed to be haemorrhage. Acquisition of a CT study should not be delayed in order to perform a FAST scan however free fluid on EFAST scan in the context of a haemodynamically unstable patient may be sufficient evidence for the surgical team to bypass CT and proceed straight to emergency laparotomy/thoracotomy.

What Do Solid Organ Injuries Look Like on CT?

Each organ should be reviewed for signs of laceration, haematoma or avulsion. The American Association for the Surgery of Trauma (AAST) grading systems for each organ describes the severity of injury and is described further in Chap. 13. Solid organ injury can be relatively subtle. A high index of suspicion should be entertained in the context of high-energy trauma, penetrating abdominal wounds and inferior rib fractures.

- **Contusion** – Non-confluent parenchymal haemorrhage. May be reflected in deranged organ function.
- **Haematoma** – The density of a haematoma changes with the evolution of the clot and degradation of blood products. Acute haemorrhage is relatively hyperdense and becomes hypodense over the course of days to weeks.
- **Laceration** – Lacerations appear as irregular linear/branching areas of hypoattenuation. Often associated with haematoma.
- **Avulsion/de-vascularisation** – catastrophic disruption of vascular supply of the organ. Often associated with haematoma or intra-abdominal haemorrhage.
- **Vascular injury** – damage to the vascular bed of an organ can lead to the formation of an arteriovenous fistula, pseudoaneurysm or venous thrombosis.

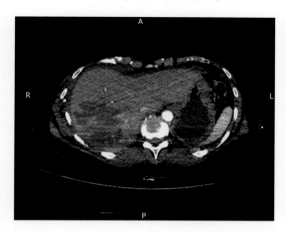

FIGURE 15.20 Contrast enhanced CT demonstrating liver laceration

Liver

80 % of liver injuries are minor and a similar proportion are associated with other abdominal injuries (Fig. 15.20).

Kidney

Renal injuries account for 10 % of abdominal trauma and 90 % are minor due to their relatively protected position. Haematuria should prompt suspicion of a renal injury. To fully characterise renal injuries a four phase study is required – non-contrast phase, an arterial phase to evaluate vascular injury, a nephrographic phase to evaluate renal parenchymal lesions and a delayed phase to evaluate bleeding and collecting system injuries. The trauma CT protocol achieves the arterial and nephrographic phases.

Spleen

The spleen is the most frequently injured organ in blunt trauma. The spleen should be homogenous in the portal

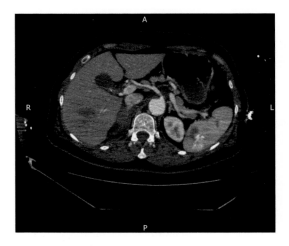

FIGURE 15.21 Contrast enhanced CT demonstrating a splenic laceration with parenchymal active extravasation of contrast

venous phase. Splenic parenchyma is heterogeneous in the
arterial phase and can fool the uninitiated (Fig. 15.21).

Can CT Detect Hollow Viscus Injury?

The bowel and mesentery are more likely to be injured in
penetrating trauma than blunt force trauma. Whilst the
defect in the bowel wall may not be seen there are stigmata
of hollow viscus injury that should raise this concern.

- **Bowel** – Positive oral contrast will not be given for a
  trauma CT. Findings include:
    - Free fluid within the abdomen and/or pelvis with no
      evidence of solid organ injury
    - Bowel contents within the abdominal cavity.
    - Extra-luminal free gas in blunt force trauma. Gas in
      penetrating trauma does not necessarily mean bowel
      perforation (Fig. 15.22).
    - Intramural haematoma

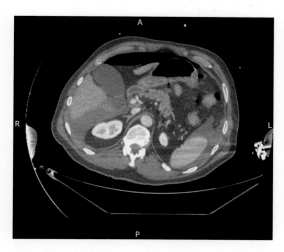

FIGURE 15.22 Contrast enhanced CT demonstrating free gas and fluid within the abdomen due to a perforating injury

- – Discontinuity in the bowel wall
- – Abnormal bowel wall enhancement

- **Mesenteric injury** – Often only soft signs that can include:
    - – Active extravasation of contrast media
    - – Intra-mesenteric free fluid or haematoma
    - – Beading and termination of mesenteric vessels
    - – Mesenteric fat stranding

CT Hypo-perfusion Complex

Most commonly described in the context of post-traumatic hypovolaemic shock but can occur in sepsis and cardiac arrest. Has superseded the term 'shock bowel'. The small bowel findings are the most commonly observed feature in CT hypotension complex. CT findings include;

- Bilateral adrenal gland hyper-enhancement
- Hypo-enhancement of the spleen and liver

388   D.A.T. Gay and J. Crighton

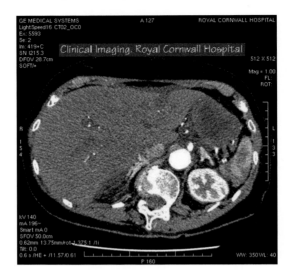

FIGURE 15.23 Contrast enhanced CT demonstrating a collapsed IVC and 'bright' adrenal glands consistent with hypoperfusion complex

- Heterogeneous enhancement of the pancreas
- Thickened bowel loops (>3 mm) with enhancing walls.
- Collapsed inferior vena cava
- Small caliber abdominal aorta (Fig. 15.23)

Part Five: Pelvic Imaging

Displaced pelvic ring injuries are a marker for high-energy trauma. They most commonly result from RTC (60%), falls from height (30%) and crush injuries (10%) [3]. Associated injuries can include;

- Venous plexus haemorrhage
- Retroperitoneal, abdominal or thigh haematoma.
- Bladder rupture
- Urethral laceration

A Trauma CT may raise the suspicion of bladder or urethral injury but dedicated retrograde contrast study is the gold standard to diagnosing urogenital injury. This is something that should be discussed with the radiologist conducting the trauma CT.

The osseous and ligamentous components of the pelvis allow it to function as a stable ring. When sufficient force is applied the pelvic ring will deform through either a fracture of the innominate bones or sacrum or through a disruption or dislocation of the pubis or SI joints. Most pelvic ring injuries include fractures or dislocations of both the anterior and posterior structures [4]. A pelvic ring injury may not involve a bony fracture.

Injuries are caused by two dominant patterns of displacement: opening and closing of the pelvis (a result of compressive rotational forces) and cephalad displacement (a result of vertical sheer forces) [5].

In a patient with a significant mechanism of injury and abnormality on plain film or CT there should be a high index of suspicion of an unstable pelvic fracture. Pelvic binders should remain in situ during the Trauma CT and if there is clinical or radiological concern of an unstable pelvic ring fracture management should be conducted with input from an appropriate pelvic surgical specialist.

What Are the Different Types of Unstable Pelvic Fracture?

Unstable fractures can be divided according to the mechanism of injury;

- **Anteroposterior compression** – Disruption of the pubic symphysis or pubic rami and the sacroiliac joints causes an 'open book' fracture (Fig. 15.24 – open book fracture).
- **Lateral compression** – Internal rotation of one iliac wing causes a unilateral sacral compression fracture with external rotation of the contralateral hemipelvis resulting in diastasis of the sacro-iliac joint resulting in a classic

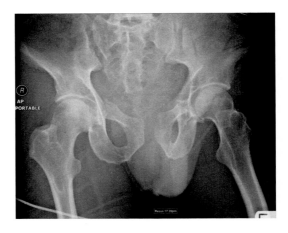

FIGURE 15.24 Open book type pelvic fracture

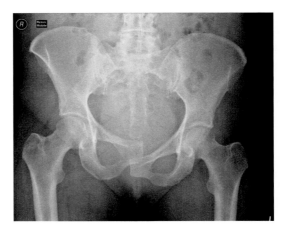

FIGURE 15.25 Lateral compression pelvic fracture

"wind-swept pelvis" appearance (Fig. 15.25- lateral compression fracture).

- **Vertical shear** – Two vertically orientated ipsilateral pelvic ring fractures i.e. disruption of the ipsilateral superior and inferior pubic rami and sacroiliac joint. Common variants involve the ilium or sacral wing rather than the sacroiliac

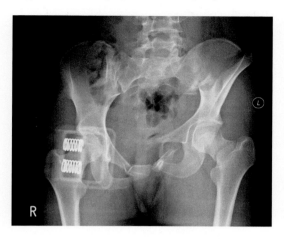

FIGURE 15.26 Vertical shear pelvic fracture

joint. This results in an unstable lateral fragment, which contains the acetabulum. Often referred to as a Malgaigne fracture (Fig. 15.26 – Vertical shear fracture).

- **Combined mechanical** – Occur when more than one force vectors are involved and results in a complex fracture pattern.

References

1. Surendran A, et al. Systematic review of the benefits and harms of whole-body computed tomography in the early management of multitrauma patients: are we getting the whole picture? J Trauma Acute Care Surg. 2014;76(4):1122–30.
2. Head injury – Triage, assessment, investigation and early management of head injury in children, young people and adults. Issued: January 2014 NICE clinical guideline 176. Available at https://www.nice.org.uk/guidance/cg176.
3. Schmal H, et al. Epidemiology and outcome of complex pelvic injury. Acta Orthop Belg. 2005;71(1):41–7.
4. Kurylo JC, Tornetta 3rd P. Initial management and classification of pelvic fractures. Instr Course Lect. 2012;61:3–18.
5. Pennal GF, Tile M, Waddell JP, Garside H. Pelvic disruption: assessment and classification. Clin Orthop Relat Res. 1980;151:12–21.

Chapter 16
Management of Sedation, Analgesia and Delirium in Critically Injured Patients

Stephen Lewis and Kate Prior

Abstract This chapter describes an integrated approach to the management of analgesia, sedation and delirium in critically injured patients. Pain is often difficult to assess especially in ventilated, unconscious patients and a dedicated assessment tool should be used. A multi-modal approach to analgesia that emphasises the early use of opiates alongside adjunctive agents is advocated. Regional analgesic techniques can be safely employed in selected major trauma patients and have been widely used by military healthcare providers. Excessive use of sedation is not indicated outside of specific circumstances, such as traumatic brain injury, as it can lead to worse outcomes. A protocolised approach to sedation has been shown to reduce the length of ICU and hospital stay. The type of sedative agent is of less importance, but an approach that uses Propofol in conjunction with an alpha 2 agonist is advocated. Delirium is common in critically

S. Lewis (✉) • K. Prior, FRCA
Department of Critical Care, King's College Hospital,
Denmark Hill, London SE5 9RS, UK
e-mail: stephen.lewis@nhs.net

S.D. Hutchings (ed.), *Trauma and Combat Critical Care in Clinical Practice*, In Clinical Practice,
DOI 10.1007/978-3-319-28758-4_16,

ill patients and is an independent marker of poor prognosis; it should be screened for and any risk factors addressed as part of an integrated approach to management.

Keywords Sedation • Sedation holds • Sedation protocols • Analgesia • Delirium • Pain • Agitation • Regional analgesia • Nerve blocks

Introduction

Historically, ventilated patients on the ICU were kept heavily sedated with a combination of drugs that favoured sedation over analgesia; little attention was given to the recognition and prevention of delirium. In recent years this has changed, with an awareness of the burden of pain in critically ill patients and the consequences of delirium on outcomes. The American College of Critical Care Medicine has produced a set of clinical practice guidelines that encourages clinicians to view pain, agitation and delirium in critically ill patients as a combined entity and to manage it with both pharmacological and non-pharmacological strategies [1].

The management of sedation and analgesia in critically injured trauma patients can present a particular challenge. On admission to the ICU, such patients are likely to be intubated and mechanically ventilated. This patient group will often require one or more returns to the operating theatre for surgical interventions and will possibly need onward transfer to a specialist trauma centre. In the short term the maintenance of deep sedation and mechanical ventilation will often seem the most humane, as well as convenient, approach.

However, sedation is a potentially hazardous intervention. There is evidence that long-term sedation increases the length of ventilation as well as ICU and hospital stay time [2]. It is also speculated that future mental health is adversely affected by a long period of deep sedation and amnesia following serious injury. The goal in most mechanically ventilated patients is therefore to create a state of comfort with minimal sedation.

The need to adequately treat pain rightly gives analgesia priority over sedation in most patients, but achieving this can be particularly problematic in the trauma patient group; injuries may lead to severe pain syndromes, in addition to non-traumatic sources of pain from routine ICU care. Accordingly, it has been necessary to develop scoring systems to assess pain severity in critically ill patients who are unable to directly communicate with medical staff. Novel analgesic techniques must often be combined with conventional analgesic regimes in a multi-modal approach to achieve the best effect.

Part One: Analgesia

What Are the Issues When Considering Analgesic Requirements in the Critically Injured Patient?

It is obvious that major trauma can lead to complex pain states. Initial injuries, subsequent surgical procedures and secondary wound infection can all contribute to the pain burden, with nerve damage adding aneuropathic component. Patients in the ICU may also experience pain from routine aspects of critical care, as shown in Table 16.1, and it is notable that the prevalence of pain is the same in medical and surgical ICUs (estimated at 50 % or higher) [3].

Anxiety, dyspnoea, delirium and sleep deprivation can also contribute to distress and may be additive or synergistic with

TABLE 16.1 Causes of non-traumatic pain in critically injured patients

Mechanical ventilation

Indwelling lines/catheters

Turning/positioning

Suctioning of the airway

pain. Successful management of pain on the ICU therefore also requires recognition of predisposing and causative factors and use of non-pharmacologic measures. In some cases there may be an acute pain team available to support in the management of complex trauma patients.

Pain has been shown to be the root cause of distress in many ICU patients and therefore requires close attention from the intensivist [4]. Aside from the direct suffering that pain causes, it can drive a stress response with autonomic and endocrine effects that result in tachycardia, hypertension, hyperglycaemia and decreased renal and splanchnic blood flow. Pain is thought to suppress natural killer cell and neutrophil phagocytic activity, potentially impairing the immune system [5]. In addition, critically ill patients who recall pain whilst on the ICU appear to have a higher incidence of chronic pain and post-traumatic stress disorder symptoms [6].

Opioids are the mainstay of analgesia in the ICU, there are a variety of agents available and these are considered in the next section. Recent experience with battlefield injuries has led the UK Defence Medical Services (UK DMS) to adopt a proactive approach to trauma pain management that effectively reverses the World Health Organisation analgesic ladder. This involves beginning with a strong opioid together with a non-opioid and adjuvant, and moving down the ladder as pain reduces over time.

How Should Pain Be Measured in Critically Injured Patients?

In order to effectively control pain it is first necessary to detect and attempt to quantify it. Where a patient is able to self report pain this should always be noted and acted upon. For patients who are unable to self report, and in whom motor function is intact, several pain measures have been developed. The most reliable and well known are the Critical Care Pain Observation Tool and the Behavioural Pain Scale (BPS). The BPS, in particular, has been validated to monitor

Behavioural Pain Scale (BPS) tool

Facial expression	Relaxed	1
	Partially tightened (e.g. eyebrow lowering)	2
	Fully tightened (e.g. eyelid closing)	3
	Grimacing	4
Upper limbs	No movement	1
	Partially bent	2
	Fully bent with finger flexion	3
	Permanently retracted	4
Compliance with ventilation	Tolerating movement	1
	Coughing with movement	2
	Fighting ventilator	3
	Unable to control ventilation	4

FIGURE 16.1 The Behavioural Pain Scale (BPS) tool

the level of pain experienced by sedated and mechanically ventilated trauma patients [7]. Frequent assessment of pain severity can be used to titrate the dose of analgesic to effect; titration is important, as there may be considerable variability in analgesic requirements between patients; Fig. 16.1 shows the BPS tool. A multitude of factors can affect a patient's sensitivity to analgesia including age, premorbid condition, prior use and genetic variability.

Which Opioid Agents Can Be Used in the Critically Injured Patient?

In addition to their analgesic properties, opioids have the added benefit of reducing respiratory drive, aiding ventilator synchronisation [8]. Their anti-sympathetic effects of reducing tachycardia and hypertension can also be useful in the trauma setting. However, given in excess, they will induce apnoea, impeding the use of patient triggered ventilation. They may also cause gastrointestinal stasis, impairing the absorption of enteral feed and causing constipation. For this reason a laxative is commonly prescribed for all sedated and

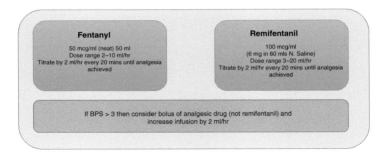

FIGURE 16.2 UK DMS ICU analgesic infusion protocol

mechanically ventilated patients, unless contraindicated. All intravenous opioid agents are equally effective when titrated to similar pain intensity endpoints. The three most commonly used agents in critically ill trauma patients are the conventional opioids Morphine and Fentanyl, and Remifentanil. The UK DMS uses Fentanyl or Remifentanil infusions for analgesia in critically injured ventilated patients as shown in Fig. 16.2.

Conventional Opioids

Morphine and Fentanyl will be familiar drugs to most clinicians working in an ICU. Morphine and its potent metabolite (Morphine-6-glucuronide) are both eliminated by the kidney and may accumulate. Fentanyl is therefore often preferred to Morphine where there is the potential for renal insufficiency. Fentanyl is particularly fat soluble and thus has a rapid onset of action. However, this property also results in an increased volume of distribution and it may also accumulate after prolonged infusion. The consequences of opioid accumulation are prolonged drug effects, risking an increase in ventilator time and length of ICU stay. Naloxone can be used to reverse opioid action in the event of excessive dosing, although the analgesia afforded by them will then be lost.

Remifentanil

Remifentanil is a short acting opioid that is metabolised by non-specific blood and tissue esterases independent of the duration of infusion or organ insufficiency. The context-sensitive half time is consistently short (3.2 min) even following a long duration of infusion (>8 h).

There is some evidence that Remifentanil may reduce the duration of mechanical ventilation. An RCT by Dahaba et al, comparing Remifentanil with Morphine in mechanically ventilated ICU patients, found that the Remifentanil group had a significantly shorter duration of mechanical ventilation and extubation time [9]. It should be noted that Remifentanil is only licensed for up to three days use in the ICU. However, even in a patient group with a short (2–3 day) anticipated ventilation time, it has been found to significantly decrease duration of mechanical ventilation and length of ICU stay. The cost of Remifentanil is high in comparison with generic Morphine and Fentanyl, which may be a factor that has limited its use on the ICU. If Remifentanil is to be used as part of a sedation regime for mechanically ventilated patients it is important that the nursing staff are familiar with it, as its pharmacokinetic behaviour is very different to that of other commonly used opioids.

Which Non-opioid Analgesics and Pain Modulation Strategies Are Available to Use in Critically Injured Patients?

Opioids are the cornerstone of analgesia in the critically ill patient but adjunctive analgesic medication and methods should be considered too. Drugs to achieve this can be divided into the non-steroidal anti-inflammatory drugs (NSAIDs), Paracetamol, Ketamine and the anti-neuropathic drugs. Local anaesthetic agents and non-pharmacological interventions may also play a useful role; these are outlined in more detail later in this chapter.

Non-steroidal Anti-inflammatory Drugs

NSAIDs (and Paracetamol) are often given alone for mild pain, but in the context of critically injured patients they are chiefly beneficial for their opioid sparing effect. There are several NSAIDs available; commonly used formulations include Ibuprofen, Diclofenac and Ketorolac. They are non sedating, have an antipyretic effect and can achieve impressive opioid dose reductions of greater than 25 % [10]. Despite this, NSAIDs are relatively contra-indicated in critically ill patients due to their potential adverse effects, in particular renal impairment and gastric ulceration. These risks seem more pronounced in elderly patients. A further risk factor to consider is a demonstrated increase in major cardiovascular events for non-selective NSAIDs. As such particular consideration should be given before prescribing them for patients with known cardiovascular disease. In general, NSAIDs should be discontinued after a short period (2–5 days) to reduce the risk of complications.

Paracetamol

Paracetamol is a non-opioid analgesic that is available in intravenous as well as enteral preparations. It too has proven opioid sparing effects as well as being an antipyretic [11]. Given intravenously in a dose of 1 g every 6 h, its well-documented hepatotoxic effects should be avoided, although some practitioners would advocate 8 hourly dosing (i.e. 3 g per day) where concerns regarding liver function exist.

Ketamine

Ketamine is a phencyclidine derivative drug that can be used as an anaesthetic induction agent. It also has impressive

analgesic effects and can be given by the enteral or parenteral routes. For ICU patients it may be administered by
intravenous infusion at a rate of 5–10 mg/h, in cases where
pain is difficult to control. Given in this way, Ketamine will
also act as an adjunct to sedation. Alternatively, it may be
included with an opioid as part of a patient-controlled analgesia (PCA) formulation. For PCA use a dose of 2 mg each
of Ketamine and Morphine with a 10-min lockout would be
a suitable initial regime for an adult. Ketamine has been
shown to reduce opioid requirement in postoperative
patients even at low doses. Concerns that it causes raised
intracranial pressure are probably unwarranted, so long as
patients are properly sedated and receiving controlled
mechanical ventilation [12].

Agents for Modulating Neuropathic Pain

Patients who have sustained critical injuries will often suffer
a degree of neuropathic pain, particularly if limb injury or
amputation has occurred. The UK DMS use a regime of
75 mg Pregabalin twice a day (increasing to 150 mg after 1
week), and Amitriptyline 20 mg at night, started immediately
on ICU admission.

Non-pharmacological Techniques

There has been increasing interest in non-pharmacological
techniques for pain management, including relaxation exercises and music therapy. Whilst there is currently little firm
evidence for their effectiveness in this particular patient
group, they are safe and relatively cheap interventions that
can be considered. Patients undergoing chest drain removal
who received relaxation therapy together with morphine
compered to morphine alone achieved significantly lower
pain scores in one study [13].

What Are the Advantages of a Regional Anaesthetic Approach to Pain Management in Critically Injured Patients?

Neuraxial, plexus and nerve blocks can play an important part in the management and the control of pain in the critically injured patient. Regional Anaesthesia (RA) can be used at any stage in the patient's care, in the pre-hospital environment, the emergency department, as intra-operative adjuncts and in the post operative period.

Regional blocks offer many attributes of an "ideal" analgesic: superior analgesia, attenuation of the stress response, increased alertness, avoidance of systemic side effects and protection against chronic pain. The increasing use of perineural catheters to provide continuous peripheral nerve blockade allows for excellent analgesia in the post operative period as well as providing anesthesia for further visits to the operating theatre.

What Are the Potential Complications/Contra Indications to Regional Anaesthetic Techniques in Critically Injured Patients?

The use of regional techniques in trauma patients has, at times, been contentious. Particular concerns have included the potential of nerve blockade to mask the development of compartment syndrome and the risk of haematoma formation in patients with trauma coagulopathy. As a result, trauma patients must be assessed for the presence of coagulopathy before a regional or neuraxial block is performed. Some blocks are deemed higher risk in this regard. For example, an epidural with an indwelling catheter would be deemed to have a relatively higher risk than a superficial plexus block which in turn would be higher risk than a superficial nerve block or infiltration of local anaesthetic.

A systematic review by Mar and colleagues showed no evidence that postoperative regional anaesthesia resulted in a delayed diagnosis of acute compartment syndrome and may in fact help facilitate the diagnosis when the patient experiences breakthrough ischaemic pain [14]. The growing evidence base from military and civilian sources is supportive of a greater role for RA in the management of patients with traumatic injury [15]. The increased use of ultrasound to identify the nerve or plexus to be blocked and the development of needles that are easier to see with ultrasound has led to more widespread adoption of these techniques in anaesthetised or sedated patients.

Careful risk/benefit analysis must be used when thinking about a regional anaesthetic technique and a list of contraindications is shown in Table 16.2. Complications of regional anaesthesia are shown in Table 16.3

What RA Techniques Can Be Used for Patients with Upper Extremity Injuries?

Upper limb injuries are particularly suited to regional techniques. Brachial Plexus Block (BPB) achieves superior analgesia, reduced opioid consumption, and earlier hospital discharge compared with general anaesthesia for ambulant upper limb trauma surgery [16]. Interscalene, supra or infraclavicular, axillary and individual nerve blocks can be performed. The choice of block will depend on the location

TABLE 16.2 Contraindications to regional analgesia

Relative contraindications	Absolute contraindications
Uncooperative patient	Patient refusal
Pre-existing neurological deficit	Local anaesthetic allergy
Mild coagulopathy	Severe coagulopathy
Infection distant to site of injection	Infection at site of injection
Distorted anatomy	Lack of equipment/training

TABLE 16.3 Complications of regional analgesia

Complication	Estimated frequency	Comments
Direct nerve injury	1:10,000–1:30,000	No effective treatment Most improve within 1–6 months
Epidural haematoma	1:150,000–1:200,000	Requires urgent surgical evacuation May cause paraplegia
Epidural abscess	1:100,000–1:150,000	Surgical evacuation and antibiotics May cause paraplegia
Drug error	Unknown	Avoidable. May be fatal
Systemic toxicity	Unknown	May be fatal unless treated
Respiratory depression	Unknown	Caution with neuraxial opioids
Hypotension	Common with neuraxial block	Treat
Confusional states	Common in the elderly	Caution with neuraxial opioids
Pruritis/urinary retention	Up to 16 %	Treat
Technical failure	5–25 % depending on technique	

of the patient's injuries, as shown in Table 16.4, and the risk/benefit ratio of the chosen block.

What RA Techniques Can Be Used for Patients with Lower Extremity Injuries?

Both neuraxial and RA techniques can be used. A lumbar epidural is very suitable if there is bilateral lower extremity

TABLE 16.4 Options for regional analgesia in the upper extremities

Site of injury	Suitable block
Shoulder	Interscalene
Upper arm	Supraclavicular or infraclavicular (upper part of humerus will be covered) Axillary (lower part of humerus will be covered)
Forearm	Axillary
Wrist and Hand	Axillary or individual nerves

TABLE 16.5 Options for regional analgesia in the lower extremities

Site of injury	Suitable block
Pelvis or acetabular fracture	Lumbar epidural Quadratus lumborum block Posterior TAP block
Proximal femur fracture	Spinal or lumbar epidural Fascia iliaca block
Femur fracture	Femoral nerve block
Lower leg injuries	Sciatic nerve block
Foot injury	Ankle block

trauma provided there are no contraindications. A decision on whether to use an opioid mixed with the anaesthetic will be made according to each patient's clinical state. In the analgesic management of trauma, a continuous infusion of local anaesthetic, rather than boluses, is most commonly used. Femoral and fascia iliaca compartment blocks for femur fractures are effective and safe and are particularly useful in the older and more frail patient. For lower leg injuries, sciatic nerve approaches facilitate analgesia and surgery. Ankle blocks allow surgery to the foot without affecting proximal sensorimotor function.

Suitable blocks for specific injury patterns are shown in Table 16.5

What RA Techniques Can Be Used for Patients with Chest Injuries?

Blunt thoracic injuries such as rib fractures and pulmonary contusions are common in major trauma and are associated with significant morbidity and mortality. Pain impairs respiratory mechanics and predisposes to atelectasis, secretion retention, and pneumonia. RA techniques include thoracic epidural analgesia, paravertebral block, intercostal block and intra-pleural catheters.

In trauma, a thoracic epidural is utilised for managing multiple and bilateral fractures, particularly in elderly patients and is considered the gold standard for analgesia after thoracotomy. There is improved analgesia and respiratory function with reduced nosocomial pneumonia rates when compared with alternative analgesic modalities [17]. However, there is no demonstrable decrease in overall mortality or ICU length of stay [18].

In trauma, multiple exclusion criteria, including spinal cord or bone injury, hypovolaemia, infection, thromboprophylaxis and coagulopathy often preclude an epidural. If a patient has a normal clotting profile on laboratory tests or normal coagulation on near patient testing (thromboelastography or thromboelastometry) and a platelet count of $>75 \times 10^9$/l, an epidural can be safely performed.

Paravertebral blocks provide unilateral segmental somatic and sympathetic block comparable with a thoracic epidural, but have fewer limitations relating to cardiovascular instability and anticoagulation. Plain local anaesthetic solutions (e.g. bupivacaine 0.25–0.5 %) or equivalent are generally used at a rate of 10–15 ml/h.

A comparison of epidural analgesia and paravertebral blocks is shown in Table 16.6.

Intercostal nerve blocks involve injection of local anaesthetic near to the posterior segment of thoracic spinal nerves. Their use is limited due to the need for multiple level, repeated injections involving palpation of painful ribs. There

TABLE 16.6 Comparison of epidural and paravertebral analgesia

Epidural	Paravertebral block
Higher failure rate	Higher success rate
Bilateral effects, more sympathetic and motor blockade	Unilateral effects, less sympathetic and motor blockade
Increased risk of hypotension	Lower risk of hypotension
Opioid often used with local anaesthetic	Plain local anaesthetic used
Risk of nerve injury	Lower risk of nerve injury
Risk of dural puncture	Lower risk of dural puncture

is also a risk of pneumothorax and injections at multiple levels carry an increased risk of local anaesthetic toxicity.

Intrapleural analgesia requires application of local anaesthetic (LA) between the visceral and parietal pleura, usually via an indwelling catheter. The analgesic effect is very variable due to unpredictable distribution of LA, which is influenced by factors including catheter site, patient position, location of injury and the presence of pleural fluid.

What RA Techniques Can Be Used for Patients with Abdominal Injuries?

Abdominal blocks include epidural, spinal, paravertebral, transversus abdominis plane (TAP), quadratus lumborum compartment and rectus sheath blocks.

TAP and rectus sheath blocks provide sensory, but not visceral, analgesia to the anterior abdominal wall. The anterior divisions of spinal nerves T7–L1 can be blocked along their course between the internal oblique and transversus abdominis muscles or as they perforate the rectus abdominis muscle (rectus sheath). The appeal of these compartmental blocks is their feasibility in patients where neuraxial analgesia is contraindicated e.g. coagulopathy or sepsis.

What Regional Anaesthetic Techniques Can Be Used for Patients with Pelvic Injuries?

Pelvic injuries leading to painful acetabular or pelvic ring fractures may benefit from a lumbar epidural for analgesia or anaesthesia. Placing the block can sometimes be challenging because it is difficult for patients with this type of injury to get in to the optimal position for siting the epidural. As a result, the lumbar epidural may be placed while the patient is under general anesthesia if the risk/benefit ratio is in favour of a neuraxial technique.

Thoracolumbar analgesia from posterior TAP or quadratuslumborum blocks may also be useful for pelvic fractures.

Part Two: Sedation

What Is the Role of Sedation in the Management of the Critically Injured Patient?

Sedative drugs are commonly used on the ICU to treat agitation and promote tolerance of an endotracheal tube. However, it is not always necessary to use a sedative provided that the patient has adequate analgesia and other reversible causes of agitation have been identified and addressed. Common causes of agitation include hypoxia, hypotension, hypoglycaemia, sepsis and drug withdrawal.

How Should Sedation Be Monitored in the Critically Injured Patient?

Just as with pain measurement, a quantifiable scale isuseful to enable meaningful titration of sedative medication. There are several scoring systems available to assess sedation in the critically ill, mechanically ventilated patient. They include the simple Ramsay Scale and the more complex Vancouver Interaction and Calmness Scale, Harris Scale and Sedation-Agitation Scale. The Richmond Agitation Sedation Scale (RASS) has emerged as a simple, reliable and valid method of monitoring sedation in ventilated adult intensive care patients [19]. Scored between +4 (combative/violent) and –5 (unrousable) it is quickly measured by bedside observation and verbal/physical stimulation.

Consensus guidelines produced by the German Medical Society recommend a minimum of 8 hourly sedation goal setting and measurement [20]. On a UK military critical care unit, 2 hourly measurements are the norm [21]. Figure 16.3 shows the RASS together with the protocol used by the UK DMS to titrate sedative therapy.

What Level of Sedation Should Be Targeted?

In general, the most desirable score is 0 (alert and calm) although a more realistic optimal target in the mechanically ventilated patient would be –1 (sustained awakening to voice). Multiple studies have demonstrated the benefits of maintaining lighter sedation levels, including shortened duration of mechanical ventilation and ICU admission, reduced delirium and reduced long-term cognitive impairment [2, 22, 23].

There are exceptions to this approach. Patients with traumatic brain injury will generally require deep sedation to manage raised intracranial pressure in the initial period following injury. Patients who are hypoxic and difficult to ventilate, and clearly those paralysed with neuromuscular blockers, should not undergo a sedation hold. Deeper sedation levels may also be considered in patients with open body cavities. Another group to consider are patients with potentially dangerous airways, for example following facial traumaor burns. In such patients an airway will be difficult to secure in an emergency and deeper levels of sedation may be initially targeted to mitigate against the risk of accidental extubation.

Richmond Agitation Sedation Scale (RASS)

Score	Term	Description
+4	Combative	Overtly combative, violent, immediate danger to staff
+3	Very agitated	Pulls or removes tube(s) or catheters(s); aggressive
+2	Agitated	Frequent non-purposeful movement, fights ventilator
+1	Restless Anxious	but movements not aggressive vigorous
0	Alert and calm	
-1	Drowsy	Not fully alert, but has sustained awakening (eye-opening/eye contact) to voice (>10 seconds)
-2	Light sedation	Briefly awakens with eye contact to voice (<10 seconds)
-3	Mod. Sedation	Movement or eye opening to voice (but no eye contact)
-4	Deep sedation	No response to voice, but movement or eye opening to physical stimulation
-5	Unarousable	No response to voice or physical stimulation

Response to RASS score

Score	Action
+4 / +3	Bolus sedative & increase infusion rate by 40 % / consider physical restraints / consider Quetiapine 25 mg twice daily
+2	Bolus sedative & increase infusion rate by 20 %
+1	Increase infusion rate by 10 %
0/-1	Optimal Sedation Score
-2/-3	Reduce sedative infusion by 20 %. Consider reducing analgesic infusion if BPS 3
-4	Reduce sedative infusion by 40 %. Consider reducing analgesic infusion if BPS 3
-5	Stop sedative infusions. Reduce analgesic infusions by 20 %

FIGURE 16.3 Richmond Agitation and Sedation Scale (RASS) tool and UK DMS protocol for titrating sedation

Finally, real-world practice means that staffing levels and skill mix on the ICU are not always optimal and it is down to the judgement of the supervising intensivist to decide what levels of sedation are safest for their patients on a given day.

Sedation and analgesia should be increased pre-emptively in anticipation of a painful or invasive procedure. Such events are the most commonly cited source of stress in ICU patients and interventions sometimes require deep 'anaesthetic' level sedation as for a surgical procedure.

Are Sedation Holds Useful?

A sedation hold involves stopping all sedative drugs, including analgesics, until there is eye opening to verbal stimuli or the patient becomes agitated. Until recently daily sedation holds were widely considered to be good practice unless contraindicated. Kress et al first showed that daily interruption of sedation in mechanically ventilated medical ICU patients led to a significantly reduced duration of mechanical ventilation and ICU stay [22]. Patients did not appear to suffer psychologically from daily sedation holds. The 'Awake and Breathing Controlled trial' (ABC) by Girard et al, which compared a daily sedation hold and spontaneous breathing trial (SBT) against SBT alone, supported this finding [23].

The SLEAP trial by Mehta and colleagues subsequently compared protocolised sedation with daily sedation holds against protocolised sedation alone [24]. Its findings appeared to be in direct conflict with those reported in previous studies. No difference was found in the time to extubation, or any other endpoint, and those patients in the interruption arm received an overall higher dose of sedation. It should be pointed out that this trial allowed an opioid/benzodiazepine combination but *not* Propofol or Dexmedetomidine. The 423 patient group was also mostly non-surgical. Nevertheless, this study has thrown some doubt over the need for a sedation hold, particularly in those units that use a sedation protocol. What seems most important is that the patient is not allowed to continuously receive sedative medication without reference to their conscious level.

Little attention is given in the literature to the de-escalation and discontinuation of sedative therapy. Withdrawal syndromes from opioids and sedatives may occur during the recovery phase of critical care illness and consideration may need to be given to alternative enteral therapy to cover withdrawal.

Which Agents Should Be Used to Achieve Sedation?

Commonly used hypnotic agents for sedation include Propofol and benzodiazepines, both of which are thought to act on the gamma-aminobutyric acid (GABA) receptor. The widely accepted theory regarding the mode of action of hypnotic drugs is that they modulate the inhibitory GABA neurotransmitter system. More recently the α_2-adrenoreceptor agonists Clonidine and Dexmedetomidine have been introduced as alternative or adjuvant sedative agents. There is little trial evidence to show clear superiority of one sedative agent over the other. Figure 16.4 shows the sedative agents used by the UK DMS for mechanically ventilated patients.

Propofol

Propofol is hydrophobic and is formulated in an oil-in-water emulsion. Its lipophilic properties allow it to cross the blood–brain-barrier rapidly. It is metabolised in the liver by conjugation, the metabolites of which are eliminated by the kidneys. Whilst hepatic and renal diseases have little impact on the pharmacokinetics of Propofol, offset of sedation varies considerably in the critical care patient population. It appears to be a function of sedation depth, duration of infusion, body mass and body composition. For a typical critically ill patient, the emergence time from light sedation (RASS −3 to −2) remains rapid (<35 mins) for Propofol infusions lasting less than 4 days. However, the emergence time from deep sedation (RASS −5 to −2) was 25 h for a 24-h infusion and 3 days for infusions lasting 7–14 days.

It is worth highlighting a rare but potentially serious complication of Propofol use, Propofol Infusion Syndrome (PriS).

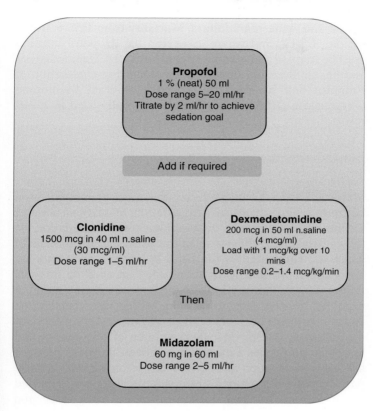

Propofol
1 % (neat) 50 ml
Dose range 5–20 ml/hr
Titrate by 2 ml/hr to achieve
sedation goal

Add if required

Clonidine
1500 mcg in 40 ml n.saline
(30 mcg/ml)
Dose range 1–5 ml/hr

Dexmedetomidine
200 mcg in 50 ml n.saline
(4 mcg/ml)
Load with 1 mcg/kg over 10
mins
Dose range 0.2–1.4 mcg/kg/min

Then

Midazolam
60 mg in 60 ml
Dose range 2–5 ml/hr

FIGURE 16.4 UK DMS sedation infusion protocol

PriS was first described in 1992 in five paediatric patients who died following sedation with high-dose Propofol [25]. PriS has since been recognized to also occur in adults, althoughless commonly.

Risk factors for PriSinclude airway infection, severe head injury, catecholamine or glucocorticoid therapy and high dose Propofol infusions (>48 h at >5 mg/kg/h) [26]. Young trauma patients who require heavy sedation, for example following traumatic brain injury, are therefore particularly at risk. Features of PriS include metabolic acidosis, myocardial failure, hyperkalaemia, hyperlipidemia, elevated creatinine kinase and acute renal failure. Mortality from PriS is in the region of 30 % and where suspected the Propofol infusion must be stopped and supportive care instituted. Haemodialysis and haemofiltration may assist by enhancing elimination of Propofol and its metabolites. Extracorporeal Membrane Oxygenation (ECMO) has been successfully used as a last resort therapy [27].

Benzodiazepines

Midazolam and Lorazepam are the most commonly used benzodiazepines in critical care sedation. Midazolam is water soluble and short acting, undergoing extensive oxidation via the cytochrome P450 system in the liver, the metabolites of which are eliminated by the kidneys. Its primary metabolite has CNS depressant activity and may accumulate in renal failure. Lorazepam is a long-acting benzodiazepine metabolized by hepatic glucuronidation to inactive metabolites. Accumulation of benzodiazepines may occur during continuous infusions due to their large volume of distribution and lipophilic properties. Lorazepam has been shown to produce less optimal sedation and have a slower emergence in comparison with Midazolam. Lorazepam has also been identified as an independent risk factor for critical care associated delirium.

A meta-analysis of 32 critical care sedation studies concluded that Propofol is at least as effective a sedative agent as Midazolam and results in a shorter period of intubation [28]. A further multi-center trial comparing sedation with Propofol and Midazolamconfirmed this but did not demonstrate earlier ICU discharge.

Whilst concerns about delirium have caused benzodiazepines to fall out of favour as the primary sedation agent of choice, there are situations when their use should be considered. Compared with benzodiazepines, Propofoland α_2 agonists carry an increased risk of hypotension. This is a particularly significant risk in hypovolaemic patients and may discourage their use where ongoing resuscitation is required. Benzodiazepines may also be used in traumatic brain injury where ICP management is problematic or when seizure activity is suspected, as they have excellent anticonvulsant properties.

α_2 Agonists

The α_2 agonist agents available for sedation on the ICU include Clonidine and Dexmedetomidine.

Clonidine is an imidazole compound that has been described as the prototype α_2 adrenoceptor agonist. Its ability to produce dose-related sedation, analgesia and anxiolysis makes it a potentially useful alternative to the more traditional sedation agents. Potential side effects include hypotension, dry mouth, constipation and the potential for rebound hypertension and tachycardia if the drug is rapidly withdrawn.

Dexmedetomidine is a sedative with high α_2-adrenoreceptor affinity that is thought to act in the locus ceruleus. In mechanically ventilated patients it has been shown to reduce the incidence of coma and delirium in comparison with lorazepam. Multicentre randomised controlled trials comparing Dexmedetomidine with Midazolam and with Propofol (named MIDEX and PRODEX respectively) have been conducted [29]. The results demonstrated improved communication and cooperation in the Dexmedetomidine group compared with both other agents and showed a reduced duration of mechanical ventilation compared with Midazolam, but not Propofol. However, there were more adverse effects (hypotension, bradycardia, 1st degree atrioventricular block) in the Dexmedetomidine groups. Overall lengths of ICU stay and mortality were similar. No difference was demonstrated in the rate of delirium as measured by the Confusion Assessment Method (CAM-ICU). Whilst currently more expensive, Dexmedetomidine has found favour over Clonidine as it is easier to titrate to a given sedation level.

Part Three: Delirium

Is Delirium an Important Issue in Critically Injured Patients?

Delirium is characterised by the acute onset of a disturbed level of consciousness with a reduced ability to focus and diminished cognition or perception. It is often associated with sleep and emotional disturbance and abnormal psychomotor activity. Two subtypes of delirium are described, between which patients may fluctuate. Patients with hyperactive delirium will appear to be clearly agitated, and this state is often associated with paranoid delusions or hallucinations. Patients with hypoactive delirium will appear calm or withdrawn, and because they are outwardly compliant, theirconfused state may often go unrecognised. Delirium is common in the ICU, affecting an estimated 65 % of sick ventilated patients in the United Kingdom.

Is Delirium a Prognostic Indicator in the Critically Unwell?

Delirium in the critically ill patient is a serious disorder. It represents an organ system failure as significant as that of any other. There is increasing evidence that delirium is associated with worse outcomes in mechanically ventilated patients and is an independent predictor of death and long-term cognitive impairment [30, 31]. It is also associated with prolonged length of stay in an ICU and in hospital [32]. All delirium is not the same. Recent evidence suggests patients with sedation related delirium, that is rapidly reversible, have fewer ventilator and hospital days and lower 1-year mortality compared with patients who have persistent delirium [33].

How Can Delirium Be Detected?

Two delirium-screening tools are available for critically ill intubated patients: the Confusion Assessment Method for the Intensive Care Unit (CAM-ICU) and the Intensive Care Delirium Screening Checklist (ICDSC) [34]. Both perform well against the gold standard diagnosis using the Diagnostic and Statistical Manual of Mental Disorders, fourth edition. CAM-ICU has the highest sensitivity and specificity and is relatively easy to perform. Daily use of a delirium-screening tool should ideally be undertaken in critically injured ICU patients, where feasible. The CAM-ICU tool is shown in Fig. 16.5.

A positive CAM-ICU assessment is associated with increased mortality and cognitive impairment [30, 35]. An assessment tool to predict the development of delirium in intensive care patients, the PRE-DELIRIC model, has also been validated [36].

How Can Delirium Be Prevented?

For critically injured patients, delirium may occur due to head injury or as an indirect consequence of trauma, for example due to pain, renal failure or sepsis. Iatrogenic causes are recognised, from sedation or other medication, as are environmental causes like sleep deprivation and prolonged immobilisation. In practice delirium is likely to be precipitated by combination of such factors. Addressing these factors is important to reduce the severity and duration of delirium.

A history of drug and alcohol abuse is frequently elicited in the trauma patient population, and should be actively searched for. Likewise, some patients may have an established dependence on their prescribed medication, or on nicotine in heavy smokers. The sudden discontinuation of

Confusion Assessment Method (CAM-ICU)

Feature 1: Acute onset or fluctuating course
Different than baseline mental status or fluctuation in past 24hrs?

Feature 2: Inattention
More than one error when slowly reading out:
S A V E A H A A R T
after asking to squeeze on hearing the letter 'A'

Feature 3: Altered level of consciousness
RASS score other than zero

Feature 4: Disorganised thinking
More than one error:
Yes/No questions: 1. Will a stone float on water?
                        2. Are there fish in the sea?
                        3. Does one kilogram weigh more than two kilograms?
                        4. Can you use a hammer to pound a nail?
Command
Say to pt: "Hold up this many fingers" (hold 2 fingers in front of pt), "Now do the same thing with the other hand" (do not repeat number of fingers) *if unable to move both arms, for 2nd part of command ask pt to "Add one more finger"
Error counted if pt unable to complete the entire command

OVERALL CAM-ICU: Feature 1 *plus* 2 *and* either 3 *or* 4 = CAM-ICU positive (delirium present)

FIGURE 16.5 The CAM-ICU tool

these substances may precipitate a withdrawal reaction that contributes to a delirious state. Common withdrawal signs include sweating, fever, tachycardia, hypertension, restlessness, vomiting and diarrhoea. Clearly these are non-specific and the intensivist should have a low threshold for instituting appropriate treatment where the history suggests substance withdrawal is possible.

However, general preventative measures should be considered too. There is little data currently available for preventative measures against delirium in intensive care patients. Most work in delirium prevention has been focused on

TABLE 16.7 Non-pharmacological measures to prevent delirium

Cognitive stimulation

Early mobilisation of mechanically ventilated patients

Listening to music

Communication and repeated reorientation of patient

Consistency of nursing staff

Television during day with daily news

Sleep hygiene measures:
    Lights off at night
    Lights on during day
    Control excess noise at night

elderly ward-based patients. These include non-drug preventative measures as shown in Table 16.7.

The early mobilisation of mechanically ventilated patients has also been found to reduce the duration of delirium, in addition to its other significant benefits [37]. Use of prophylactic antipsychotics such as Haloperidol has previously been suggested in some older guidelines, but current evidence does not support their use for this indication.

How Can Delirium Be Treated?

Where identified, the treatment of delirium must be primarily directed at removing the cause. This will include the identification and treatment of sepsis and metabolic derangement, provision of analgesia for pain, consideration of a drug withdrawal syndrome and possible discontinuation of deliriogenic drugs. Common culprit agents that can cause delirium are shown in Table 16.8.

After considering and treating potential causes of delirium it may be decided to commence the patient on an antipsychotic, especially when sedative agents are being tapered off. A

TABLE 16.8 Commonly prescribed
drugs that may contribute to delirium

Benzodiazepines
Steroids

Anticholinergics
  Metoclopramide
  H2 blockers

Cochrane review has concluded that there is some evidence for the efficacy of antipsychotics in delirium [38]. The atypical antipsychotic Quetiapine had a demonstrable benefit on duration of delirium in a single RCT in ICU patients [39]. It is given via the enteral route at an initial dose of 25 mg twice daily, which may be doubled every 24–48 h up to a maximum dose of 100 mg twice daily. Although previously recommended, there is currently no good quality evidence to suggest that Haloperidol reduces the duration of delirium. Both Quetiapine and Haloperidol can prolong the QTc interval and daily ECGs should be performed to monitor for this whilst patients are receiving these drugs. They should be not be used in patients at significant risk of developing torsades de pointes.

Where a continuous infusion of sedative medication is required to manage delirium, Dexmedetomidine is preferred over a benzodiazepine. Trial evidence suggests that Dexmedetomidine is superior to benzodiazepines with regard to reducing the prevalence of delirium [40]. Whether this is due to a positive effect of Dexmedetomidine or a negative effect of benzodiazepines on delirium is unclear.

How Can an Integrated Approach to Analgesia, Sedation and Delirium Be Practically Applied?

There is no single best approach to managing analgesia, sedation and delirium in critically injured patients, but an integrated approach is recommended. Such an integrated approach, used by the UK DMS is shown in Fig. 16.6.

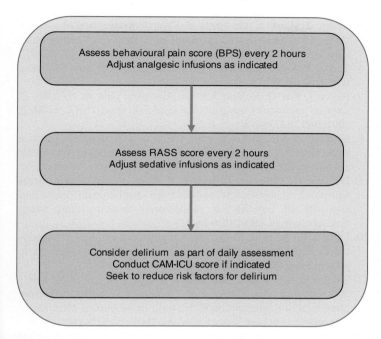

FIGURE 16.6 An integrated approach to analgesia, sedation and delirium in critically injured patients used by theUK DMS

References

1. Barr J, Fraser G, Puntillo K, et al. Clinical practice guidelines for the management of pain, agitation, and delirium in adult patients in the intensive care unit. Crit Care Med. 2013;41:263–306.
2. Kollef M, Levy N, Ahrens TS, et al. The use of continuous IV sedation is associated with prolongation of mechanical ventilation. Chest. 1998;114:541–8.
3. Chanques G, Sebbane M, Barbotte E, et al. A prospective study of pain at rest: incidence and characteristics of an unrecognized symptom in surgical and trauma versus medical intensive care unit patients. Anesthesiology. 2007;107:858–60.
4. Chanques G, Jaber S, Barbotte E, et al. Impact of systematic evaluation of pain and agitation in an intensive care unit. Crit Care Med. 2006;34:1691–9.

5. Beilin B, Shavit Y, Hart J, et al. Effects of anesthesia based on large versus small doses of fentanyl on natural killer cell cytotoxicity in the perioperative period. Anesth Analg. 1996;82:492–7.

6. Scragg P, Jones A, Fauvel N. Psychological problems following ICU treatment. Anaesthesia. 2001;56:9–14.

7. Payen J, Bru O, Bosson J, et al. Assessing pain in critically ill sedated patients by using a behavioral pain scale. Crit Care Med. 2001;29(12):2258–63.

8. Soliman H, Melot C, Vincent J. Sedative and analgesic practice in the intensive care unit: the results of a European survey. Br J Anaesth. 2001;87:186–92.

9. Dahaba A, Grabner T, Rehak P, et al. Remifentanil versus Morphine analgesia and sedation for mechanically ventilated critically ill patients: a randomized double blind study. Anesthesiology. 2004;101:640–6.

10. Gillis J, Brogden R. Ketorolac: a reappraisal of its pharmacodynamic and pharmacokinetic properties and therapeutic use in pain management. Drugs. 1997;53:139–88.

11. Sinatra R, Jahr J, Reynolds L, et al. Efficacy and safety of single and repeated administration of 1 gram intravenous acetaminophen injection (paracetamol) for pain management after major orthopaedic surgery. Anesthesiology. 2005;102:822–31.

12. Himmelseher S, Durieux M. Revising a dogma: ketamine for patients with neurological injury? Anesth Analg. 2005;101:524–34.

13. Friesner S, Curry D, Moddeman G. Comparison of two pain-management strategies during chest tube removal: relaxation exercise with opioids and opioids alone. Heart Lung. 2006;35:269–76.

14. Mar GJ, Barrington MJ, McGuirk BR. Acute compartment syndrome of the lower limb and the effect of postoperative analgesia on diagnosis. Br J Anaesth. 2009;102:3–11.

15. Beard D, Wood P. Pain in complex trauma: lessons from Afghanistan. BJA Education. 2015;15(4):207–12. doi:10.1093/bjaceaccp/mku035.

16. O'Donnell BD, Ryan H, O'Sullivan O, Iohom G. Ultrasound-guided axillary brachial plexus block with 20 milliliters local anesthetic mixture versus general anesthesia for upper limb trauma surgery: an observer-blinded, prospective, randomized, controlled trial. Anesth Analg. 2009;109:279–83.

17. Bulger EM, Edwards T, Klotz P, Jurkovich GJ. Epidural analgesia improves outcome after multiple rib fractures. Surgery. 2004;136(2):426–30.

18. Carrier FM, et al. Effect of epidural analgesia in patients with traumatic rib fractures: a systematic review and meta-analysis of randomized controlled trials. Can J Anaesth. 2009;56(3):230–42.
19. Sessler C, Gosnell M, Grap M, et al. The Richmond agitation-sedation scale: validity and reliability in adult intensive care patients. Am J Respir Crit Care Med. 2002;166:1338–44.
20. Martin J, Heymann A, Basell K, et al. Evidence and consensus-based German guidelines for the management of sedation and delirium in intensive care. Ger Med Sci. 2010;8:Doc02.
21. Defence Medical Services Critical Care Clinical Guidelines for Operations. Department of Military Anaesthesia and Critical Care, Royal Centre for Defence Medicine. 1st Revision. 2012.
22. Kress J, Pohlman A, O'Connor M, et al. Daily interruption of sedative infusions in critically ill patients undergoing mechanical ventilation. N Engl J Med. 2000;342:1471–7.
23. Girard T, Kress J, Fuchs B, et al. Efficacy and safety of a paired sedation and ventilator weaning protocol for mechanically ventilated patients in intensive care (Awakening and Breathing Controlled trial): a randomized controlled trial. Lancet. 2008;371(9607):126–34.
24. Mehta S, et al. Daily sedation interruption in mechanically ventilated critically ill patients cared for with a sedation protocol: a randomized controlled trial. JAMA. 2012;308(19):1985–92.
25. Parke T, Stevens J, Rice A, et al. Metabolic acidosis and fatal myocardial failure after propofol infusion in children: five case reports. Br Med J. 1992;305:613–6.
26. Motsch J, Roggenbach J. Propofol infusion syndrome. Anaesthesist. 2004;53:1009–22.
27. Culp K, Augoustides J, Onchroch A, Milas B. Clinical management of cardiogenic shock associated with prolonged propofol infusion. Anesth Analg. 2004;99:221–6.
28. Ostermann M, Keenan S, Seiferling RA, et al. Sedation in the intensive care unit: a systematic review. JAMA. 2000;283:1451–9.
29. Jakob S, Ruokonen E, Grounds R, et al. Dexmedetomidine vs midazolam or propofol for sedation during prolonged mechanical ventilation. Two randomised controlled trials. JAMA. 2012;307(11):1151–60.
30. Ely E, Shintani A, Truman B, et al. Delirium as a predictor of mortality in mechanically ventilated patients in the intensive care unit. JAMA. 2004;291:1753–62.
31. Girard T, Jackson J, Pandharipande P, et al. Delirium as a predictor of long-term cognitive impairment in survivors of critical illness. Crit Care Med. 2010;38:1513–20.

32. Ely E, Gautam S, Margolin R, et al. The impact of delirium in the intensive care unit on hospital length of stay. Intensive Care Med. 2001;27:1892–900.

33. Patel S, Poston J, Pohlman A, Hall J, Kress J. Rapidly reversible, sedation-related delirium versus persistent delirium in the intensive care unit. Am J Respir Crit Care Med. 2014;189:658–65.

34. Ely E, Inouye S, Bernard G, et al. Delirium in mechanically ventilated patients: Validity and reliability of the confusion assessment method for the intensive care unit (CAM-ICU). JAMA. 2001;286:2703–10.

35. Lat I, McMillian W, Taylor S, et al. The impact of delirium on clinical outcomes in mechanically ventilated surgical and trauma patients. Crit Care Med. 2009;37:1898–905.

36. Boogaard M, Pickkers P, Slooter A, et al. Development and validation of PRE-DELIRIC (PREdiction of DELIRium in ICu patients) delirium prediction model for intensive care patients: observational multicentre study. BMJ. 2012;344:e420.

37. Schweickert W, Pohlman M, Pohlman A, et al. Early physical and occupational therapy in mechanically ventilated, critically ill patients: a randomised controlled trial. Lancet. 2009;373:1874–82.

38. Lonergan E, Britton A, Luxenberg J. There is some evidence from RCTs that antipsychotics are effective, in varying doses, for different presentations of delirium. Cochrane Summ. 2009.

39. Devlin J, Roberts R, Fong J, et al. Efficacy and safety of quetiapine in critically ill patients with delirium: a prospective, multicenter, randomized, double-blind, placebo-controlled pilot study. Crit Care Med. 2010;38:419–27.

40. Riker R, Shehabi Y, Bokesch P, et al. SEDCOM (Safety and Efficacy of Dexmedetomidine Compared with Midazolam) Study Group: Dexmedetomidine vs midazolam for sedation of critically ill patients: A randomized trial. JAMA. 2009;301:489–99.

Chapter 17
Nutrition in the Critically Injured Patient

Stephanie R. Strachan and Karen Friend

Abstract Critically ill patients with severe traumatic injuries require precise attention to their nutrition in order to achieve rapid recovery and rehabilitation. Nutritional management can often be difficult in these patients and requires consideration of their baseline nutritional state as well as identification of the phase of critical illness. A key component of nutritional assessment is an accurate measure of the patient's weight, either ideal or actual. In the absence of indirect calorimetry body weight is required to estimate energy requirements through use of predictive equations. In addition to energy, protein is an essential component of the nutritional provision, with protein requirements elevated following traumatic injury. A number

S.R. Strachan, MBBS, MMedEd, MRCP, FRCA, DICM (✉)
Critical Care Department, King's College Hospital NHS Trust,
Denmark Hill, London SE5 9RS, UK
e-mail: stephanie.strachan@nhs.net

K. Friend, BSc, PgDip
Nutrition and Dietetics Department, King's College Hospital NHS
Trust, Denmark Hill, London SE5 9RS, UK

S.D. Hutchings (ed.), *Trauma and Combat Critical Care
in Clinical Practice*, In Clinical Practice,
DOI 10.1007/978-3-319-28758-4_17,
© Crown Copyright 2016

of nutritional supplements, including glutamine, have been purported to improve outcome in critically ill trauma patients although evidence is conflicted. There has been much debate with regard the route of feeding in critically ill patients and studies have compared enteral and parenteral feeding; both routes appear safe but there seems to be no particular advantage in the early institution of parenteral feeding. A protocol-based approach to feeding ensures its early commencement and helps to achieve optimal nutritional goals. Finally, re-feeding syndrome is an important phenomenon in critically ill patients who present with a background of malnutrition.

Keywords   Energy • Calories • Protein • Re-feeding syndrome • Parenteral nutrition • Enteral nutrition • Feeding protocols

What Is the Importance of Nutrition in the Critically Injured Patient?

The aim of nutritional support in the critical care setting is to provide patients with the ingredients they require to recover quickly and successfully from a wide spectrum of disorders. With regards to recovering from traumatic insults, patients need to heal damaged tissue, often undergo further surgical insults, overcome infective and other complications, and then rehabilitate to an optimal level of functional status. Both a good nutritional state at the time of admission and the receipt of adequate nutritional support whilst in intensive care are associated with improved outcomes for patients [1–3]. Table 17.1 highlights some of the recognised sequelae of mismatched energy provision.

There are numerous observational studies in the field of critical care nutrition which suggest potentially advantageous nutritional strategies. Unfortunately, few subsequent randomised controlled trials have provided clarity on what is the ideal nutritional practice in critical illness. The reasons for

TABLE 17.1 Overfeeding and underfeeding – why we need to get energy delivery right

Underfeeding

An energy deficit of ~1200 kcal/day is associated with an independent likelihood of ICU death [4]

Evidence suggests that an accumulation of energy/protein deficits is linked to poorer patient outcomes including an increased length of hospital stay, prolonged time needing mechanical ventilation and increased risk of infections [5, 6]

Poor outcomes may also extend to an increased risk of mortality and a decreased functional status at the time of hospital discharge [7]

Overfeeding

Hypercapnia – delayed ventilatory weaning, increased length of stay

Hyperglycaemia

Hypertriglyceridemia and fatty liver

Refeeding syndrome

Uraemia

Metabolic acidosis

this lack of clarity are primarily due to the inherent heterogeneity of critically ill patients, but also because the ability of a patient to maintain nutritional integrity whilst critically ill is, in itself, an exquisite indicator of their ability to recover. Researchers are continuing to study the metabolic response to critical illness and investigating which macro- and micro-nutrients are required during critical illness. They are also exploring how nutritional interventions may influence the adaptive and mal-adaptive pathways that occur as a consequence of insult or injury in order to enhance the recovery process [8].

Adequate nutrition is fundamental to survival but feeding is often challenging in the critical care population. The manipulation of nutrition is also laden with questions; as with every drug we use in the context of critical illness, the questions for nutrition are how much, of what, when and in whom? This chapter aims to highlight current best practice in nutritional support in the critically ill with a particular emphasis on patients with severe traumatic injury.

What Factors Influence Critical Care Nutritional Support Decisions?

There are a number of factors which may influence the nutritional requirements of a critically injured patient. While it is important to consider these factors, it is important to note that the evidence-base does not always provide clear guidance on how best to manage them.

Baseline Nutritional Status

Defining the patient's baseline nutritional status is probably the most important consideration in planning the nutritional support of any patient. There are a number of options for screening patients and measuring their nutritional status. Measures such as Body Mass Index (BMI) and specific anthropometric measurements are in use both in and out of hospital and can help in the assessment of nutritional status. Screening tools designed specifically for the critically ill patient, such as the (NUTritionRisk In the Critically Ill) NUTRIC score [9], are in the early stages of use in the clinical setting and may have the potential to help identify those at high nutritional risk. The merits of these tools will be discussed later in the chapter. Figure 17.1 highlights some of the issues that need to be taken into consideration for patients commencing their critical care journeys from different baseline nutritional states.

Phase of Critical Care Illness

The journey through critical care can be thought of as occurring in metabolic phases [10] as shown in Fig. 17.2. When a primary insult occurs there is an acute 'ebb' phase response

Malnutrition	Aim to minimise further loss of lean body mass and replenish micro-nutrient stores Potential risk of r efeeding syndrome Underfeeding may occur due to excess caution Overfeeding is also a risk and deleterious Micro-and macro-nutritional deficiencies are present at baseline Hypoglycaemia risk due to the loss of liver nutrition stores Fluid handling may be problematic (due to cardiac dysfunction and other altered protein sequelae from malnourishment) Increased risk of the development of pressure sores and delayed wound healing Increased morbidity and mortality
Normal nourishment	Aim to minimise the degree of nutritional deterioration by ensuring prescribed feed is delivered Note the micronutrient state cannot be reliably measured due to acute phase mobilisation
Obesity	Aim to minimise nutritional deterioration by careful assessment of patient's needs, additional logistical challenges are present Obese patients may be malnourished despite increased non-lean body mass Calorie estimates should be based on ideal or adjusted body weight in order to prevent overfeeding (the fat mass does not require nourishment) Critical illness is not an opportunity for intentional weight loss ("dieting"), as weight loss during critical illness is largely from lean body mass (which needs preserving) and not fat stores Difficulties with anthropometric measurements, access and mobilisation Bariatric beds and mattresses may be required Increased insulin resistance (as with diabetes) more likely Drug dosing challenges Increased morbidity and mortality

FIGURE 17.1 Nutritional status considerations

which lasts approximately 24–48 h and is characterised by a drop in body temperature and oxygen consumption. This is soon followed by the flow or acute phase which is marked by a period of hyper-metabolism. Hyper-metabolism leads to a catabolic state and is characterised by a rapid breakdown of protein, hyperglycaemia and fluid accumulation. This catabolic phase may last from days to weeks, depending upon the degree and severity of injury. Eventually, if the patient survives their critical illness, there is a recovery phase and with rehabilitation, anabolism.

Each metabolic phase has different nutritional implications which need to be taken into account in order to achieve optimal nutritional provision. However, it can be difficult to define what phase a patient is in, with patients often moving forwards and backwards though the metabolic phases depending on secondary insults and complications.

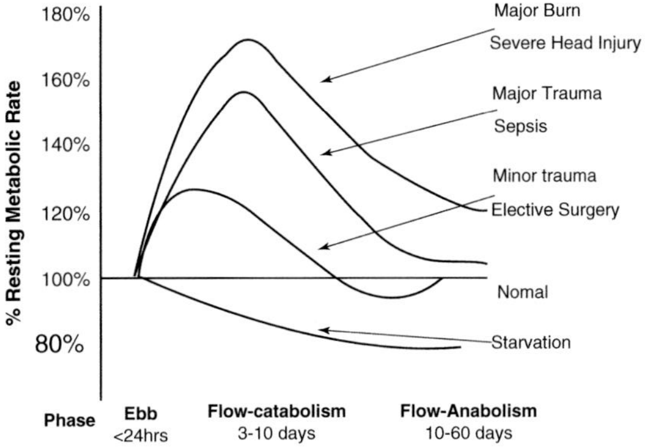

	Ebb	Flow-Catabolism	Flow-Anabolism
Overview	Shock, hypovolaemia, tissue hypoxia and hypothermia	Acute phase response, hormonal and immune response	Recovery decreased inflammatory markers
Hormone response	Catecholamines Cortisol Aldosterone ADH Glucagon Insulin resistance	Insulin Glucagon Cortisol Catecholamines Greater insulin resistance	Growth hormone IGF Anabolic steroids
Metabolism	Reduced metabolic rate Reduced oxygen consumption	Increased metabolic rate Increased oxygen consumption	Increased metabolic rate (returning to baseline)
Macro-nutrients	Hyperglycaemia Increased FFA	Hyperglycaemia Increased FFA Rapid breakdown of protein Amino acids released from muscle tissues for the synthesis of acute phase proteins Negative nitrogen balance (Exogenous protein sources are poorly utilized)	Resolving hyperglycaemia Replenishing fat and CHO stores Rebuilding lean muscle mass Positive nitrogen balance (Exogenous protein can now be utilised for muscle gain)
Fluid		Fluid accumulation	Fluid mobilisation

Graph (% Resting Metabolic Rate vs Phase):

% Resting Metabolic Rate: 180%, 160%, 140%, 120%, 100%, 80%

Curves labelled: Major Burn, Severe Head Injury, Major Trauma, Sepsis, Minor trauma, Elective Surgery, Normal, Starvation

Phase: Ebb <24hrs | Flow-catabolism 3-10 days | Flow-Anabolism 10-60 days

FIGURE 17.2 Metabolic response to stress varies with critical care condition and phase of critical care illness

Nature of Illness/Injury

Different pathological conditions may require different nutritional approaches; in addition, specific treatments and management strategies may influence nutritional requirements. Critical care nutrition research is therefore often performed in specific groups of patients because of their different postulated requirements. This chapter focuses on the patient with traumatic, including thermal injury. Some of the specific nutritional issues relevant to these patients are shown in Fig. 17.3.

What Are the Components of a Nutritional Assessment for Critically Ill Patients?

A full nutritional assessment incorporates a nutritional history from the patient or relatives where possible as well as examination findings. Dietitians and nutritionists take anthropometric measurements to enhance the assessment and monitoring of patients [11]. However, there are barriers to these tools in critical care (Table 17.2). Screening tools e.g., The Malnutrition Universal Screening Tool (MUST), are promoted for all in-patient populations in the UK, but have not been validated for specific use in the ICU patient [12]. The NUTRIC score has been specifically developed for the ICU patient as a way to help discriminate which ICU patients may benefit from aggressive protein-energy provision. The NUTRIC model components include: severity of illness (by SOFA and APACHE II scores); presence of inflammation (IL-6); number of co-morbidities; patient age and the length of hospital stay prior to ICU admission. Recording such scores in critical care research and utilising scores to enable evidence based best practice is not yet performed consistently [9].

The measurement of body weight is the most widely used tool in the assessment and monitoring of nutritional status in

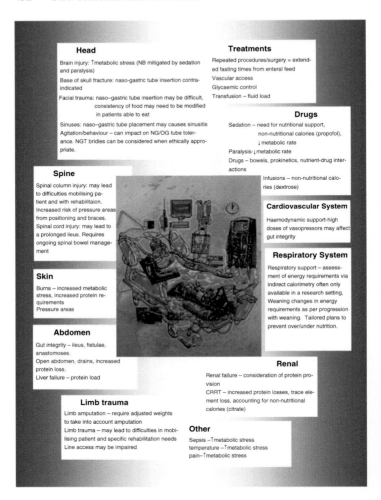

Head

Brain injury: ↑metabolic stress (NB mitigated by sedation and paralysis)

Base of skull fracture: naso-gastric tube insertion contra-indicated

Facial trauma: naso–gastric tube insertion may be difficult, consistency of food may need to be modified in patients able to eat

Sinuses: naso–gastric tube placement may causes sinusitis

Agitation/behaviour – can impact on NG/OG tube tolerance. NGT bridles can be considered when ethically appropriate.

Spine

Spinal column injury: may lead to difficulties mobilising patient and with rehabilitaion. Increased risk of pressure areas from positioning and braces. Spinal cord injury: may lead to a prolonged ileus. Requires ongoing spinal bowel management

Skin

Burns – increased metabolic stress, increased protein requirements
Pressure areas

Abdomen

Gut integrity – ileus, fistulae, anastomoses.
Open abdomen, drains, increased protein loss.
Liver failure – protein load

Limb trauma

Limb amputation – require adjusted weights to take into account amputation
Limb trauma – may lead to difficulties in mobilising patient and specific rehabilitation needs
Line access may be impaired

Treatments

Repeated procedures/surgery = extended fasting times from enteral feed
Vascular access
Glycaemic control
Transfusion – fluid load

Drugs

Sedation – need for nutritional support, non-nutritional calories (propofol), ↓ metabolic rate
Paralysis-↓ metabolic rate
Drugs – bowels, prokinetics, nutrient-drug interactions
Infusions – non-nutritional calories (dextrose)

Cardiovascular System

Haemodynamic support-high doses of vasopressors may affect gut integrity

Respiratory System

Respiratory support – assessment of energy requirements via indirect calorimetry often only available in a research setting, Weaning changes in energy requirements as per progression with weaning. Tailored plans to prevent over/under nutrition.

Renal

Renal failure – consideration of protein provision
CRRT – increased protein losses, trace element loss, accounting for non-nutritional calories (citrate)

Other

Sepsis –↑metabolic stress
temperature –↑metabolic stress
pain–↑metabolic stress

FIGURE 17.3 Influences on approach to nutrition in critical care

the non-critically ill patient. However, this basic measurement becomes complex in the setting of critical care. Estimates of body weight are frequently used in clinical practice due to the barriers in obtaining accurate readings, some of which are outlined in Table 17.3. Some experts promote the use of Ideal

TABLE 17.2 Anthropometric measurements frequently used in clinical practice

Anthropometric measurements frequently used in clinical practice		
Weight	BMI	Mid-upper-arm circumference
Height	Subjective global assessment	Triceps skinfold thickness

These measurements are often estimates only

Due to barriers including oedema, fluid retention and patient positioning, the use of anthropometric measurements such as ulna length and mid upper arm circumference are not validated tools in the critical care setting

If these measurements are used they should be considered as a guide only and used in conjunction with clinical judgement

TABLE 17.3 Barriers to obtaining accurate measurements of body weight

Patients may be unable to provide a history and have no previous medical documentation of weight, height or nutritional history

Weighing scales and equipment may not be available in the intensive care unit; bed weighing scales when present are frequently not calibrated

If actual weight can be measured, it may fluctuate dramatically due to fluid shifts. ICU patients can increase their weight by 10–20 % in 24 h making readings potentially inaccurate [14]

Critically ill patients are often immobile. It may not be possible for a patient to be moved onto scales if they are haemodynamically compromised or have unstable injuries in the context of trauma

Equipment such as traction, casts and braces provide logistic difficulties and need to be accounted for in resultant measurements

Adjusting body weight in amputees can add additional scope for errors

TABLE 17.4 Adjusting body weight in amputees [11]

	Percentage of total body weight of limb components					
	Upper arm	Forearm	Hand	Thigh	Leg	Foot
Women	2.55	1.38	0.56	14.78	4.81	1.29
Men	2.71	1.62	0.61	14.16	4.33	1.37

Body Weight (IBW) when using formulae to calculate nutritional requirements or drug dosing due to the problems in acquiring an Actual Body Weight (ABW) [13]. Using IBW may have an advantage in preventing overfeeding, but it is a static measurement and is not therefore particularly useful when making a baseline nutritional assessment or for monitoring. There is currently limited evidence to advocate the use of either IBW or ABW and practice will often depend on the clinical setting and the amount of input available from a dietitian/nutritionist or clinician.

Trauma and surgery, new or old, are processes that can add to the complexity of calculating patient body weight. If large volumes of fluid are drained, tissue excised or if there has been an amputation there will be an impact on patient weight. Table 17.4 illustrates a useful tool for estimating the necessary adjustment of bodyweight in patients with a new amputation [15].

What Are the Nutritional Requirements of the Critically Injured Patient?

Energy Requirements

Determining the energy requirements of a critically ill patient is a significant challenge and many equations and formulae have been created to attempt to best-estimate requirements (Table 17.5). There are pros and cons associated with each predictive equation and a lack of clinical evidence supporting the use of one particular method. The method chosen may be

TABLE 17.5 Predictive equations for energy requirements in critically ill patients

Equation (reference)	Advantages	Disadvantages
20–25 kcal/ kg (catabolic phase) [19, 20] 25–30 kcal/ kg (anabolic phase)	Quick and easy Avoids harmful overfeeding	Does not account for age, gender or condition Based on consensus opinion rather than clinical evidence No clear guidance on what weight should be used Low accuracy when compared to momentary energy expenditure (MEE) Does not incorporate physiological factors Difficult to define what phase a patient is in
Henry equation [21]	Accounts for age, gender and weight Used in conjunction with stress (disease state) and activity factors	Use of stress factors adds substantial error Does not incorporate physiological factors Data based on healthy populations
Penn State University [22–24]	Accounts for age, gender and height Incorporates physiological factors e.g. temperature, ventilator mode ICU specific Adjusted formula for obese and >60 years 67 % accuracy within 10 % of MEE in 202 patients	Time required Complex equations 24 h variability due to changes in temperature and ventilation Does not account for activity

(continued)

TABLE 17.5 (continued)

Equation (reference)	Advantages	Disadvantages
Ireton-Jones [25]	ICU specific Accounts for age and gender Includes factors for trauma and burns	Developed on burns and trauma patients Overestimates in non-obese and underestimates in obese patients 46 % accuracy when compared with MEE
Faisy [22, 26]	Age, height specific Incorporates physiological factors e.g. temperature, ventilator mode	Developed on medical critical care patients only Mean age 61 years Does not account for gender 53 % accuracy when compared with MEE
Harris – Benedict [27]	Accounts for gender, age, weight and height Used in conjunction with stress (disease state) and activity factors	Use of stress factors adds substantial error Does not incorporate physiological factors 34 % accuracy when compared with MEE

Adapted from Gandy [18] *with permission*

affected by the choice and availability of expert staff as well as access to the "gold standard" indirect calorimetry.

Indirect calorimetry is the most accurate method for measuring energy requirements. It is most frequently used in a research setting and, as evidenced in NutritionDay data, it is rarely available in most clinical settings [16]. Recent work has been done to improve the future availability of indirect calorimetry however standardised equations remain the primary tool for estimating energy requirements for most [17].

The main problem with all the formulae is their predictive accuracy. Patient energy requirements are influenced by several factors such as illness type, pyrexia, ventilation modes, activity, paralysis and sedation which are not all considered by the formulae available. Essentially, the formulae have an inherent degree of inaccuracy which results in patients frequently receiving either more or less energy than their actual requirements as determined by indirect calorimetry. *Frankenfield* carried out a large validation study comparing nine different metabolic rate calculations to indirect calorimetry; results showed that the Penn State equation was the most accurate equation being able to predict Energy Expenditure (EE) within a 10 % range in 67 % of occasions [22].

Protein Requirements

During critical illness, protein turnover is increased resulting in a net negative balance [28]. Skeletal muscle loss can be mitigated by sufficient nutrition; however optimal nutritional support cannot totally eliminate muscle wasting [29]. Several studies have investigated the influence of differing levels of protein intake on protein metabolism [30–32]. *Rooyackers* demonstrated improved whole body protein balance from enteral feeding and amino acid infusions [33, 34]. However, post hoc analyses of the results of three trials suggest better outcomes in patients who received less protein whereas some observational studies demonstrate improved outcomes from increased protein prescriptions [35–38].

Current guidelines suggest different protein targets for different patient populations, as shown in Table 17.6. The predicted physiological and pathophysiological changes as well as the impact of interventions need to be considered when studying protein dosing in critical care and may provide some explanation for the conflicting study results.

Traumatic injury, as with other types of critical illness, induces catabolism and muscle breakdown.; losses of 13–16 % of total body protein stores over a 21 day admission have been seen in both trauma and severely septic surgical patients [42–44]. The majority of these losses come from skeletal muscle and muscle loss is a key contributing factor to the

TABLE 17.6 Protein requirements in critically ill patients

Patient group (reference)	Protein target (g/kg/ABW)
General ICU [20]	1.2–1.5
Trauma [20]	1.3–1.5
Burns [39]	1.5–2.0
Continuous renal replacement therapy [40]	1.5–1.7
Obese [41]	2.0–2.5 (g/kg/IBW)

development of ICU acquired weakness, which has been reported in 50 % of patients receiving mechanical ventilation for more than 7 days [45]. ICU-acquired weakness is associated with delayed recovery, prolonged weaning from mechanical ventilation, increased length of ICU and hospital stay, increased healthcare costs and is an independent risk factor for death [36].

Protein intake targets are set higher in the context of trauma, but to fully understand actual requirements, studies are needed that consider nutritional constituents (including protein) alongside objectively measured retention of muscle strength. In addition, more relevant outcome measures such as rehabilitation time and quality of life indices are needed in addition to those only considering the usual critical care and hospital endpoints [46].

What Is the Role of Trace Elements, Vitamins and Other Supplements?

Critical illness following injury is characterised by oxidative stress, with micronutrients being immensely important for redox balance and antioxidant function, as well as the prevention of clinical deficiency states. Critically ill patients are at risk of both overt and sub-clinical trace element and vitamin deficiencies. However, these deficiencies are difficult to diagnose or confirm as plasma levels and enzyme functions tend to change in the acute phase following injury. Supplementation studies have been performed in different critically ill patient populations utilising different collections of trace elements and vitamins for their redox properties; selenium, zinc, vitamin C and vitamin E have dominated these studies either alone or in combination. Optimal composition, dose, timing, and duration of therapy are key factors that still need to be established. Generally, replacement studies utilising low doses of trace elements and vitamins trend towards benefit; stressing the importance of replacing likely deficits and providing balanced nutrition. To ensure recommended daily amounts of trace elements and vitamins are delivered, additional prescription will be needed if the patient is receiving less than 50 % of prescribed enteral nutrition or if the supplied parenteral nutrition does not already include the addition of these micronutrients. There is no evidence from the literature for supra-physiological doses or pharmaconutrition [47–49].

Glutamine

Glutamine is required for immune function and in conditions of oxidative stress. Glutamine supplementation was recommended in all patients receiving parenteral nutrition for a number of years following a small number of positive outcome studies and meta-analyses [20]. The weight of evidence supporting supplementation first came under doubt when the SIGNET trial showed no mortality benefit from intravenous administration of glutamine in patients receiving parenteral nutrition [50]. Then in 2013, the REDOXS trial signalled harm from glutamine supplementation [51]. This large study used high doses of parenteral and enteral glutamine and produced more questions than answers. It caused a paradigm shift in the utilisation of glutamine towards one of much greater caution. Research in this area is on going, but routine glutamine supplementation is currently not recommended in the critically ill or injured patient [52].

Fish Oil and Omega-6 Fatty Acids

Immune-modulating diets using different oils with varying omega 6:3 ratios have been studied and suggest possible benefit in patients with ARDS. More work is required to understand whether this strategy has a clinically relevant advantage for critically ill patients.

Beta-Blockers

The use of beta-blockers to counter the exaggerated sympathetic response seen in some patients has been studied in a number of different critically ill patient populations including those with severe traumatic injury [53]. However, adoption into clinical practice has not been widespread with the exception of critically ill patients with thermal injury [39].

Oxandrolone

Oxandrolone, an anabolic steroid, has been studied for its effect on switching off catabolism and its use is accepted in patients suffering from severe burns during the rehabilitation phase. There is some evidence that oxandrolone also halts the catabolism associated with polytrauma but this has not led to any measured outcome benefit. Further research is on going in this area [39, 54].

When Should Feeding Be Established Following Critical Injury?

There is clear consensus in both national and international guidelines for the commencement of early feeding (24–48 h after admission) for the critically ill patient [55–57]. If a patient is at high risk of nutritional deficiency e.g., NUTRIC score >6, then the patient is especially likely to benefit from early feeding; including by the parenteral route if necessary. Early nutritional support is associated with a significant reduction in hospital length of stay and a trend towards reduced mortality [58].

What Is the Preferred Method of Feeding the Critically Injured Patient?

The enteral route is consistently promoted when experts debate the methods of feeding the critically ill and the psychological benefits of eating should never be forgotten when this is a feasible route. However, in the context of critical illness, appetite is often suppressed and the oral route is often not feasible due to ventilation and sedation. If patients cannot achieve optimal nutrition via the oral route then guidelines recommend enteral feeding as the preferred route of nutrition [55–57].

Benefits of the enteral route are also thought to include the maintenance of gut integrity and the prevention of bacterial translocation. As a result, trophic feeding of Enteral Nutrition (EN) should be considered in order to help maintain gut integrity even if the aim is not to meet full nutritional requirements.

Despite the clear recommendations advocating enteral feeding, the scientific literature surrounding the topic of route of nutrition in the critically ill can appear confusing and conflicting. Despite the well-established pros and cons to both EN and Parenteral Nutrition (PN) as shown in Table 17.7, and the overwhelming advocacy for EN where possible, there has still been research undertaken recently examining the benefits of one route over the other [59]. Other studies either directly compare the use of EN alone with PN alone, or compare the use of EN alone with EN and supplemental PN [60]. Three meta-analyses of these comparison trials have been

TABLE 17.7 Comparison of enteral and parenteral nutrition

	Enteral	**Parenteral**
Access	Minimally invasive procedure Can be placed under guidance in patients with challenging anatomy	Invasive procedure Always placed under guidance

Duration	Short/medium term
	  Nasogastric
	  Orogastric
	  Nasojejunal
	Medium/long term
	  Jejunostomy
	  Gastrostomy
	  (PEG/RIG)
		Short term (<14 days)
		  Dedicated central venous catheter line
		  PICC
		  Dedicated single lumen
		Long term (>14 days)
		  PICC lines (up to 4 weeks)
		  Hickman lines (months or years)

Administration	Bolus Continuous Supplementary	Continuous Cyclical Supplementary
Formulations	Pre-prepared formulations Contain trace elements and vitamins	Pre-prepared formulations +/− ability to manipulate components Scratch bags Restrictions on products for peripheral route Trace elements and vitamins usually require adding
Cost	~ £4–10 per day	~ £40–80 per day
Indications	Functioning gastrointestinal tract but unable to achieve an adequate or safe oral intake	Inaccessible or non-functioning gastrointestinal tract Unable to achieve an adequate enteral intake

TABLE 17.7 (continued)

Possible complications	Tube positioning (misplaced tube) Accidental tube removal Tube blockage Aspiration Gastrointestinal disturbances Nasal ulceration Stoma site problems (e.g. buried bumper syndrome) Mechanical faults with feeding pump	Insertion of line related problems Catheter related sepsis Thrombosis, catheter occlusion, thrombophlebitis Fluid overload Hyperglycaemia Electrolyte disturbances Deranged liver functions tests Specific nutritional deficiencies Mechanical faults with infusion devices

published with varying findings regarding superiority of approach [61–63]. The most recent interpretation of the EN/PN debate is discussed later in this chapter.

How Should Enteral Feeding Be Established?

Enteral nutrition is most frequently administered via a NasogastricTube (NGT). Alternative routes such as an OrogastricTube (OGT) can be used when NG tubes are contra-indicated e.g., base of skull fracture. The enteral route can also be accessed through naso-jejunal tubes, feeding jejunostomies, and percutaneous gastrostomies.

Evidence suggests that the use of appropriate feeding protocols in critical care improves the number of patients receiving nutrition support and promotes early feeding [64, 65]. As a result, this may also impact on other important outcomes, with evidence showing a trend towards a reduction in gastric residual volumes, less time to reach goal feeding rates, a significant reduction in length of hospital stay, and a reduction in hospital mortality.

Common elements of feeding protocols include recommendations on the timing of EN, the type of enteral formula, titration rate and the monitoring of gastric tolerance through the measurements of Gastric Residual Volumes (GRV). Protocols often also include guidance for optimizing the delivery of enteral nutrition through recommendations on the use of prokinetics and the timing of parenteral nutrition if clinically indicated.

Most centres commence feeding at reduced rates with a gradual increase in the volume of feed until the target rate has been reached as per patient tolerance. Studies have shown no difference in outcome for continuous compared with bolus feeds and so commonly continuous feeding is used. As well as there being a logistical advantage, in terms of nursing workload, this strategy may also promote more effective glycaemic control. Figure 17.4 shows an example of an enteral feeding protocol.

Novel Feeding Protocols

Due to the challenges of delivering optimal nutrition to critically ill patients, various groups have looked at the impact of novel protocols; two of which are outlined in Table 17.8. Consistent elements of these protocols are the early commencement (within 72 h) of feeding, targeting delivery of specific volumes, monitoring delivery and calorie balances, compensation for lost delivery of feed (catch up feeding within a 24 h period), quantified GRV influencing the delivery of feed and maximum infusion rates.

What Enteral Feeds Should Be Used for the Critically Injured Patient?

Enteral feeds are commercially available and produced by a variety of manufacturers. They typically contain varying proportions of carbohydrates, fat and protein together with

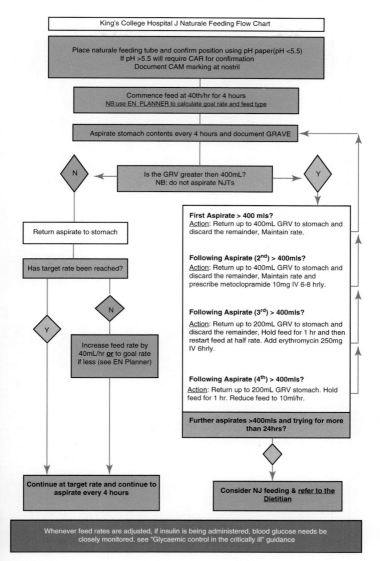

FIGURE 17.4 Example of a feeding protocol for use in a critical care unit

TABLE 17.8 Novel approaches to nutrition protocols

	Usual practice	PeP UP [66]	FEED ME [67]
Initiation rate of feed	10–40 ml/h	Target rate	As per standard practice
Target rate achievement	Build up every 4 h, target usually reached within 24 h	At commencement of feed	As per standard practice
Approach	Rate based	Volume based	Volume based
Product	Variety, frequently 1 kcal/mL	Semi-elemental 1.5 kcal/mL	Variety (1–2 kcal/mL)
GRV accepted	200–500 mL	350 mL	250 mL
Pro-kinetics	Not routinely, added with high GRV	Yes	No
Maximum infusion rate	Not stated	150 mL/h	120 mL/h
Monitoring energy delivery	No	Yes	Yes
Protein	Not considered	Supplemented	Monitored
Compensation of lost delivery of energy/protein	Not considered	Based on EN volume prescribed for a 24 h period, volume held, and hours remaining in a 24 h period to deliver the missed volume – new rate calculated	Based on EN rate prescribed, hours held and hours remaining read from a look up table

electrolytes, trace elements and vitamins. There will be slight variations between different manufacturers; however most companies will produce a type of feed that falls into each of the categories outlined in Table 17.9.

As a result of the elevated protein requirements of the trauma patient, high protein feeds are frequently used in this population. High protein feeds can vary in energy concentration (1.2–1.3 kcal/mL) and in protein provision (5.5–8 g protein/100 mL). The choice of feed type within the high protein sub-group will largely depend on issues surrounding availability of feed resources in each differing clinical environment. In instances where protein requirements cannot be met by the chosen feed alone, then the use of additional protein supplements, either powder or liquid, can also be administered enterally.

What Options Are There for Patients in Whom Enteral Feeding Has Failed or in Whom It Is Contra Indicated?

Gastro-intestinal symptoms are frequent in critically ill patients and can include diarrhoea, delayed gastric emptying with high GRV, vomiting, abdominal distention and aspiration. EN delivery can be hampered by slow gastric emptying in the trauma patient and specifically in the head injured patient as a result of sedation, paralysis, raised ICP, cooling or a raised sodium [68]. The initiation of PN should be considered in patients with poor gastric tolerance only once strategies to optimise the enteral route of delivery have been explored, unless the patient is malnourished on presentation.

Gastric Residual Volumes (GRV)

Protocols should incorporate strategies for promoting enteral feeding, including the use of prokinetic agents and post-pyloric feeding. The use of these strategies is based on GRV

TABLE 17.9 Range of commercially prepared enteral feeds and indications for use

Feed category	Content Energy (kcal/mL)	Content Protein (g/100 mL)	Use	Brand (manufacturer) examples
Standard formula	1	4	Normal requirements Free of fibre Used with new/high output stomas/following GI surgery/severe diarrhoea	Nutrison (Nutricia) Osmolite (Abbott) Fresubin Original (Fresenius Kabi)
Standard formula with fibre	1	4	Normal requirements Fibre containing	NutrisonMultifibre (Nutricia) Jevity (Abbott) Fresubin Original Fibre (Fresenius Kabi)
Energy formula	1.5	6	Normal requirements Fibre/fibrefree Reduced volume	Nutrison Energy/Multifibre (Nutricia) Jevity/Osmolite 1.5 (Abbott) Fresubin Energy (Fresenius Kabi)
Protein plus formula	1.2–1.25	5.5–6.3	High protein/energy requirements e.g. catabolic ICU patients Can be fibre or fibre free	Nutrison protein plus (Nutricia) Jevity plus (fibre)/Osmolite plus (non-fibre) (Abbott)

High protein formula	1.28–1.3	7.5–8	High protein requirements e.g. burns, trauma, traumatic head injury, CVVH, obesity Can be fibre or fibre free	Nutrison Advanced Protison (*Nutricia*) Jevity Plus HP (fibre)/Osmolte Plus HP (non-fibre) (*Abbott*)
Concentrated (low volume)	2	7.5–8.4	Normal requirements Fluid restriction	Nutrison Concentrate (*Nutricia*) TwoCal (*Abbott*)
Low electrolyte	1.8–2	7.5–8.1	High energy Low electrolyte Renal failure not needing filtration/ intermittent filtration	Nepro HP (*Abbott*) Nutrison Concentrate (*Nutricia*)
Semi-elemental	1–1.5	5.5–6.3	Range of energy to protein ratio Malabsorption Pancreatic insufficiency	Nutrison MCT (*Nutricia*) Peptisorb (*Nutricia*) Peptamen (*Nestle*) Vital 1.5 (*Abbott*)
Protein supplements	**Per 100 g powder: 368 kcal, 87.2 g protein Per 100 ml liquid: 333 kcal, 33 g protein**		**Patients unable to meet full protein requirements from feed alone e.g. trauma, burns, bariatric** **Variety of powder or liquid forms**	**Protifar** (*Nutricia*) **ProSource Liquid** (*Nutrinovo*)

measurements in the majority of intensive care units. GRV, usually by 4 hourly aspirates, is used as a marker of gastric emptying and is assumed to reflect tolerance and absorption of feed. Ultrasound estimation of stomach volume is being trialled in some centres, however this method is not widely used [69]. With patient safety paramount, studies have looked at the relationship between size of GRV and the occurrence of vomiting, aspiration of gastric contents and development of pneumonia. McClave et al. (2005) and Montejo et al. (2010) both found that increasing the GRV cuff off value to 400 mL and 500 mL respectively in comparison to a standard cut off value of 200 mL did not increase the incidence of aspiration or ICU acquired pneumonia [70, 71]. Montejo (2010) also found that the mean enteral delivery was significantly greater in the intervention (increased GRV) group. As a result of these findings most centres now tolerate higher GRVs, with some experts questioning the need for measuring GRV at all [72].

Pro-kinetic Agents

Prokinetic agents are commonly used in critically ill patients with high GRV or delayed gastric emptying despite the evidence base being poor. Both metoclopramide and erythromycin are used "off label" as prokinetic drugs and combination therapy, utilising these two agents together, has been demonstrated to increase the rate of successful feeding compared with monotherapy in critically ill patients intolerant of enteral feeding [73]. There are concerns for patient safety in utilising these drugs with tachyphylaxis and side-effects reported for both agents. It is recommended that metoclopramide is utilised first line; with a maximum dose of 10 mg four times daily and if intolerance persists, to add erythromycin for a further 24–48 h. The overall maximum duration for the use of prokinetics suggested is 7 days with a move to altering the route of feeding if unsuccessful [74].

Post-pyloric Feeding

Post-pyloric feeding may be considered in patients with gastroparesis; evidenced by high GRV, as an alternative method of successfully delivering enteral nutrition and preventing the need for parenteral nutrition. Jejunal feeding can be given either via a Naso-jejunalTube (NJT) or via a surgically inserted jejunostomy. NJTs can be inserted with endoscopy or radiology assistance or at the bedside with the use of specialist equipment, which can make the post-pyloric route easily accessible with a minimally invasive intervention [75, 76].

Parenteral Nutrition

PN can either be as a supplemental parenteral source of nutrition (SPN) or as an exclusive source of nutrition, termed as total parenteral nutrition (TPN). There is no contention that if the gut is inaccessible, non-functioning or enteral nutritional support is inadequate then provision of nutrition should be considered via the parenteral route. However, the decision of when to initiate parenteral nutrition is not always clear-cut, particularly in the rapidly changing environment of critical care nutrition research and, as always, these decisions need to be made based on an individual patient's clinical status at that point in time. Clinicians are unable to predict the likelihood of success of the enteral route so it should always be trialled in the first instance unless contraindicated. Specific indications for PN are listed in Table 17.10.

Debate remains regarding the optimal timing of commencement of PN with prominent differences between the European and American guidelines. The more recent American Society for Parenteral and Enteral Nutrition (ASPEN) and Society of Critical Care Medicine (SCCM) guidance recommends tolerating hypocaloric feeding for 7 days in patients who are not malnourished on ICU admission. Whereas the European Society for Parenteral and

TABLE 17.10 Indications for parenteral nutrition

Gastrointestinal failure e.g. ischaemic gut, prolonged ileus, obstruction, severe inflammatory bowel disease, high output fistula, severe diarrhoea for >7 days

Post-major abdominal surgery where significant malnourishment prior to surgery is present and enteral feeding is not possible or prolonged gut rest is absolutely necessary (for more than 5 days)

Prolonged mucositis, radiation enteritis or severe nausea and vomiting

Severe acute pancreatitis where EN has failed

Severe trauma or burns where EN has failed

Other "non-critical care" indications e.g. congenital gut malformation, short bowel syndrome or scleroderma

Enteral Nutrition (ESPEN) recommend commencing PN within 2 days of ICU admission for those unable to establish adequate EN [55, 57]. This conflict is understandable when bearing in mind that many of the same research works that underpin these guidance documents resulted in the conflicting meta-analyses in the early 2000s [61–63]. A number of further studies have been performed since these guidelines were produced that are now also informing practice in this area.

Most recently, the CALORIES trial (2014), a large multi-centre RCT carried out in 33 adult critical units in the UK, has demonstrated that starting parenteral feeding early in critical care is neither superior nor inferior to the enteral route [59]. PN was shown to be safe and this provided evidence to support the parenteral route being considered early if the enteral route is unsuccessful. There is little doubt that PN should be used when there are clear contra-indications to EN, such as mechanical bowel obstruction, acute bowel ischaemia or infarction, and bowel perforation, but maintaining gut integrity is also important where possible. Trophic feeding is one approach previously mentioned that is used with the intention of maintaining gut function, improving immune status and to help the prevention of an ileus [77].

The EPaNIC trial (2011) compared the two strategies, "early" versus "late" PN by randomising patients to receive either late or early supplemented PN [35]. Results found that withholding PN was associated with fewer ICU infections, shorter duration of mechanical ventilation, shorter length of ICU stay, a slight increase in hypoglycaemic episodes and shorter hospital stay. There were no significant differences in 90 day mortality between the groups. There are design limitations, however, from this single-centre study that make it questionable whether results are applicable to a contrasting ICU population e.g. the trauma patient. A subsequent cost analysis was performed on the EPaNIC trial population, which concluded the use of early PN in critically ill patients could not be recommended for both clinical (no benefit), and cost-related reasons [78].

Heidegger (2012) studied the provision of supplementary PN for 5 days from day 3 of ICU admission to patients receiving suboptimal EN (<60 % of requirements) [60]. The supplemented PN group were shown to have less antibiotic days and decreased infection rates. In light of their findings the authors made a recommendation to consider PN from day 4 onwards in those poorly nourished and failing to achieve EN goals.

Doig (2013) concludes from his study that the provision of early PN to critical care patients with relative contraindications to early EN, compared with standard care, did not result in a difference in day-60 mortality. Whilst the early PN strategy resulted in more ventilator-free days it did not significantly reduce ICU or hospital stay [29].

Whilst initially confusing, there is some clarity emerging from these studies. PN is no longer thought to be "dangerous" – and indeed PN formulations have been manipulated over the past decade particularly with respect to their lipid content as studies have shown different fatty acid sources to be more beneficial [79]; and, if not malnourished, critical care patients can safely wait a week for the gut to start working. Patient-safe and cost-effective care would therefore currently conclude that PN should be given at about 5–7 days if EN is

Do:
- Make a nutrition assessment.
- Collaborative working with the nutrition team – a multi-professional and inter-disciplinary team, whose expertise can be used to aid nutrition decision-making, help review complex cases and facilitate and monitor appropriate nutrition care plans (81).
- Develop a clear plan with all stakeholders regarding the rationale for the enteral route not being utilised and the expected length of time for this.
- Consider early (during first 48 hours of a critical care admission) PN for malnourished patients in whom enteral route contra-indicated, receiving trophic feeding or failing to achieve optimal EN goals.
- Consider PN for other critical care patients who are not receiving adequate EN at day 5-7.
- PN is not an emergency drug and commencement can usually be planned for within normal working days.
- Electrolytes can be manipulated in PN manufacturing – communicate with your provider as to what manipulation has been required in ICU.
- Trace elements and vitamins need adding to PN – check if they have been added by your provider.

Don't:
- PN is unlikely to be beneficial where it is required for less than 7 days.
- PN should not be initiated in the context of end-of-life care.

FIGURE 17.5 The do's and don'ts of parenteral nutrition

unsuccessful at this point, but if a patient is malnourished on admission then PN should be commenced earlier. In either case PN is rarely an emergency drug that requires an ill-informed, non-specialist, out-of-hours prescription. Some further practical advice for clinicians considering the use of PN is given in Fig. 17.5.

Is the Prescribed Nutrition Always Delivered?

Results from the International Nutrition Survey (2011), show that critically ill patients typically only receive 53.6 % of prescribed calories and 53 % of prescribed protein when fed by the enteral route [81]. Multiple barriers occur in the ICU setting, outlined in Table 17.11, which prevent the delivery of optimal nutrition. Monitoring energy balances can help ensure calories that are prescribed are delivered, or precipitate action to optimise calorie delivery if a patient is being over- or under- fed. Where critical care units have a computer information system, such a system can be programmed to calculate energy and protein balances and highlight when there is deviation from the prescription. A simple method for monitoring and calculating daily energy balances is shown in Fig. 17.6.

TABLE 17.11 Barriers to delivering prescribed feed

Modifiable (usually logistical)	Non-modifiable (usually patient factors)
Time taken to	Ileus
Insert feeding tubes	GI intolerance –
Check positioning of feeding tubes	vomiting, high
To commence feed	gastric aspirates
Interruptions to feeding and unnecessary starvation for procedures	Fasting for a procedure
Longer periods than required	
Postponed procedures	
Protocols that do not consider whether there is a need for starvation in the intubated critical care setting	
Miscalculations when feed is not administered over 24 h (e.g. drug administration requiring an empty stomach)	
Unit variations on GRV cut off values	
Unit variations on protocols of when and by how much NG feeds should be reduced or ceased in relation high GRVs	

- Keep an hourly record of the amount and type of feed delivered
- At the end of each day/ chart, the total amount of feed prescribed will be recorded
- At the end of each day/ chart, the total amount of feed delivered will be recorded
- Each day/ chart, the energy balance for the day i.e. the amount delivered *minus* the amount prescribed *(NB if all the feed prescribed was not delivered this will be a negative number)*
- The energy balance for the patient should be amended to incorporate non-nutritional calories at this stage:
  Propofol 1% contains 1.1 kcal per mL (as lipid)
  5% glucose contains 0.2 kcal per mL
  10% glucose contains 0.4 kcal per mL
  Citrate 0.59 kcal per mmol but energy provision also influenced by removal during CRRT(83)

FIGURE 17.6 Simple method for calculating energy balance

What Is Refeeding Syndrome, Who Is at Risk and How Should It Be Managed?

Refeeding syndrome is a rare, potentially life threatening condition that may occur in malnourished or starved patients on the re-introduction of nutrition. It is characterised by

Starvation	
Body	**Cellular level**
Glycogenolysis reduces glycogen stores from liver and muscle	Intracellular minerals (phosphate, potassium and magnesium) are utilised and depleted.
Gluconeogenesis – protein catabolism leads to glucose for the brain and red blood cells; lipolysis produces FFA and ketone bodies for non-glucose dependent tissues	Vitamins and trace element co-enzymes are also depleted
Protein catabolism reduces to preserve protein once ketone levels rise and CNS switches to utilising ketones for fuel.	
Refeeding	
Body	**Cellular level**
Glycaemia occurs with the introduction of food which stimulates insulin production	Phosphate, potassium and magnesium are moved into cells with glucose
Insulin stimulates reversal of the above starvation pathways and encourages CHO, protein and fat storage	Sodium moves extracellularly
Insulin also causes renal retention of sodium and water	Further depletion of vitamins and trace elements occurs, especially thiamine

FIGURE 17.7 Pathophysiology of refeeding syndrome

severe intracellular electrolyte shifts and acute circulatory fluid overload; organ failure may also occur. The hallmark biochemical feature of refeeding syndrome is hypophosphataemia, but hypokalaemia and hypomagnesaemia as well as other electrolyte disturbances may also occur alongside changes in glucose, protein, and fat metabolism [83]. The pathophysiological mechanisms for these changes are outlined in Fig. 17.7.

Refeeding syndrome is potentially preventable and criteria for identifying those at risk are shown in Fig. 17.8. Novel biomarkers are being studied to aid prediction of the condition [84].

When a patient is identified as being at risk, steps are taken to prevent the development of refeeding syndrome through careful reintroduction of nutrition combined with vitamins and electrolytes. NICE guidelines are available which recommend a nutritional prescription for commencing feeding in these patients as shown in Fig. 17.9.

At risk:
Malnourished patients – chronic alcohol abuse, elderly, poorly controlled diabetes, chronic malabsorption diseases (e.g. cystic fibrosis, Crohn's disease), chronic organ impairment conditions (e.g. COPD, CCF, liver cirrhosis)
Any patient who has had very little or no food intake for > 5 days

High risk:
Patient has one or more of the following:
BMI less than 16kg/m^2
Unintentional weight loss greater than 15% within the last 3–6 months
Little or no nutritional intake for more than 10 days
Low levels of potassium, phosphate or magnesium prior to feeding
Or patient has two or more of the following:
BMI less than 18.5 kg/m^2
Unintentional weight loss greater than 10% within the last 3–6 months
Little or no nutritional intake for more than 5 days
A history of alcohol abuse or drugs including insulin, chemotherapy, antacids or diuretics

Extremely High risk:
Patients in a starved state with BMI less than 14 kg/m^2
Very little or no nutritional intake for more than 15 days

FIGURE 17.8 Patients at risk of refeeding syndrome (Adapted from NICE clinical guideline 32 [85])

All Patients
- Circulatory and fluid management need to be considered
- Thiamine (200-300 mg daily) and vitamin B tablets, compound, strong (1 or 2, three times a day) or the full dose of a daily intravenous vitamin B preparation, for the first 10 days of feeding
- A multivitamin supplement for the first 10 days of feeding
- Monitor appropriate biochemistry and supplement as indicated
- Provide oral, enteral or intravenous supplements of
  - potassium (likely requirement 2–4 mmol/ kg/ day),
  - phosphate (likely requirement 0.3–0.6 mmol/ kg/ day), and
  - magnesium (likely requirement 0.2 mmol/ kg/ day intravenous, 0.4 mmol/ kg/ day oral)

At risk:
Commence feeding at a maximum of 50% total energy requirements for the first 2 days before increasing to meet full requirements.

High risk:
Start nutritional support at a maximum 10 kcal/ kg/ day, increasing slowly to meet full needs by 4–7 days.

Extremely high risk:
Consider starting feed at 5 kcal/ kg, increasing slowly to meet full needs by 4-7 days.
N.B. Pre-feeding correction of low plasma levels of electrolytes is unnecessary

FIGURE 17.9 Commencing feeding in at risk patients (Adapted from NICE clinical guideline 32 [85])

References

1. Giner M, Laviano A, Meguid MM, Gleason JR. In 1995 a correlation between malnutrition and poor outcome in critically ill patients still exists. Nutrition. 1996;12:23–9.
2. Alberda C, Gramlich L, Jones N, Jeejeebhoy K, Day AG, Dhaliwal R, Heyland DK. The relationship between nutritional intake and clinical outcomes in critically ill patients: results of an international multicenter observational study. Intensive Care Med. 2009;35(10):1728–37.
3. Robinson MK, Mogensen KM, Casey JD, McKane CK, Moromizato T, Rawn JD, Christopher KB. The relationship among obesity, nutritional status, and mortality in the critically ill. Crit Care Med. 2015;43(1):87–100.
4. Faisy C, Lerolle N, Dachraoui F, Savard JF, et al. Impact of energy deficit calculated by a predictive method on outcome in medical patients requiring prolonged acute mechanical ventilation. Br J Nutr. 2009;101:1079–87.
5. Guidelines for the Provision of Intensive Care Services (GPICS). 2015. http://www.ficm.ac.uk/sites/default/files/GPICS%20-%20Ed.1%20%282015%29.pdf. Accessed 4 Oct 2015.
6. Schetz M, Casaer MP, Van den Berghe G. Does artificial nutrition improve outcome of critical illness? Crit Care. 2013;17:302.
7. Tremblay B. Impact of body mass index on outcomes following critical care. Chest. 2003;123(4):1202–7.
8. Preiser JC, et al. Metabolic and nutritional support of critically ill patients: consensus and controversies. Crit Care. 2015;19:35.
9. Heyland DK, Dhaliwal R, Jiang X, Day AG. Identifying critically ill patients who benefit the most from nutrition therapy: the development and initial validation of a novel risk assessment tool. Crit Care. 2011;15(6):R268.
10. Cuthbertson DP. The physiology of convalescence after injury. Br Med Bull. 1945;3:96–102.
11. Simpson F, Doig GS. Physical assessment and anthropometric measures for use in clinical research conducted in critically ill patient populations: an analytic observational study. J Parenter Enteral Nutr. 2013;39(3):313–21.
12. The Malnutrition Universal Screening Tool. http://www.bapen.org.uk/screening-for-malnutrition/must/introducing-must. Accessed 4 Oct 2015.
13. Berger MM, Pichard C. Best timing for energy provision during critical illness. Crit Care. 2012;16:215.

14. Lowell JA, Schifferdecker C, Driscoll DF, et al. Postoperative fluid overload: not a benign problem. Crit Care Med. 1990;18:728–33.

15. Adjusting body weight in amputees. http://www.amputee-life.org/2012/10/14/amputee-weight-loss/. Accessed 4 Oct 2015.

16. NutritionDay. http://www.nutritionday.org/. Accessed 4 Oct 2015.

17. Pichard C, Oshima T, Berger MM. Energy deficit is clinically relevant for critically ill patients: yes. Intensive Care Med. 2015;41(2):335–8.

18. Gandy J. Manual of dietetic practice. 5th ed. Chichester: Published by Wiley-Blackwell on behalf of the BDA; 2014.

19. Cerra F, Benitez M, Blackburn G, Irwin R, Jeejeebhoy K. Applied nutrition in ICU patients. A consensus statement of the American College of Chest Physicians. Chest. 1997;111:769–78.

20. Singer P, et al. ESPEN guidelines on parenteral nutrition: intensive care. Clin Nutr. 2009;28:387–400.

21. Henry CJ. Basal metabolic rate studies in humans: measurement and development of new equations. Public Health Nutr. 2005;8(7A):1133–52.

22. Frankenfield DC, Coleman A, Alam S, Cooney RN. Analysis of estimation methods for resting metabolic rate in critically ill adults. J Parenter Enteral Nutr. 2009;33:27–36.

23. Frankenfield DC, Ashcraft CM. Estimating energy needs in nutrition support patients. J Parenter Enteral Nutr. 2011;35(5):563–70.

24. Frankenfield DC. Validation of an equation for resting metabolic rate in older obese critically ill patients. J Parenter Enteral Nutr. 2011;35:264–9.

25. Ireton-Jones CS, Turner WW, Liepa GU, Baxter CR. Equations for estimation of energy expenditure of patients with burns with special reference to ventilator status. J Burn Care Rehabil. 1992;13:330–3.

26. Faisy C, Guerot E, Diehl JL, Labrousse J, Fagon JY. Assessment of resting energy expenditure in mechanically ventilated patients. Am J Clin Nutr. 2003;78:241–9.

27. Harris JA, Benedict FG. A biometric study of the basal metabolism in man. Washington, DC: Carnegie Institution of Washington; 1919. p. 279; Publication no. 279.

28. Genton L, Pichard C. Protein catabolism and requirements in severe illness. Int J Vitam Nutr Res. 2011;81:143–52.

29. Doig GS. Early parenteral nutrition in critically ill patients with short-term relative contraindications to early enteral nutrition: a randomized controlled trial. JAMA. 2013;309:2130–8.

30. Larsson J, et al. Nitrogen requirements in severely injured patients. Br J Surg. 1990;77(4):413–6.
31. Shaw JH, et al. Whole body protein kinetics in severely septic patients. The response to glucose infusion and total parenteral nutrition. Ann Surg. 1987;205:288–94.
32. Ishibashi N, Plank LD, Sando K, Hill GL. Optimal protein requirements during the first 2 weeks after the onset of critical illness. Crit Care Med. 1998;26(9):1529–35.
33. Liebau F, Wernerman J, van Loon LJC, Rooyackers O. Effect of initiating enteral protein feeding on whole-body protein turn-over in critically ill patients. Am J Clin Nutr. 2015;101:549–57.
34. Liebau F, Sundström M, van Loon LJV, Wernerman J, Rooyackers O. Short-term amino acid infusion improves protein balance in critically ill patients. Crit Care. 2015;19:106.
35. Casaer MP, Mesotten D, Hermans G, Wouters PJ. Early versus late parenteral nutrition in critically ill adults. N Engl J Med. 2011;365:506–17.
36. Puthucheary Z, Montgomery H, Moxham J, Harridge S, Hart N. Structure to function: muscle failure in critically ill patients. J Physiol. 2010;588:4641–8.
37. Singer P, Anbar R, Cohen J, Shapiro H. The tight calorie control study (TICACOS): a prospective, randomized, controlled pilot study of nutritional support in critically ill patients. Intensive Care Med. 2011;37(4):601–9.
38. Allingstrup MJ, Esmailzadeh N, Wilkens Knudsen A, Espersen K. Provision of protein and energy in relation to measured requirements in intensive care patients. Clin Nutr. 2012;31(4):462–8.
39. Rousseau AF, Losser MR, Ichai C, Berger MM. ESPEN endorsed recommendations: nutritional therapy in major burns. Clin Nutr. 2013;32:497–502.
40. Cano N, Fiaccadori E, Tesinsky P, Toigo G, Druml W. ESPEN guidelines on enteral nutrition: acute renal failure. Clin Nutr. 2006;25:295–310.
41. Choban P, et al. ASPEN clinical guidelines. Nutrition support of hospitalised adult patients with obesity. J Parenter Enteral Nutr. 2013;37:714–44.
42. Streat SJ, Beddoe AH, Hill GL. Aggressive nutritional support does not prevent protein loss despite fat gain in septic intensive care patients. J Trauma. 1987;27:262–6.
43. Plank LD, Hill GL. Similarity of changes in body composition in intensive care patients following severe sepsis or major blunt injury. Ann N Y Acad Sci. 2000;9:592–602.

44. Monk DN, Plank LD, Franch-Arcas G, Finn PJ, Streat SJ, Hill GL. Sequential changes in the metabolic response in critically injured patients during the first 25 days after blunt trauma. Ann Surg. 1996;223:395–405.
45. De Jonghe B, Sharshar T, Lefaucheur JP, Authier FJ. Paresis acquired in the intensive care unit: a prospective multicenter study. JAMA. 2002;288:2859–67.
46. Rafferty G, Moxham J. Assessment of peripheral and respiratory muscle strength in ICU. In: Stevens R, Hart N, Herridge M, editors. Textbook of post-ICU medicine: the legacy of critical care. Oxford: Oxford University Press; 2014.
47. Manzanares W, Langloisb PL, Hardy G. Update on antioxidant micronutrients in the critically ill. Curr Opin Clin Nutr Metab Care. 2013;16:719–25.
48. Manzanares W, Dhaliwal R, Jiang X, Murch L, Heyland DK. Antioxidant micronutrients in the critically ill: a systematic review and meta-analysis β-blockers in critically ill patients: from physiology to clinical evidence. Crit Care. 2012;16:R66.
49. Reddell L, Cotton BA. Antioxidant and micronutrient supplementation in critically ill trauma patients. Curr Opin Clin Nutr Metab Care. 2012;15(2):181–7.
50. Andrews PJ, Avenell A, Noble DW, Campbell MK, Croal BL, Simpson WG, Vale LD, Battison CG, Jenkinson DJ, Cook JA, Scottish Intensive care Glutamine or seleNium Evaluative Trial Trials Group. Randomised trial of glutamine, selenium, or both, to supplement parenteral nutrition for critically ill patients. BMJ. 2011;342:d1542.
51. Heyland D, Muscedere J, Wischmeyer PE, Cook D, Jones G, Albert M, Elke G, Berger MM, Day AG, Canadian Critical Care Trials Group. A randomized trial of glutamine and antioxidants in critically ill patients. N Engl J Med. 2013;368(16):1489–97.
52. Wernerman J. How to understand the results of studies of glutamine supplementation. Crit Care. 2015;19:385.
53. Coppola S, Froio S, Chiumello D. β-blockers in critically ill patients: from physiology to clinical evidence. Crit Care. 2015;19:119.
54. Gervasio JM, Dickerson RN, Swearingen J, Yates ME, Yuen C, Fabian TC, Croce MA, Brown RO. Oxandrolone in trauma patients. Pharmacotherapy. 2000;20(11):1328–34.
55. Kreymann KG, Berger MM, Deutz NE, Hiesmayr M. ESPEN guidelines on enteral nutrition: intensive care. Clin Nutr. 2006;25(2):210–23.

56. Clinical practice guideline for nutrition support in the mechanically ventilated, critically ill adult patient. www.criticalcarenutrition.com. Accessed 4 Oct 2015.
57. McClave SA, et al. Guidelines for the provision and assessment of nutrition support therapy in the adult critically ill patient: Society of Critical Care Medicine (SCCM) and American Society for Parenteral and Enteral Nutrition (A.S.P.E.N.). J Parenter Enteral Nutr. 2009;33(3):277–316.
58. Martin CM, Doig GS, Heyland DK, Morrison T, Sibbald WJ, Southwestern Ontario Critical Care Research Network. Multicentre, cluster-randomized clinical trial of algorithms for critical-care enteral and parenteral therapy (ACCEPT). CMAJ. 2004;170:197–204.
59. Harvey SE, Parrott F, Harrison DA, Bear DE. Trial of the route of early nutritional support in critically ill adults. N Engl J Med. 2014;371(18):1673–84.
60. Heidegger CP, Berger MM, Graf S, Zingg W. Optimisation of energy provision with supplemental parenteral nutrition in critically ill patients: a randomised controlled clinical trial. Lancet. 2013;381(9864):385–93.
61. Heyland DK, Dhaliwal R, Drover JW, Gramlich L, Dodek P. Canadian clinical practice guidelines for nutrition support in mechanically ventilated, critically ill adult patients. J Parenter Enteral Nutr. 2003;27:355–73.
62. Simpson D. Parenteral vs. enteral nutrition in the critically ill patient: a meta-analysis of trials using the intention to treat principle. Intensive Care Med. 2005;31(1):12–23.
63. Gramlich L, Kichian K, Pinilla J, Rodych NJ, Dhaliwal R, Heyland DK. Does enteral nutrition compared to parenteral nutrition result in better outcomes in critically ill adult patients? A systematic review of the literature. Nutrition. 2004;20:843–8.
64. Compton F, et al. Use of a nutrition support protocol to increase enteral nutrition delivery in critically ill patients. Am J Crit Care. 2014;23(5):369–403.
65. Mackenzie S, et al. Implementation of a nutrition support protocol increases the proportion of mechanically ventilated patients reaching enteral nutrition targets in the adult intensive care unit. J Parenter Enteral Nutr. 2005;29:74–80.
66. Enhanced protein-energy provision via the enteral route feeding protocol in critically ill patients: The PEP uP protocol. http://www.criticalcarenutrition.com/docs/tools/NIBBLE_Issue8_Generic.pdf=refPepup. Accessed 4 Oct 2015.

67. Taylor B, Brody R, Denmark R, Southard R, Byham-Gray L. Improving enteral delivery through the adoption of the "Feed Early Enteral Diet Adequately for Maximum Effect (FEED ME)" protocol in a surgical trauma ICU: a quality improvement review. Nutr Clin Pract. 2014;29(5):639–48.
68. Ott L, Young B, Phillips R, McClain C, Adams L, Dempsey R, Tibbs P, Ryo UY. Altered gastric emptying in the head-injured patient: relationship to feeding intolerance. J Neurosurg. 1991;74(5):738–42.
69. Hamada SR, Garcon P, Ronot M, Kerever S, Paugam-Burtz C, Mantz J. Ultrasound assessment of gastric volume in critically ill patients. Intensive Care Med. 2014;40:965–72.
70. McClave SA, Lukan JK, Stefater JA, Lowen CC. Poor validity of residual volumes as a marker for risk of aspiration in critically ill patients. Crit Care Med. 2005;33(2):324–30.
71. Montejo JC, et al. Gastric residual volume during enteral nutrition in ICU patients: the REGANE study. Intensive Care Med. 2010;36(8):1386–93.
72. Reignier J, Mercier E, Le Gouge A, Boulain T, Desachy A, Bellec F, Clavel M, Frat JP, Plantefeve G, Quenot JP, Lascarrou JB, Clinical Research in Intensive Care and Sepsis (CRICS) Group. Effect of not monitoring residual gastric volume on risk of ventilator-associated pneumonia in adults receiving mechanical ventilation and early enteral feeding: a randomized controlled trial. JAMA. 2013;309(3):249–56.
73. Nguyen NQ, Chapman MJ, Fraser RJ, Bryant LK, Holloway RH. Erythromycin is more effective than metoclopramide in the treatment of feed intolerance in critical illness. Crit Care Med. 2007;35:483–9.
74. Gert van der Meer Y, Venhuizen WA, Heyland DK, van Zanten ARH. Should we stop prescribing metoclopramide as a prokinetic drug in critically ill patients? Crit Care. 2014;18(5):502.
75. Niv E, Fireman Z, Vaisman N. Post-pyloric feeding. World J Gastroenterol. 2009;15:1281–8.
76. Zhang Z, Xu X, Ding J, Ni H. Comparison of postpyloric tube feeding and gastric tube feeding in intensive care unit patients: a meta-analysis. Nutr Clin Pract. 2013;28:371–80.
77. Sertaridou E, Papaioannou V, Kolios G, Pneumatikosa I. Gut failure in critical care: old school versus new school. Ann Gastroenterol. 2015;28:309–22.
78. Vanderheyden S, et al. Early versus late parenteral nutrition in ICU patients: cost analysis of the EPaNIC trial. Crit Care. 2012;16:R96.

79. Grimble R. Fatty acid profile of modern lipid emulsions: scientific considerations for creating the ideal composition. Clin Nutr Suppl. 2005;1:9–15.
80. NCEPOD: parenteral nutrition: a mixed bag. http://www.ncepod.org.uk/2010pn.html, http://www.ncepod.org.uk/2010report1/downloads/PN_report.pdf.
81. International Nutrition Survey. http://www.criticalcarenutrition.com/index.php?option=com_content&view=article&id=146&Itemid=50. Accessed 4 Oct 2015.
82. Oudemans-van Straaten HM, Ostermann M. Bench-to-bedside review: citrate for continuous renal replacement therapy, from science to practice. Crit Care. 2012;16:249. DOI: 10.1186/cc11645. © BioMed Central Ltd 2012. Published 7 December 2012.
83. Mehanna HM, Moledina J, Travis J. Refeeding syndrome: what it is, and how to prevent and treat it. BMJ. 2008;336:1495–8.
84. Goyale A, Ashley SL, Taylor DR, Elnenaei MO, et al. Predicting refeeding hypophosphataemia: insulin growth factor 1 (IGF-1) as a diagnostic biochemical marker for clinical practice. Ann Clin Biochem. 2015;52:82–7.
85. NICE clinical guideline 32. 2006. http://www.nice.org.uk/guidance/cg32/resources/guidance-nutrition-support-in-adults-pdf. Accessed 4 Oct 2015.

Chapter 18
Venous Thromboembolism in Critically Injured Patients

Ian Ewington

Abstract Critically ill trauma patients present a range of particular challenges with respect to prevention and treatment of venous thromboembolism (VTE). The incidence of VTE is high in trauma patients. Prevention should be through combined mechanical and chemical methods unless there are contraindications. There is a small amount of evidence to indicate superiority of low molecular weight heparin over unfractionated heparin in the prevention of pulmonary embolism. Patients with head and spinal injuries are particularly at risk from VTE but it is extremely difficult to provide definitive guidance as to the timing of thromboprophylaxis initiation. VTE should be diagnosed using multiple modalities, including Duplex and cardiac ultrasound as well as CT. Patients with pulmonary embolism (PE) should have their risk stratified depending on the presence of absence of right ventricular

I. Ewington, MBChB, MML, MRCP, FRCA, FFICM
Department of Anaesthesia, Royal Centre for Defence Medicine,
Queen Elizabeth Hospital Birmingham,
Mindelsohn Way, Edgbaston, Birmingham B15 2WB, UK
e-mail: ianewington1@nhs.net

S.D. Hutchings (ed.), *Trauma and Combat Critical Care in Clinical Practice*, In Clinical Practice,
DOI 10.1007/978-3-319-28758-4_18,
© Crown Copyright 2016

(RV) strain. Those with RV strain should be considered for thrombolytic treatment or catheter embolectomy. The use of inferior vena caval filters may offer a solution to prevention of VTE in high risk patients, particularly those with contra indications to chemical thromboprophylaxis.

Keywords   Venous thromboembolism • Deep venous thrombosis • Pulmonary embolism • Trauma • Thromboprophylaxis • Inferior vena cava filter • Unfractionated heparin • Low molecular weight heparin

What Is the Incidence of Venous Thromboembolism in the Critically Injured Patient Population?

Venous thromboembolism (VTE) is an important cause of mortality and morbidity in critically ill patients and is particularly prevalent in those who have suffered severe traumatic injury. This is, in part, due to the pathophysiological processes which follow major trauma and lead to abnormal coagulation profiles as well as direct mechanical effects on the venous system. Combined with periods of prolonged immobility these factors put such patients at increased risk of VTE following major traumatic injury. Delayed initiation of prophylaxis and prolonged immobilisation also seem to have significance in the critically injured patient population [1, 2]. In one epidemiological study of 7937 trauma patients the reported incidence of VTE was 1.8 %; however, 81 % of these patients were receiving either mechanical and/or chemical prophylaxis [3]. The reported incidence of VTE varies widely depending on the study population, the injuries sustained and the presence or absence of specific risk factors and has been reported to be as high as 58 % [3].

Pulmonary embolism (PE) remains relatively common after trauma and a significant proportion occur early, within the first 5 days [4]. Specific risk factors within this cohort include advancing age, long bone fracture, pelvic fracture, traumatic brain injury and spinal cord injury [5]. PEmay occur in the absence of spinal or lower limb fractures andthere is some evidence to suggest that deep vein thrombosis (DVT) is not always present. In a study of 1872 severely injured blunt trauma patients only 5.7 % of those who had a PE also had evidence of DVT [5].

What Mechanical Methods Should Be Used to Prevent DVT?

The UK Defence Medical Services (UK DMS) guidelines for prevention of VTE in critically ill patients is shown in Fig. 18.1

Combination therapy with mechanical and pharmacological elements is likely to provide the most comprehensive reduction in risk of VTE, where there are no contraindications. For those at high risk of bleeding then mechanical methods aloneshould be considered. This may include the use of graduated compression stockingsand intermittent pneumatic compression (IPC) devices where appropriate. However, the American College of Physicians guidelines (2011) [6] for prevention of VTE in medical patients suggests that mechanical devices be avoided. In a systematic review of three trials, there was no statistical difference between those who had mechanical prophylaxis and those that did not. One of the major concerns they noted was lower limb skin breakage. This was statistically significant at 39 events per 1000 patients treated (RR 4.02 [CI 2.34–6.91] [6]).

A Cochrane Database publication did suggest there was evidence for the use of compression stockings however the review predominantly looked at data from surgical patients [7]. Therefore in the absence of an obvious contraindication, the use of compression stockings would seem advisable in critically ill trauma patients until there is any evidence to the contrary.

Effectiveness of graduated compression stockings has also not been reported in the trauma population. Intermittent pneumatic compression devices however, have been studied in a randomized trial comparing IPC to the venous foot pump

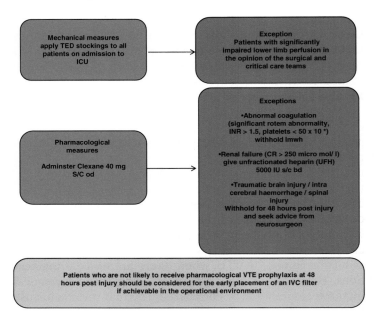

FIGURE 18.1 UK DMS guideline for prevention of VTE in critically ill patients

(VFP) in injured patients. After randomisation of 149 patients without lower extremity fractures, the authors demonstrated a statistically significant decrease in the incidence of DVT using IPC when compared to VFP (6.5 % vs 21 %). This would suggest that VFP should play no role in DVT prophylaxis in trauma patients [8].

What Pharmacological Methods Should Be Used to Prevent VTE?

Coagulation abnormalities often cause pharmaceutical prophylaxis to be withheld due to the assumption that there is an increased bleeding risk. However this may not always be the case, indeed there may be a pro-coagulant state in the first 48 hours following trauma and massive transfusion; possibly due to a decrease in anti-thrombin III levels and suppression of fibrinolysis [9]. There are of course special circumstances related to head and spinal injuries, these will be discussed later.

A retrospective review of 513 coagulopathic (INR >1.5 or platelets <100,000 per microlitre) critically ill surgical patients where chemical prophylaxis had either been given or withheld showed no significant difference between the two groups when comparing the incidence of VTE. This led the authors to conclude that in the critically ill patient with evidence of coagulopathy chemical prophylaxis may not be of benefit [10]. Further work is needed in this complex area with the aim of trying to identify which patients require early chemical thromboprophylaxis. Thromboelastography may be helpful here as a more sensitive marker of coagulation defects than traditional lab based assays. UK Defence Medical Services guidelinesrecommend the early introduction of chemical thromboprophylaxis as soon as thromoboelastography results have normalised which often occurs faster than the normalisation of other variables, such as the INR.

When considering which form of heparin is most appropriate for VTE prophylaxis, there appears to be little difference between low molecular weight heparin (LMWH) and low dose subcutaneous unfractionated heparin (UFH) in meta-analyses of randomised controlled trials. Bleeding risks are also comparable [11, 12]. Neither agent requires therapeutic monitoring in adults though it is possible to measure anti-Xa levels as a guide to LMWH therapy. The dose of LMWH will need to be reduced, or UFH substituted, if there is significant renal impairment [13].

In trauma there is evidence that there is an increased risk of heparin induced thrombocytopaenia (HIT) and the risk increases with the severity of trauma; there was a correlation between a higher Abbreviated Injury Score (AIS) and development of HIT (P=0.03) [14].

A recent multicentre trial of 3764 patients compared LMWH and UFH in the critically ill patient population. One group received dalteparin, the other UFH. The incidence of proximal leg DVT was not significanty different between the two groups. However, the incidence of PE was significantly lower in those receiving dalteparin (1.3 % vs 2.3 %) [15].

The use of once daily dosing of low molecular weight heparin (743 patients, average ISS 19.5) was studied prospectively and found to be safe and effective in high risk trauma patients, including in those with head injury. Compliance with the once daily dosing protocol was maintained in 74 % of the patients. DVT was detected in 3.9 % and PE in 0.8 % [16].

What Are the Special Considerations for VTE Prophylaxis in Patients with Head and Spinal Trauma?

Traumatic brain injury (TBI) is associated with an increased risk of VTE. A recent study which prospectively looked for evidence of proximal DVT using daily Duplex scanning found an incidence of 17 % in patients with moderate or severe TBI [17]. However the difficulty comes in knowing when it is safe to administer prophylactic anticoagulation in the presence or risk of intracranial haemorrhage (ICH). Previous research seems to suggest that it is safe to administer early LMWH prophylaxis in selected patients with ICH [18, 19]. However the decision of when to commence treatment will have to remain at the discretion of the treating clinicians given the multiple factors to take into account. The important elements to consider are the increased risk of VTE in the first four days following injury and the previous evidence suggesting safety of LMWH prophylaxis in some patients with ICH.

Higher dose anticoagulation holds a greater risk of bleeding and therefore for those patients with proven DVT or PE then further difficult decisions may become necessary. As earlier, the decisions will have to rest with the treating clinicians as the nature of the condition does not allow for definitive advice.

VTE is a common complication following spinal cord injury, however much like head injury there is often a reticence to administer chemical prophylaxis due to perceived risks of exacerbating bleeding and injury. Analysis of data from 18,302 patients with spinal cord injury concluded that those with a high thoracic injury (T1-T6) were at greatest risk of VTE (rate of 6.3 %) and those with a high cervical spinal injury were at lowest risk (rate of 3.4 %) [20].

If there is radiological evidence of spinal haematoma then it is appropriate to use mechanical methods alone initially as the VTE risk in isolated spinal injury is low for the first 3 days. The difference between administration before and after 72 h has been reported as significant (incidence of DVT of 2 % and 26 % respectively) [21].

How Can VTE Be Diagnosed?

Clinical diagnosis of DVT in trauma can be difficult due to associated tissue damage which means the classical symptoms of thigh pain, swelling and redness may be masked. This may also be the case for PE, particularly if the patient has associated chest trauma. This means clinicians need to consider the use of other diagnostic tests.

D-dimer

When venous thrombosis occurs, the coagulation and fibrinolytic systems are activated. Fibrin monomers are cross-linked into a polymer chain and these chains are subsequently degraded during the fibrinolytic process by plasmin. One of the terminal products of this process is the D-dimer fibrin fragment. This can be tested for using a monoclonal antibody assay with high sensitivity for VTE.

The main problem with using this test in polytrauma patients is that the presence of clot from the original injuriesare likely to cause elevated levels of D-dimer antigen thus making it a poor diagnostic tool in this group with a low specificity for VTE [22].

Ultrasound

Duplex ultrasound combines real-time B-mode ultrasound with pulsed Doppler and colour flow imaging allowing an assessment of physiological flow to be made. During the examination, non-compressibility of the vein is highly suggestive of DVT. Echogenic thrombus maybe visualised within the lumen and there maybe evidence of venous distension. However, duplex ultrasound cannot reliably image the iliac veins and patient factors such as pain or swelling may limit the test. In a review of high risk asymptomatic patients, duplex ultrasound imaging was not accurate as a screening method for DVT when compared with venography [23].

Chest Radiograph

There are several non-specific findings of pulmonary embolism which may be seen on a chest radiograph including pleural effusion, consolidation, atelectasis and cardiomegaly. Effusions may be seen in around a quarter of cases and these are usually exudative. Focal lucency beyond an occluded vessel, which may be accompanied by mild dilatation of the central pulmonary vessels known as Westermark's sign, was seen in 7–14 % of cases in the PIOPED I study [24]. It is thought to be secondary to embolic obstruction of the pulmonary artery or hypoxic vasoconstriction secondary to ventilation of poorly perfused lung. Therefore although not helpful in providing a firm diagnosis these are signs that may allow the clinician to target subsequent investigations.

Electrocardiography and Echocardiography

The ECG may show some of the common signs of right ventricular overload including sinus tachycardia, T-wave inversion (V1-V4, III and aVF), right bundle branch block (complete or partial), P pulmonale (II and III) and atrial fibrillation.

Echocardiography should be readily available and is a useful tool in assisting with diagnosis. Signs include: Increased RV/LV ratio; hypokinesia or akinesia of the RV free wall; RV dilatation; pulmonary artery dilatation and regurgitant flow through the tricuspid valve of >2.8 m/s [25].

Computed Tomographic Pulmonary Angiography (CTPA)

CT scans are now widely available and this modality has become the test of choice for clinicians in diagnosing PE. It allows the thrombus to be visualised directly both for central and, with the advent of multiple slice scans, for sub-segmental PEs. CTPA has been shown to be more sensitive than ventilation-perfusion (V/Q) scanning [26].

CTPA also has the advantage that it may diagnose pathology that presents in a similar way to PE. It can also demonstrate an enlarged right ventricle which has been shown to be associated with poor outcome following PE [27].

Ventilation-Perfusion Scanning

Ventilation-perfusion scans have formed the mainstay of PE diagnosis for over 30 years. Whilst CTPA has supplanted this, in many institutions V/Q scanning is still performed. The disadvantage of the scans comes from the interpretation of the images and the utility of the result passed to the clinician.

The criteria for 'high probability' and 'low probability' scans vary with the interpreter but depend on size and number of perfusion defects as well as relationship to the chest radiograph. The probability from the scan must be combined with the clinical probability in order to arrive at a diagnosis. Unfortunately, most scans are indeterminate and those of 'low probability' do not equate to a normal scan. Lower extremity ultrasound may be beneficial in such patients but only a negative result can assist with excluding VTE.

Cardiac Markers

Myocardial injury in patients with PE can be demonstrated using troponin (I or T). There is a strong association between elevated troponin I and right ventricular dysfunction in normotensive patients with PE. The presence of either is associated with a higher mortality which may be of benefit in risk stratification [28].

What Is the Management of DVT in Critically Ill Trauma Patients?

In terms of definitive treatment for DVT, LMWH is at least as safe and effective as UFH and has the major advantage that it is easier to administer and monitor [29]. Enoxaparin has been proven effective in treating venous thromboembolism [30]. A dose regimen for enoxaparin of 1 mg/kg twice daily or 1.5 mg/kg once daily was proven to be equally effective and as safe as continuously infused UFH [31]. The treatment of isolated calf DVT has remained a controversial subject area [32]. The timing and type of anticoagulation will be significantly influenced by the need for subsequent surgical procedures as well as the type of injuries sustained. Therefore this will need to be weighed up by the treating clinician against the risks of withholding anticoagulation. As with considerations for VTE prophylaxis, therapeutic management may be influenced by head injuries, spinal injuries and non-operatively managed spleen or liver lacerations. The guideline used by the UK DMS for the treatment of VTE in critically injured patients is shown in Fig. 18.2.

There is potential for an incidental asymptomatic calf vein thrombosis to be diagnosed on imaging in the trauma patient. In a small retrospective analysis of symptomatic isolated calf

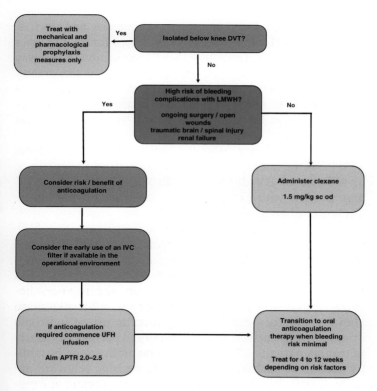

FIGURE 18.2 UK DMS guideline for treatment of VTE in critically ill patients

DVT it was suggested that the risk of progression is minimal and that observation only should be performed followed by a subsequent scan 1–2 weeks later [33]. When one considers the additional risks of anti-coagulating a trauma patient this would seem appropriate.

What Is the Presentation and Management of PE?

PE is commonly defined as massive, sub massive and low risk. The American Heart Association definitions for the sub types of PE are shown in Table 18.1 [34]. Classification in this way is of limited use when considering mortality as the greater influence is co-morbidities. In the case of trauma patients, a low risk PE in someone with multiple injuries and obstructive airways disease for example may still lead to significant complications.

The critical factor affecting the prognosis of patients with PE is the haemodynamic impact; in effect the presence or absence of RV dysfunction. Patients with massive PE may present with cardiac arrest, shock and hypotension. Occlusion of greater than 30–50 % of the pulmonary vascular bed will result in haemodynamic disturbance [35]. Around 10 % will die suddenly from acute obstruction of the pulmonary bed. Acute massive PE leads to cor pulmonale which may result in acute RV dilatation, hypokinesis, tachycardia, presence of gallop rhythm and signs of elevated central venous pressure. As per the AHA definition above, circulatory instability requires the use of inotropic or vasopressor support to maintain organ perfusion. Clearly in trauma patients other causes of haemodynamic instability need to be excluded. This is where bedside echocardiography may be especially useful in acute assessment and risk stratification.

TABLE 18.1 AHA definitions of types of PE with associated mortality risks

PE related early mortality risk and classification	Shock or hypotension SBP <90 mmHg for >15 min	RV dysfunction	Myocardial injury	Treatment implications
High >15 % massive PE	+	+	+	Thrombolysis or embolectomy
Intermediate 3–15 % sub-massive PE	–	+	+	Hospital admission
		+	–	
		–	+	
Low <1 % low risk PE	–	–	–	Potentially managed at home

Adapted from Torbicki et al. [36]

Initial Treatment

Those who present in cardiac arrest should be managed accordingly and where PE is the likely diagnosis, consideration should be given to targeted therapy as outlined below (See Fig. 18.3 for suggested treatment algorithm adapted

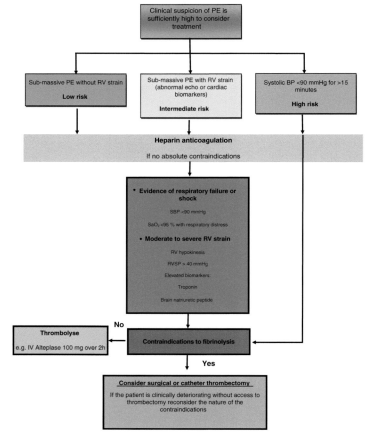

FIGURE 18.3 Suggested treatment algorithm for Pulmonary Emoblism (Adapted from Jaff et al. [34])

from AHA scientific statement 2011). Supportive treatment may become necessary for both cardiovascular and respiratory failure. Norepinephrine has been demonstrated to improve RV function via a direct positive inotropic effect as well as coronary perfusion and increase in systemic blood pressure. If this fails the addition of other inotropic drugs will be required.

If mechanical ventilation is required or has already been instituted, then there is a potential for worsening RV failure secondary to reduced venous return from the positive intra-thoracic pressure. Lung protective strategies should be employed but positive end expiratory pressure (PEEP) applied cautiously.

Anticoagulation and Thrombolytic Therapy

Trauma patients with confirmed PE should ideally receive prompt anticoagulation with low molecular weight heparin. Those with intermediate or high risk of PE should be anti-coagulated whilst awaiting diagnosis. If there are contraindications, these need to be weighed up by the treating clinician. Considerations include those discussed earlier with regard to head and spinal injuries. However, the requirement for further surgery as well as the propensity to bleed from wounds particularly in the liver and spleen will likely influence clinicians decision making. This may also mean that shorter acting agents such as UFH may be more appropriate compared to fully anti-coagulating with LMWH. Once patients are clinically stable then they should be considered for oral therapy such as warfarin or rivaroxaban.

Thrombolytic therapy carries a significant risk of bleeding therefore in the majority of trauma patients the use of it has to be weighed up very carefully. The fibrinolytic drugs will actively break down clot by converting circulating plasminogen into plasmin. This splits the fibrin resulting in breakdown products including D-dimer fragments. Summative data from a number of randomised trials across all types of patients suggests a 13 % cumulative rate of major bleeding and a 1.8 % of intracranial or fatal haemorrhage [36]. In life threatening PE some trauma patients with a bleeding risk may still benefit from thrombolysis if for example cardiac arrest is imminent and there is no time or ability to remove the clot by other methods such as surgical thrombectomy.

Around 92 % of patients can be classified as responding to thrombolysis based on clinical improvement within the first 36 h [37]. Whilst treatment should be initiated within 48 h of the onset of symptoms, thrombolysis maybe beneficial for up to 14 days depending on the clinical circumstances [38].

Surgical Embolectomy

Surgical removal of clots under direct vision was in the past reserved for those patients who required cardiopulmonary resuscitation. However it has been shown to be potentially beneficial in those high risk cases where thrombolysis is contraindicated. It is dependent on rapid diagnosis to clarify clot burden on CT scan and right ventricular dysfunction on echocardiogram [39]. Previous thrombolysis is not considered a contraindication to surgical embolectomy when it has failed to result in clinical improvement. Prolonged periods of cardiopulmonary bypass may be a necessity following the procedure whilst right ventricular function recovers.

Catheter Assisted Pulmonary Embolectomy

Catheter based techniques should be widely available in most centres where interventional radiology is practiced. They are better tolerated and allow thrombolytics to be directed into the pulmonary circulation at a fraction of the dose required for systemic administration. In addition, fragmentation is often possible which allows redistribution of clot and reduction of the RV afterload. The disadvantage to the technique is that the clot needs to be accessible in proximal pulmonary vessels. The availability of endovascular devices for the pulmonary vasculature is limited but new ultrasonic systems have been introduced to enhance clot dissolution.

When Should Sub Massive PE Be Treated and What Strategies Are Available?

Patients who are normotensive with evidence of RV dysfunction or myocardial necrosis would be regarded as having a sub massive PE. In most cases treatment with LMWH would be the strategy of choice after consideration for the potential bleeding risk. Data from six trials suggest that this group do not benefit from thrombolysis and if they are trauma patients then it is highly likely that the risk will outweigh the benefit [40].

What Is the Role of Inferior Vena Cava Filters in the Prevention of VTE?

If there are contraindications to chemical thromboprophylaxis in high risk patients or in the case of proven DVT, to treatment, then it may be beneficial to consider the use of an inferior vena cava (IVC) filter an example of which is shown in Fig. 18.4. The benefits that may be gained from the use of the filter needs to be weighed against the risks associated with their use including caval occlusion, infection and migration. However in recent years the use of retrievable filters has mitigated these risks to some degree.

The use of filters can be either considered prophylactic where there is a risk of VTE or therapeutic when there is proven VTE. The use of prophylactic IVC filters is controversial; a meta-analysis suggested that the incidence of PE was statistically lower in the group with IVC filters in place, however the strength of evidence is low [41]. There are published

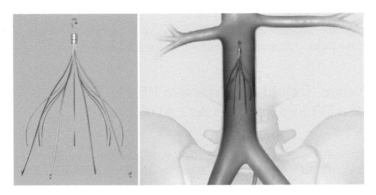

FIGURE 18.4 Retrievable IVC filter – paramagnetic filter with platinum markers (Celect Platinum Vena Cava filter, William Cook Europe ApS, Bjaeverskov, Denmark, *reproduced with permission*)

guidelinesthat suggestfilters should be inserted prophylactically in trauma where there is a contraindication to anticoagulation or a complex and severe injury pattern [42]. Once the contraindication to anticoagulation has passed it should be instituted and continued until the filter has been removed. However, removal is not always possiblealthough this has improved in recent years with the development of retrievable filters.

There was a review of the usage of IVC filters in US military trauma patients published in 2009 [43]. Of theseventy 2 cases reviewed over a 4 year period, 23 were placed for prophylactic reasons and 49 were therapeutic. There were no cases of breakthrough PEs, migration or occlusion. However anticoagulation was continued in both groups. Retrieval rates were only 18 % due to contraindications to removal, loss to follow-up or in some cases technical issues; the mainsuch issue being incorporation of the filter into the caval wall which was most frequently seen in those filters left in place for over 90 days.

The development of the IVC filter-catheter offers clinicians the ability to place a caval filter at the bedside on the ICU. The Angel® catheter (Fig. 18.5) combines a triple

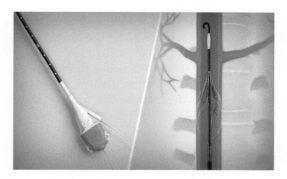

FIGURE 18.5 Angel IVC filter-catheter – external catheter hub when filter is positioned and expanded in the IVC

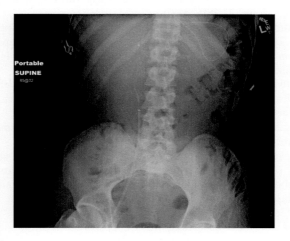

FIGURE 18.6 Radiographic appearance of an appropriately deployed filter inserted via the right femoral vein (biO2 Medical, San Antonio, Texas, reproduced with permission)

lumen central venous catheter and a self-expanding IVC filter. It is designed to be placed without fluoroscopy via femoral venous access (Fig. 18.6) and it should be removed once the contraindication to anticoagulation is no longer present. There have been several small published studies using these devices clinically which have suggested they can successfully prevent PE [44, 45]. However a larger trial is necessary to compare them with other filters and therapies. A trial, comparing the safety and effectiveness of these catheters against standard pharmacological therapy began recruitment in 2015 [45].

References

1. Geerts WH, Bergqvist D, Pineo GF, et al. Prevention of venous thromboembolism: American College of Chest Physicians Evidence-Based Clinical Practice Guidelines (8th Edition). Chest. 2008;133:381S–453.
2. Knudson MM, Ikossi DG, Khaw L, Morabito D, Speetzen LS. Thromboembolism after trauma: an analysis of 1602 episodes from the American College of Surgeons National Trauma Data Bank. Ann Surg. 2004;240:490–6.
3. Paffrath T, Wafaisade A, Lefering R, et al. Venous thromboembolism after severe trauma: incidence, risk factors and outcome. Injury. 2010;41(1):97–101.
4. Menaker J, Stein DM, Scalea TM. Incidence of early pulmonary embolism after injury. J Trauma. 2007;63:620–4.
5. Brakenridge SC, Henley SS, Kashner TM, et al. Comparing clinical predictors of deep venous thrombosis versus pulmonary embolus after severe injury: a new paradigm for posttraumatic venous thromboembolism? J Trauma Acute Care Surg. 2013;74(5):1231–7.
6. Qaseem A, Chou R, Humphrey LL, et al. Venous thromboembolism prophylaxis in hospitalized patients: a clinical practice guideline from the American College of Physicians. Ann Intern Med. 2011;155(9):625–32.
7. Sachdeva A, Dalton M, Amaragiri SV, Lees T. Elastic compression stockings for prevention of deep vein thrombosis during a hospital stay. Cochrane Database of Systematic Reviews. 2010;(7):CD001484.
8. Elliott CG, Dudney TM, Egger M, Orme JF, Clemmer TP, Horn SD, Weaver L, Handrahan D, Thomas F, Merrell S, Kitterman N, Yeates S. Calf-thigh sequential pneumatic compression compared with plantar venous pneumatic compression to prevent

deep-vein thrombosis after non-lower extremity trauma. J Trauma. 1999;47:25–32.

9. Enderson BL, Chen JP, Robinson R, Maull KI. Fibrinolysis in multisystem trauma patients. J Trauma. 1991;31(9):1240–6.

10. Edwards M, Felder S, Ley E, et al. Venous thromboembolism in coagulopathic surgical intensive care unit patients: is there a benefit from chemical prophylaxis? J Trauma. 2011;70(6): 1398–400.

11. Koch A, Ziegler S, Breitschwerdt H, Victor N. Low molecular weight heparin and unfractionated heparin in thrombosis prophylaxis: meta-analysis based on original patient data. Thromb Res. 2001;102(4):295–309.

12. Koch A, Bouges S, Ziegler S, Dinkel H, Daures JP, Victor N. Low molecular weight heparin and unfractionated heparin in thrombosis prophylaxis after major surgical intervention: update of previous meta-analyses. Br J Surg. 1997;84(6):750–9.

13. Boneu B. Low molecular weight heparin therapy: is monitoring needed? Thromb Haemost. 1994;72(3):330–4.

14. Hinz P, Thomaschewski S, Lietz T, et al. The severity of trauma determines the immune response to PF4/heparin and the frequency of heparin-induced thrombocytopenia. Blood. 2010; 115(9):1797–803 1.

15. The PROTECT Investigators for the Canadian Critical Care Trials Group and the Australian and New Zealand Intensive Care Society Clinical Trials Group. Dalteparin versus unfractionated heparin in critically Ill patients. N Engl J Med. 2011;364:1305–14.

16. Cothren CC, Smith WR, Moore EE, Morgan SJ. Utility of once-daily dose of low-molecular-weight heparin to prevent venous thromboembolism in multisystem trauma patients. World J Surg. 2007;31(1):98–104.

17. Nichol A, French C, Little L, The EPO –TBI Investigators. Erythropoietin in traumatic brain injury (EPO-TBI): a double-blind randomised controlled trial. Lancet. 2015;386(10012): 2499–506.

18. Norwood SH, Berne JD, Rowe SA, Villarreal DH, Ledlie JT. Early venous thromboembolism prophylaxis with enoxaparin in patients with blunt traumatic brain injury. J Trauma. 2008;65:1021–7.

19. Koehler D, Shipman J, Davidson M, et al. Is early venous thromboembolism prophylaxis safe in trauma patients with intracranial hemorrhage. J Trauma. 2011;70(2):324–9.

20. Maung AA, Schuster KM, Kaplan LJ, et al. Risk of venous thromboembolism after spinal cord injury: not all levels are the same. J Trauma. 2011;71(5):1241–5.
21. Aito S, Pieri A, D'Andrea M, Marcelli F, Cominelli E. Primary prevention of deep venous thrombosis and pulmonary embolism in acute spinal cord injured patients. Spinal Cord. 2002;40: 300–3.
22. Wells PS, Anderson DR, Ginsberg J. Assessment of deep vein thrombosis or pulmonary embolism by the combined use of clinical model and non-invasive diagnostic tests. Sem Thromb Hemost. 2000;26(6):643–56.
23. Agnelli G, Radicchia S, Nenci GG. Diagnosis of deep vein thrombosis in asymptomatic high-risk patients. Haemostasis. 1995;25:40–8.
24. Worsley DF, Alavi A, Aronchick JM, Chen JT, Greenspan RH, Ravin CE. Chest radiographic findings in patients with acute pulmonary embolism: observations from the PIOPED Study. Radiology. 1993;189(1):133–6.
25. Kreit JW. The impact of right ventricular dysfunction on the prognosis and therapy of normotensive patients with pulmonary embolism. Chest. 2004;125:1539–45.
26. Anderson DR, Kahn SR, Rodger MA, et al. Computed tomographic pulmonary angiography vs ventilation-perfusion lung scanning in patients with suspected pulmonary embolism: a randomized controlled trial. JAMA. 2007;298(23):2743–53.
27. Kang DK, Thilo C, Schoepf UJ, Barraza Jr JM, Nance Jr JW, Bastarrika G, et al. CT signs of right ventricular dysfunction: prognostic role in acute pulmonary embolism. JACC Cardiovasc Imaging. 2011;4:841–9.
28. Keller K, Beule J, Schulz A, Coldewey M, Dippold W, Balzer JO. Cardiac troponin I for predicting right ventricular dysfunction and intermediate risk in patients with normotensive pulmonary embolism. Neth Heart J. 2015;23(1):55–61.
29. Quinlan DJ, et al. Low-molecular-weight heparin compared with intravenous unfractionated heparin for treatment of pulmonary embolism: a meta-analysis of randomized, controlled trials. Ann Intern Med. 2004;140:175–83.
30. The Columbus Investigators. Low-molecular-weight heparin in the treatment of patients with venous thromboembolism. The Columbus Investigators. N Engl J Med. 1997;337:657–62.
31. Merli G, Spiro TE, Olsson CG, et al. Subcutaneous enoxaparin once or twice daily compared with intravenous unfractionated

heparin for treatment of venous thromboembolic disease, Ann Intern Med. 2001;134(3):191–202.

32. Righini M, Paris S, Grégoire LG, Laroche JP, Perrier A, Bounameaux H. Clinical relevance of distal deep vein thrombosis. Review of literature data. Thromb Haemost. 2006;95: 56–64.

33. Sule AA, Chin TJ, Handa P, Earnest A. Should symptomatic, isolated distal deep vein thrombosis be treated with anticoagulation? Int J Angiol. 2009;18(2):83–7.

34. Jaff MR, McMurtry MS, Archer SL, et al. Management of massive and submassive pulmonary embolism, iliofemoral deep vein thrombosis, and chronic thromboembolic pulmonary hypertension: a scientific statement from the American Heart Association. Circulation. 2011;123:1788–830.

35. McIntyre KM, Sasahara AA. The hemodynamic response to pulmonary embolism in patients without prior cardiopulmonary disease. Am J Cardiol. 1971;28:288–94.

36. Torbicki A, Perrier A, Konstantinides S, et al. Guidelines on the diagnosis and management of acute pulmonary embolism: the Task Force for the Diagnosis and Management of Acute Pulmonary Embolism of the European Society of Cardiology (ESC). Eur Heart J. 2008;29:2276–315.

37. Meneveau N, Seronde MF, Blonde MC, Legalery P, Didier-Petit K, Briand F, et al. Management of unsuccessful thrombolysis in acute massive pulmonary embolism. Chest. 2006;129:1043–50.

38. Daniels LB, Parker JA, Patel SR, Grodstein F, Goldhaber SZ. Relation of duration of symptoms with response to thrombolytic therapy in pulmonary embolism. Am J Cardiol. 1997;80:184–8.

39. Leacche M, Unic D, Goldhaber SZ, Rawn JD, Aranki SF, Couper GS, et al. Modern surgical treatment of massive pulmonary embolism: results in 47 consecutive patients after rapid diagnosis and aggressive surgical approach. J Thorac Cardiovasc Surg. 2005;129:1018–23.

40. Wan S, Quinlan DJ, Agnelli G, Eikelboom JW. Thrombolysis compared with heparin for the initial treatment of pulmonary embolism: a meta-analysis of the randomized controlled trials. Circulation. 2004;110:744–9.

41. Haut ER, Garcia LJ, Shihab HM, et al. The effectiveness of prophylactic inferior vena cava filters in trauma patients: a systematic review and meta-analysis. JAMA Surg. 2014; 149(2):194–202.

42. Rogers FB, Cipolle MD, Velmahos G, et al. Practice management guidelines for the prevention of venous thromboembolism in trauma patients: the EAST practice management guidelines work group. J Trauma. 2002;53(1):142–64.
43. Johnson ON, Gillespie DL, Aidinian G, et al. The use of retrievable inferior vena cava filters in severely injured military trauma patients. J Vasc Surg. 2009;49(2):410–6.
44. Taccone FS, Bunker N, Waldmann C, et al. A new device for the prevention of pulmonary embolism in critically ill patients: results of the European Angel Catheter Registry. J Trauma Acute Care Surg. 2015;79(3):456–62.
45. Cadavid CA, Gil B, Restrepo A, et al. Pilot study evaluating the safety of a combined central venous catheter and inferior vena cava filter in critically ill patients at high risk of pulmonary embolism. J Vasc Interv Radiol. 2013;24(4):581–5.

Chapter 19
Aeromedical Evacuation and Transfer of the Critically Injured Patient

Ian Ewington

Abstract Aeromedical evacuation employs the enduring characteristics of air power in order to save lives: height, speed and reach. It has a long history in both military and civilian arenas and developments in pre-hospital and critical care retrievals during recent combat operations have contributed to improved survival rates.

There are several key elements to aeromedical evacuation that are vital to ensure success. This includes correctly trained personnel, appropriate aircraft, robust medical equipment, together with comprehensive administrative and logistic processes. There are unique characteristics of the aviation environment that can affect the patient, therefore the implications of these must be understood in order to prevent clinical deterioration during the flight.

I. Ewington, MBChB, MML, MRCP, FRCA, FFICM
Department of Anaesthesia, Royal Centre for Defence Medicine,
Queen Elizabeth Hospital Birmingham,
Mindelsohn Way, Edgbaston, Birmingham B15 2WB, UK
e-mail: ianewington1@nhs.net

S.D. Hutchings (ed.), *Trauma and Combat Critical Care in Clinical Practice*, In Clinical Practice,
DOI 10.1007/978-3-319-28758-4_19,
© Crown Copyright 2016

Keywords   Critical care • Transfer • Retrieval • Aeromedical
• Military • Trauma

Introduction

Aeromedical evacuation has a long and notable history. In the Franco-Prussian war of 1870–1871, 160 casualties were flown out of Paris [1]. The French launched 66 observation balloons which were subsequently referred to as 'air ambulances'. In the United States of America in 1909, two Army officers Captain George Gosman and Lieutenant Albert Rhoades designed a patient transport aircraft; it was unsuccessful and crashed on the test flight but nevertheless highlighted the great potential for transporting military casualties away from the battlefield by air [2].

In 1913, French Army medical officer M. Gautier suggested *"we shall revolutionise war surgery if the aeroplane can be adapted as a means of transport for the wounded"* [3]. It was not until 1917 that French surgeons Chassang and Godart modified the fuselage of the Dorant AR II in order to carry stretchers. By the late 1920s, the US military had agreed that the air ambulance should become 'a means of normal evacuation in modern wars' [4]. This evolution continued through the Second World War and the Korea and Vietnam conflicts culminating in the incredible successful aeromedical evacuation chain used in the Iraq and Afghanistan conflicts of the first decade of the twenty-first century [5].

The term 'Aeromedical Evacuation' (AE) within the military generally refers to evacuation of casualties by air with escorting medical personnel who can provide treatment as required. This may be as a primary transfer from the battlefield to an initial medical facility for damage control surgery or a secondary transfer away from the operational theatre, usually back to the home base. In the USA, the terms CASEVAC and MEDEVAC generally refer to evacuation of casualties by air from the point of injury to field medical treatment facilities. The latter will have personnel who provide medical care during the process, the former does not. That is not to say casualties will not be treated on a CASEVAC but it may be provided by their fellow soldiers on a non-medical air asset, rather than by dedicated medical personnel.

There have been significant developments in contemporary aeromedical evacuation that have positively impacted on mortality and morbidity of combat soldiers. This has included rapid evacuation from the point of injury by highly-skilled teams such as the UK Medical Emergency Response Team (MERT) in Afghanistan. Following stabilisation in the operational theatre, critically injured patients were evacuated back to the UK by the Critical Care Air Support Team (CCAST) with the ability to provide in flight intensive care to an extremely high standard. The United States (US) military, in addition to their critical care teams (CCAT), also have the ability to provide extra-corporeal membrane oxygenation (ECMO) in flight with the development of their Landstuhl Acute Lung Rescue Team [6].

What Types of Aeromedical Evacuation Are There?

In the United Kingdom (UK), military AE is classified into three types: Forward, Tactical and Strategic. Forward AE tends to be from the point of injury to a hospital within the theatre of operation. A recent example of this is MERT in Afghanistan. Tactical AE moves patients between medical facilities usually within or just outside the operational theatre. This is usually for specialist care not available locally, e.g., neurosurgery or to facilitate onward movement out of theatre. Strategic AE usually involves repatriation of the patient to their home base. In the case of the UK, all overseas operational casualties are flown to the Queen Elizabeth Hospital, Birmingham.

What Personnel Are Required?

The skill set required by personnel making up an AE team will vary depending on the anticipated requirements of the patient. It is therefore imperative that initial clinical assessments are as accurate as possible in order to ensure the appropriate personnel are utilised. This could include the use of mental health nurses, specialist physicians or in the case of critically ill patients, an intensive care team.

The Royal Air Force CCAST consists of a consultant anaesthetist, two critical care nurses, an equipment technician and a flight medic. This is often augmented by those in training for these roles such as a specialty registrar in anaesthesia. Whilst typically caring for 1–2 patients the team can be expanded to look after a further 4–6 should it be necessary. The team can also be augmented with specialist physicians, such as a cardiologist, if deemed necessary. During the 2015 West African Ebola epidemic, CCAST also augmented specialist teams transporting Ebola patients in the Air Transportable Isolator (ATI) in order to assist with advanced vascular access, sedation, or to take part in discussions about escalation of care.

A United States Air Force (USAF) CCAT is made up of a critical care physician, critical care nurse and a cardiopulmonary technician and is designed to care for three ventilated patients. There is the option to expand the number of nurses with the use of an 'extender team' to care for more.

It is essential that the personnel making up the team are able to maintain their skill set including non-technical skills when not undertaking transfers. The RAF CCAST have chosen to do this by a combination of classroom based practical teaching in the form of an annual medical equipment course and a validation exercise at the start of the CCAST duty period. The simulation exercise involves assessment of critical incident management in the aviation environment.

There should be an identified team leader who will be responsible for the flow of the overall mission including liaising with the air and ground crews. This should not usually be the doctor as if there are significant clinical issues their focus will be on the patient.

What Are the Key Elements of Aeromedical Evacuation?

The Request

For the critically injured patient, timely transfer with appropriate levels of care is essential; on the battlefield, availability of air assets and skilled personnel will determine what can be provided. Accordingly, medical planning for any military operation and therefore the evacuation process should be clear before the need arises.

The request for AE should be done using a standardised method which ensures accurate clinical and geographical information. In the case of combat casualties this must include information regarding ongoing hostilities on the ground which could affect the incoming AE aircraft and team. A common method used by several armed forces on the battlefield is the 'nine liner' request which gives the requesting combat unit a clear format in which to provide information to the dispatching AE unit. This will include clinical priority, special equipment required, method of marking the pick-up site and hostile activity.

For tactical and strategic AE, it is usual to provide more detail than is available on the 'nine liner'. This takes the form of a patient movement request. This will usually be written either by a doctor or nurse with AE training who will aim to ensure all relevant clinical details are passed to the AE team. For the ICU patient, this should include detailed clinical information such as ventilator settings, sedation requirements and blood gas analysis results.

The Aircraft

The aircraft tasked to carrying out the evacuation of patients will be dependent on the environment, patient factors, types of aircraft and their availability. In the forward environment, rotary wing aircraft will usually be employed in order to facilitate retrieval from a potentially hostile environment. It may even be an aircraft expressly designated for AE as was the case in Afghanistan with MERT. In such situations, the medical team work with a regular aircrew which allows for targeted training to optimise human factors [7].

Tactical AE may utilise rotary or fixed wing aircraft. As with forward AE, it is imperative that the aircraft and team are prepared to deal with hostile forces during the course of the retrieval. The tactical team will often be moving patients who have already had some form of surgical intervention but may need additional specialist care such as neurosurgery or ophthalmology. Both forward and tactical AE are usually within the theatre of operations but this may be to an off-shore medical facility such as the Royal Navy Primary Casualty Receiving Facility.

The strategic AE team is usually responsible for transferring patients back to their home base or another allied country. Due to the often long distances covered, they will often utilise larger aircraft such as the Boeing C17-A Globemaster III or the Airbus A330-200. The C17-A (see Fig. 19.1) offers a very flexible aeromedical platform and in practice could transfer at least four intensive care patients as shown in Fig. 19.2.

The Receiving Medical Facility

It is essential that there is a clear pathway of care from the referring facility through the aeromedical team to the receiving facility. In order to ensure effective communication the referring unit will often speak directly to clinicians at the

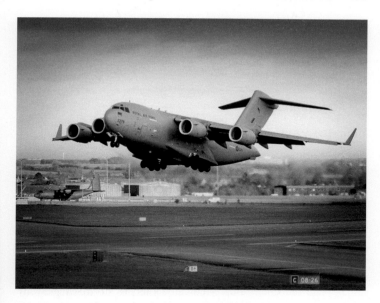

FIGURE 19.1 A Royal Air Force C17 taking off from RAF Brize Norton. It has a short airfield capability allowing it to operate in austere environments. It is very versatile in the aeromedical role providing the speed and reach necessary for transferring critically injured patients long distances (Crown Copyright 2015)

receiving unit. The aeromedical evacuation team is also responsible for ensuring all the relevant clinical details are passed on including copies of all clinical notes and images. Ongoing communication between all parties regarding the progress of the patient has proved vital for clinical governance, research and education. A good example of this is the weekly UK Joint Theatre Clinical Case Conference (JTCCC) involving amongst others, clinical personnel in several overseas theatres of operation, AE teams and the Role 4[1] Hospital in Birmingham [8].

---

[1] [Explain Role 4].

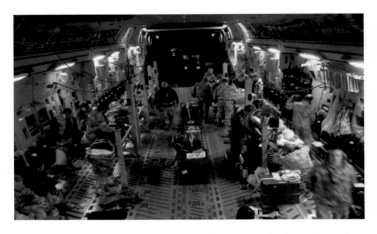

FIGURE 19.2 A Royal Air Force C17 in aeromedical configuration. The patient at the far right rear of the aircraft is ventilated. The other patients are of a lower dependency. The ambulance is visible just beyond the open ramp. Medical Iacons are stropped centrally for ease of access with black roll bags containing consumables hanging at the side (Reproduced with permission: Sgt Chris Andrews, Tactical Medical Wing, RAF Brize Norton)

What Equipment Is Required for Aeromedical Evacuation?

The medical equipment used during AE is essentially similar to that used in hospitals. The main difference is that it aeromedical equipment has been tested and cleared for use in the aviation environment. This is essential to ensure there is no interaction between the avionics and the medical kit which could cause dysfunction in either system. It is also important to know what will happen to the equipment in the event of an aircraft emergency such as emergency landing or rapid decompression. Ideally, any equipment should be robust, compact and lightweight and must continue to work accurately and dependably despite changes in pressure, temperature and humidity.

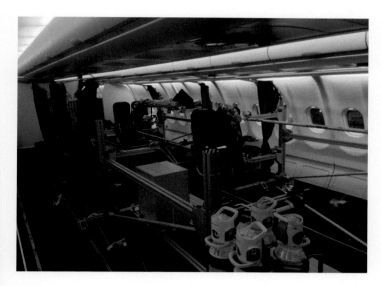

FIGURE 19.3 The stretcher stanchions on the RAF Voyager aircraft (Airbus A330-200). The oxygen cylinders can be seen secured at the head end. This central stanchion is designed for critical care patients with all round access. Some of the stretcher fits in the background have privacy curtains fitted. The seats would be allocated to the AE team

Stretchers

Stretchers must have the capability to be secured to the floor of the aircraft or to bespoke stretcher stanchions depending on the aircraft design (Fig. 19.3). They should also be tested to determine survival of the structure and harness from a significant impact; the UK DMS commonly use the NATO standard stretcher. If injuries allow, the use of an appropriate backrest permits the patient to be nursed at 30° in order to optimise ventilation and if required, intracranial pressure. The addition of a vacuum mattress provides a further level of security during the transfer as well as spinal support.

The use of a stretcher bridge provides a useful support in order to secure kit away from the patient however they also add to the equipment burden. During Strategic AE transfers the RAF CCAST tend to use a second stretcher at least 30 cm beneath the patient to accommodate the aeromedical equipment.

Aircraft Loading

In the military environment, loading the patient is often done via the rear ramp of the aircraft or in the case of some helicopters via the side door. If the aircraft is a standard airliner as is the case with the RAF Voyager, then consideration must be made as to how to get the patient safely aboard. Most airfields will have some form of high lift and this is usually adequate, however there maybe cases where this is not available, in which case other options may include a scissor lift or cherry picker. Whatever is chosen the safety of the patient and crew is paramount and it is essential that the risks of using alternative devices are weighed up carefully.

Ventilator

The principles and modes of mechanical ventilation are well known and well described. In the aviation environment patients and the ventilators are subject to variations in pressure, partial pressure of oxygen, vibration, acceleration and deceleration. The ventilator must be sufficiently portable to allow for ease of transfer yet robust enough to tolerate the potentially austere environment it has to function in. It is essential to have an alternative method of ventilation secured near the patients head in order to take over respiratory support quickly in the event of equipment failure.

An important consideration is the delivery of tidal volume (V_T) which can vary in the hypobaric environment with the potential for both volutrauma and inadequate ventilation. It is therefore essential to monitor end-tidal carbon dioxide and arterial blood gases. The V_T rises with the fall in the environmental pressure with greater rises seen during the descent of the aircraft [9].

The LTV 1000 series ventilator (CareFusion, San Diego, CA) currently used by the RAF is extremely versatile and lightweight. It is turbine based and can be connected to either high or low pressure oxygen. This provides some flexibility should the aircraft be delayed or diverted.

Physiological Monitoring

As with all critically injured patients continuous monitoring of clinical parameters allows for rapid intervention where appropriate. In the AE patient this is crucial as they are also subject to variations in acceleration, pressure and partial pressure of oxygen which can impact on physiology. Standard parameters which should be monitored include heart rate, oxygen saturation, blood pressure (either invasively or non-invasively), end-tidal carbon dioxide and temperature. Additional measurements include central venous pressure (CVP) and intra-cranial pressure (ICP). The latter can be done with a ventriculostomy catheter and the pressure transduced in the same way as the blood pressure and CVP. Intraparenchymal catheters usually require a dedicated monitor which may not be cleared for flight on all aircraft.

Recent developments in wireless technology mean that the patient can be monitored remotely either locally or in some cases at a distance. The Corpuls (GS ElektromedizinischeGerate G. Stemple GmbH, Kaufering, Germany) is a patient monitor with integrated defibrillator/pacer which can be modularised for ease of transfer. This allows the patient to be monitored by a clinician separately when the patient is being moved around on the stretcher.

Syringe Drivers and Fluid Administration Devices

Continuous drug delivery devices are often essential in the critically ill patient for sedation, inotropes and fluids. Newer pumps, whilst having a wider range of useful functions such as the ability to perform drug calculations, also have the potential to be less robust than older, simpler versions. However, they offer clinicians greater versatility and reassurance as they often have expanded alarm functions as well as the ability to subsequently interrogate the memory in the case of a clinical incident. The use of pumps for fluid administration should avoid the potential for pressure variations affecting the flow as well as the ability to monitor for air in the lines.

Blood Analysis

On longer flights, it is useful to have a point of care system for core assays. The iStat hand held analyser (Abbott, Illinois) can analyse blood gases and electrolytes as well as haemoglobin, creatinine, lactate and activated clotting time.

Power Supply

Whilst many aircraft can provide a source of electricity for the medical equipment, it offers greater flexibility for the medical team if they have their own independent power supply. This allows them to quickly change aircraft should the need arise as well as continuing to power equipment if grounded due to problems with the aircraft. Such power sources usually take the form of light weight batteries for transfer and larger batteries secured near the patient on the aircraft; lead-acid batteries are commonly used.

Oxygen

Some aircraft, may be able to supply therapeutic oxygen, however as with power, it is best not to be reliant on it. The larger cylinders (UK ZX) hold 3040 l and can be secured on the stretcher stanchions for use during flight. The smaller cylinders (UK CD) hold 460 l and are ideal for transfer between aircraft and hospital. The oxygen consumption will depend on clinical need and the set-up of the ventilator. As a rough estimate the ZX cylinder will last around 2–3 h and the CD cylinder around 30–45 mins.

Drugs

The choice of drugs taken on AE ultimately rests with the clinician and may be influenced by the information provided by the initial medical request. However, there should be a basic list of relevant critical care drugs routinely carried including those needed quickly in an emergency. One important consideration with respect to drugs used outside of hospital are those that require strict temperature control and how best to achieve that within the logistic or environmental limitations [10]. Continuous temperature monitoring allows for documentation of extremes of temperature, which in recent UK military operations was not unusual. Response to temperature extremes depends on the drug and environmental context however one potential course is to dispose of the drugs within a shorter time frame than the actual expiry date, for example 6 months.

Who and What Determines Fitness for AE?

It is important that the AE patient is thoroughly assessed prior to emplaning to ensure that the correct personnel, drugs and equipment are available should there be clinical deterioration during the flight. Initially this may be an AE trained doctor, nurse or medic who has seen the patient to assess their 'fitness to fly'. For the critically ill patient this will occur in close liaison with an intensive care specialist.

In the RAF, the final decision on fitness to fly rests with a doctor who has advanced training in aviation medicine, usually the duty Medical Officer at the Aeromedical Evacuation Control Centre (AECC) at RAF Brize Norton. In the case of overseas military operations, there may be a deployed equivalent.

Considerations include potential for deterioration and whether any intervention is necessary prior to the flight that will improve stability. Examples of such interventions include invasive ventilation, insertion of a chest drain or external fixation of a fractured pelvis. If the patient requires prolonged AE, not addressing these prior to emplaning could result in significant deterioration in the austere aviation environment.

What Are the Environmental Considerations During AE and What Are the Potential Clinical Implications?

Pressure

Variations in ambient pressure can have significant deleterious consequences for the critically ill patient. Long range aircraft, cruising at around 30,000 ft will typically pressurise the cabin to around 8000 ft, but how this is achieved can vary and therefore there may be periods of variable pressure on ascent and descent. The clinical implications for the patient are due to the physical properties of gas. If the nature of the injury has resulted in gas trapped in an enclosed space then the reduction in the ambient pressure will result in a relative expansion of this gas. If the gas is unable to escape this could cause an increase in pressure within the relevant body cavity resulting in further instability and injury. A change from sea level to 8000 ft will typically cause gas to expand by 35 % [11].

Typical examples include: Pneumothorax, which if it expands may cause respiratory or cardiovascular compromise; traumatic head injury resulting in or potential for pneumocephalus with increasing intracranial pressure and penetrating injuries to the globe of the eye. If the patient has had definitive surgery resulting in anastomosis of the bowel then expansion of gas within the lumen of the gut could potentially threaten the repair leading to a leak.

Consideration should also be given to the pressure within the cuff of the endotracheal tube which can rise significantly on ascent to altitude. This could potentially cause necrosis of the tracheal mucosa if not monitored and corrected appropriately. A fall in the pressure in the cuff could increase the risk of micro aspiration.

The consequences of gas expansion may be difficult to recognise and difficult to reverse during flight. If there is a risk to the patient then the AE team will discuss cabin altitude restrictions with the aircraft captain – for example ground level or ground level plus 2000 ft. The aircraft will usually have to fly at a lower altitude to achieve a restricted cabin pressure and this adds to fuel consumption, decreases the range, may alter the flight plan and increases the risk of turbulence.

Hypoxia

Hypoxia secondary to altitude should not be a major issue for the patients receiving invasive ventilation as the FiO_2 can be titrated with ease. However, for the spontaneously breathing patient, there is a risk that the resultant fall in partial pressure of oxygen could be significant enough to cause problems. The PIO_2 decreases from 150 mmHg at sea level to 107 mmHg at 8000 ft. For the healthy individual, this will result in a fall of oxygen saturations to around 90 %.

A patient with a chest injury following trauma may have an acceptable level of oxygenation at sea level but develop significant hypoxia when exposed to the reduced PIO2 at 8000 ft. This may respond to simple oxygen therapy but in some situations may require invasive ventilation. Anticipation of this with appropriate intervention prior to the flight is essential.

Acceleration

During take off, acceleration will produce horizontal gravitational force on the supine patient. If loaded head first this will cause pooling of blood in the lower extremities potentially causing transient haemodynamic compromise. The critically ill patient may not be able to mount an adequate sympathetic response to counteract this and a pre-emptive strategy of fluid loading or vasopressors may be appropriate.

If the patient is loaded feet first then there may be some elevation in intracranial pressure during take-off which, for the head injured patient, may be significant. Many fixed-wing aircraft, including the C17, will also cruise with the nose angled slightly upwards. This may also adversely impact on the force exerted on the head of the patient if loaded feet first.

Noise and Vibration

These can be significant and consideration should be given to protecting the patient's ears in the same way as the crew's. Gravitational forces, turbulence and the nature of the environment mean that it is essential that the patient is adequately secured to the stretcher, usually by way of a five-point harness. This may be released temporarily to enable patient care. The positioning and security of all lines and tubes is also paramount to prevent events such as inadvertent extubation or dislodgement of vascular access.

Noise can also interfere with communication between the AE team therefore the use of headsets which are independent from the aircrew can vastly improve on this. Their use during clinical emergencies is invaluable.

What Are the Key Considerations When Moving from the Aircraft to the Receiving Unit?

Transfer to Receiving Unit

The onward move from the airhead to the hospital must be meticulously planned in advance by the aeromedical ground support staff in liaison with the AE team. This should include communication to the ground ambulance crew of clinical priorities and the potential need for additional resources, such as extra oxygen. Advance communication with the receiving unit should allow for seamless transfer of care. Any clinical deterioration in flight that may warrant either early surgical intervention or urgent imaging should be highlighted prior to arrival.

Handover

If the patient is stable it is often better to verbally handover the patient prior to transfer to the bed and the new equipment. This ensures all parties are aware of the issues should there be any subsequent problems. It is essential at this stage that all the relevant paperwork is passed on as well as any clinical imaging.

Recovery to Base

Aeromedical evacuation missions can potentially take several days. Due to the nature of the missions, the working environment and the sometimes trans-meridian distances travelled, fatigue can be a major problem for the AE team [12]. It is therefore vital that adequate rest is achieved prior to re-tasking.

It is helpful if a debrief is held after every mission. This allows each team member to highlight things that went well and areas that could be improved on. There should also be the opportunity for team members to express any issues they have experienced personally with the nature of the mission. This type of reflection is beneficial for future professional development as well as for the longer term health of the team.

References

1. Howard M. The Franco-Prussian war: the German invasion of France, 1870–1871. New York: Macmillan; 1962. p. 325–6.
2. Dorland P, Nanney J. Dust off: army aeromedical evacuation in Vietnam. Washington, DC: Center of Military History United States Army; 1982. p. 6–7.
3. Haller JS. Battlefield medicine: a history of the military ambulance from the Napoleonic Wars through World War I. Carbondale: Southern Illinois University Press; 1992. p. 193–4.
4. Ibid., 197
5. Patterson CM, Woodcock T, Mollan IA, Nicol ED, McLoughlin DC. United Kingdom military aeromedical evacuation in the post-9/11 era. Aviat Space Environ Med. 2014;85:1005–12.
6. Fang R, Allan P, Womble SG, et al. Closing the "care in the air" capability gap for severe lung injury: the Landstuhl Acute Lung Rescue Team and extracorporeal lung support. J Trauma. 2011;71(1):S91–7.
7. Mercer SJ, Whittle CL, Mahoney PF. Lessons from the battlefield: human factors in defence anaesthesia. Br J Anaesth. 2010;105(1):9–20.
8. Willdridge D, Hodgetts TJ, Mahoney PF. The Joint Theatre Clinical Case Conference (JTCCC): clinical governance in action. J R Army Med Corps. 2010;156(2):79–83.
9. Hernandez Abadia de Barbara A, LópezLópez JA. Mechanical ventilation in hypobaric environment: aeromedical transport of critically ill patients. Crit Care. 2004;8(S1):19.

10. Madden JF, O'Connor RE, Evans J. The range of medication storage temperatures in aeromedical emergency medical services. Prehosp Emerg Care. 1999;3:27–30.
11. Essebag V, Halabi AR, Churchill-Smith M, Lutchmedial S. Air medical transport of cardiac patients. Chest. 2003;124(5):1937–45.
12. Myers JA, Haney MF, Griffiths RF, et al. Fatigue in air medical clinicians undertaking high-acuity patient transports. Prehosp Emerg Care. 2015;19(1):36–43.

Index

Printed in the United States
By Bookmasters